Methods in Clinical Pharmacology—
Central Nervous System

Methods in Clinical Pharmacology— Central Nervous System

Edited by
M. H. Lader & A. Richens

Reprinted from *British Journal of Clinical Pharmacology*
Volume 10, 1980
Volume 11, 1981

ISBN 978-1-349-06040-5   ISBN 978-1-349-06038-2 (eBook)
DOI 10.1007/978-1-349-06038-2

First published in 1981, by THE MACMILLAN PRESS LTD
London and Basingstoke
Associated companies in Delhi Dublin
Hong Kong Johannesburg Lagos Melbourne
New York Singapore and Tokyo

CONTENTS

Preface   Alan Richens &
Malcolm Lader   1

Neuroendocrine markers of CNS drug effects   E. C. Johnstone &
I. N. Ferrier   3

Tests of autonomic function in assessing
centrally-acting drugs   Paul Turner   21

Psychomotor function and psychoactive drugs   Ian Hindmarch   29

Sleep studies in clinical pharmacology   Ian Oswald   51

Measurement of serum drug levels in the
assessment of antidepressants   Stuart A. Montgomery   61

Biochemical assessment of antidepressive drugs   Karabi Ghose   67

The clinical assessment of depression   Malcolm Lader   79

Assessment of extrapyramidal disorders   C. D. Marsden &
M. Schachter   89

Assessment of anti-psychotic drugs   A. V. P. Mackay   113

The clinical assessment of analgesic drugs   D. W. Littlejohns &
D. W. Vere   125

Methods of assessment of antiepileptic drugs   Norman Milligan &
Alan Richens   139

Clinical assessment of neuromuscular
transmission   J. P. Payne &
R. Hughes   153

PREFACE

Clinical pharmacology is an area of study which is heavily dependent on the excellence of its methods of investigation, its techniques and assessments. Evaluation of the effects of drugs on the central nervous system has suffered somewhat from the difficulties of developing valid and reliable techniques to assess functions as disparate as tremor of the fingers or subtleties of feelings. However, such techniques have become available in the last few years and few aspects of central nervous system function remain inaccessible to quantification. Accounts of these methods are widely scattered in the literature and it was thought useful to commission a series of review articles for publication in the British Journal of Clinical Pharmacology which would bring together the various techniques. These articles were well-received by researchers and clinicians so it was decided to publish the review articles as a separate book.

We made no attempt in commissioning these articles to distinguish between neuropharmacology and psychopharmacology. Indeed, the distinction is spurious as shown by the example of the dopaminergic systems, important in extrapyramidal disorders and in psychoses. But some areas of this topic do have particular problems. The diagnosis and classification of psychiatric syndromes is a notoriously controversial subject and the assessment of subjective phenomena raises epistemological questions which have never been satisfactorily resolved.

Our first review deals with neuroendocrine markers of central drug effects and the technical advances in hormone assays. Autonomic functions of centrally-acting drugs form the topic of the next review with its particular importance for the unwanted effects of these drugs. Psychomotor function effects and sleep studies form the areas for the next two chapters.

Drug levels have been of especial interest in the use of antidepressants and a chapter is devoted to this topic. Biochemical assessment of antidepressant drugs forms a complementary chapter. The final review in this group deals with the clinical assessment of depression. Extrapyramidal disorders and antipsychotic drugs are next reviewed.

The final three chapters deal with analgesic drugs, antiepileptic drugs and drugs affecting neuromuscular transmission. Thus, a wide area is covered and it is hoped that these accounts of available techniques will prove useful both to the tyro setting up new studies and to the expert moving into new areas.

Alan Richens

Malcolm Lader

July, 1981

NEUROENDOCRINE MARKERS OF CNS DRUG EFFECTS

E.C. JOHNSTONE & I.N. FERRIER

Division of Psychiatry, Clinical Research Centre, Watford Road, Harrow HA1 3UJ

Introduction

The idea that there is a relationship between symptoms referable to the nervous system and endocrine effects has its origins in antiquity. The direct investigation of such relationships is, of course, of much more recent origin and the principal focus of such investigation has tended to be anterior pituitary hormone secretion (APHS) (Martin, Reichlin & Brown, 1977). Such studies have been greatly aided by the development of specific and sensitive radio immunoassays for anterior pituitary hormones (Berson & Yallow, 1968). Neuro-pharmacological studies, allied with histochemical and immuno-fluorescence techniques, have established that biogenic amines and other neurotransmitters play a crucial role in the modulation of APHS through an action on the hypothalamic hypophysiotrophic neurones (Fuxe & Hokfelt, 1969).

There is a complex system of innervation of the hypothalamus by monoaminergic neurones. Noradrenergic and serotonergic nerves cells are mainly situated in the brain stem (caudal medulla and raphe nuclei respectively) and terminate in several hypothalamic nuclei. The dopaminergic system is situated mainly in the medial basal hypothalamus (the so-called tubero-infundibular dopaminergic system). It has been shown that there is a close anatomical relationship between these monoamine systems and the hypothalamic neurones containing releasing factors for APHS (Martin, 1973; McNeill & Sladek, 1978). The role of monoamines and other putative neurotransmitters in modulating APHS is outlined in Table 1.

It has been hypothesised that schizophrenia (Randrup & Munkvad, 1972), affective illness (Schildkraut, 1965; Lapin & Oxenkrug, 1969), Huntington's chorea (Bird & Iversen, 1974) and Parkinson's disease (Bernheimer, Mirkmayer, Hornykiewicz, Jellinger & Seitelberger, 1973) are all disorders of neurotransmission. On the basis that any disturbance of neurotransmission underlying these disorders might also involve hypothalamic neuro-transmission much research has been focused upon APHS in these conditions. Furthermore, if drugs which have therapeutic actions in these conditions do so because of their effects upon neurotransmitters it is possible that these effects would be associated with changes in APHS which could be used as an index of clinical effects. It is obvious that the investigation of APHS in association with the clinical study and treatment of the above diseases has considerable potential. There are, however, certain limitations to the study of APHS as an index of more central events. These include the following—

(A) APHS varies widely in relation to temporal factors, e.g.

   (1) Luteinising hormone (LH), follicle stimulating hormone (FSH), adrenocorticotrophic hormone (ACTH) and growth hormone (GH) have markedly episodic secretory patterns (Martin et al., 1977).

   (2) LH, FSH and prolactin (PRL) vary considerably in relation to the state of maturity of the individual and with the menstrual cycle (Yen, 1977).

   (3) PRL, ACTH and GH have sleep-related secretions which may respond differently to pharmacological stimuli (Rubin, 1977).

(B) Feedback effects from target organ hormone secretion are of major importance in APHS e.g. gonadotrophins—oestrogen/testosterone, and $TSH–T_4/T_3$.

(C) There is a wide variation in normal levels of these hormones even when (A) and (B) are taken into account. Thus, direct comparison with a normal range may lead to problems of interpretation.

(D) Non-specific stimuli may be the important determinant affecting APHS at the time of the study, e.g. stress on PRL and ACTH, nutritional status on LH and glucose intake on GH (Noel, Suk, Stone & Frantz, 1972; Himsworth, Carmel & Frantz, 1972; Strain & Strain, 1978).

If indeed, the functional psychoses are disorders of neurotransmission it might be expected that the clinical states might be reflected in changes in APHS. Such findings have been reported in the affective disorders (Ettigi & Brown, 1977). In schizophrenia LH has been found to be low in unmedicated chronic patients (Brambilla, Guerrini, Guastalla, Rovere & Riggi, 1975; Johnstone, Crow & Mashiter, 1977) and relationships between FSH and prolactin secretion and clinical state have been found (Johnstone et al., 1977).

(E) The systemic administration of neuropharmacological agents provides little evidence as to their site of action (Grahame-Smith, 1976).

In spite of these limitations, there is a considerable body of work concerning the relationship between endocrine effects and drugs acting upon the central nervous system.

It may be classified as follows:—

(a) Endocrine effects of drugs used to treat psychiatric disorders.

(b) Endocrine effects of drugs used to investigate psychiatric disorders.

(c) Endocrine effects of drugs of abuse.

Endocrine effects of drugs used to treat psychiatric disorders

Neuroleptics

Neuroleptics have the effect of reducing the florid 'positive' symptoms of schizophrenia such as delusions and hallucinations. This group of drugs includes the phenothiazines, butyrophenones and thioxanthenes. They have several properties such as α-noradrenergic receptor blocking and anticholinergic activity but the principal property which they share is blockade of dopaminergic transmission by an action on postsynaptic dopamine receptors. It appears that the dopamine blocking ability of these drugs relates closely to their clinical efficacy in the treatment of acute schizophrenia (Creese, Burt & Snyder, 1976) and is the major factor in inhibiting pituitary lactotrophic cells (Muller, Nistico & Scapagini, 1977). There is evidence to suggest that dopamine may act directly as the primary prolactin inhibiting factor (PIF) (Ben-Jonathan, Oliver, Weiner, Mical & Porter, 1977). It has been shown that PRL secretion is elevated after neuroleptic administration in animals (de Wied, 1967), in normal subjects (Kleinberg, Wharton & Frantz, 1971, Friesen, Guyda, Hwang, Tyson & Barbeau, 1972) and in schizophrenic patients (Beumont, Corker, Friesen, Gelder, Harris, Kolakowska, MacKinnon, Mandelbrote, Marshall, Murray & Wiles, 1974, Wilson, Hamilton, Boyd, Forrest, Cole, Boyns & Griffiths, 1975). With two possible exceptions, all drugs which are known to be effective neuroleptics cause an elevation of prolactin secretion. Clozapine

Table 1 Role of monoamines, other putative neurotransmitters and physiological stimuli in regulating the secretion of anterior pituitary hormones

| Pituitary hormone | Hypothalamic releasing hormone | Physiological stimuli | Role of putative neurotransmitters | | | | |
			Dopamine	Noradrenaline α	β	5-HT	Others
Prolactin	Prolactin inhibiting factors, PIF	Suckling +ve Stress +ve sleep +ve Pregnancy +ve	−ve	—	—	+ve	opiates +ve ? ACH
	? Prolactin releasing factor/?TRH						
Growth hormone	Growth hormone release inhibiting factor (somatostatin)	Stress +ve Sleep +ve	+ve	+ve	−ve	+ve	opiates +ve GABA −ve
	Growth hormone releasing factor	Glucose↑ −ve					
ACTH	Corticotrophin releasing factor (CRF	Sleep +ve Stress +ve Cortisol ↑ −ve	—	+ve	−ve	−ve +ve	?ACH opiates −ve ?GABH
LH	Luteinizing hormone releasing hormone (LHRH)	Puberty +ve Testosterone/oestrogen −ve	−ve (?)	+ve (?)	—	−ve (?)	opiates −ve −ve ACh
FSH	? LHRH	Menopause +ve					
TSH	Thyrotrophin releasing hormone (TRH) (somatostatin −ve)	Cold +ve, cortisol↑ −ve Stress +ve, oestrogen +ve −ve T4/T3↑ −ve	—	—	—	−ve	opiates −ve

References: Muller *et al.* (1977), Martini & Besser (1977).

elevates prolactin to only a slight extent (Gruen, Sachar, Altman, Leifer, Frantz & Halpern, 1978a; Gruen, Sachar, Altman, Langer, Tabrizi & Halpern, 1978b; Meltzer, Goode, Schyre, Young & Fang, 1979). This drug does appear to have anti-psychotic activity (Meltzer *et al.,* 1979) but clinical studies have been limited by the fact that its administration is associated with the development of agranulocytosis (Idanpaan-Hakkila, Alhava & Olkinvora, 1977) and it has therefore been withdrawn from some European countries. Propranolol is a β-adrenergic receptor blocking agent which has been used in very high dosage in the treatment of schizophrenia (Yorkston, Gruzelier, Zaki, Hollander, Pitcher & Sergeant, 1977). Because of the cardiovascular effects of this drug double-blind studies are difficult to achieve and its anti-psychotic efficiency is not certainly established. It has been suggested that at the dosages used in the treatment of psychoses, propranolol does elevate prolactin secretion (Nasrallah, Freed, Rogol & Wyatt, 1977) but the evidence on this matter is conflicting (Hanssen, Heyden, Sundberg, Wetterburg & Enroth, 1978; Ridges, Lawton, Harper, Ghosh & Hindson, 1977).

It is generally held that the action of neuroleptics on PRL secretion is a direct one on the pituitary. Stereospecific dopamine receptors are found in the pituitary (Friend, Brown. Jawahir, Lee & Seeman, 1978) but not in the hypothalamic median eminence (Brown, Seeman & Lee, 1976). *In vitro* studies show that neuroleptics elevate prolactin secretion from cultured pituitary cells and block dopamine induced inhibition (McLeod & Lehemeyer, 1974). Domperidone (a drug with dopamine receptor blocking activity which does not cross the blood brain barrier) is a powerful inducer of prolactin secretion (Cocchi, Gil-ad, Parenti, Stefanini, Locatelli & Muller, 1980).

It has been shown that the administration of neuroleptics leads to a reproducible and dose-dependent elevation of PRL secretion in the individual subject (Langer, Sachar, Gruen & Halpern, 1977) but these relationships are much weaker if groups of patients are studied. A positive relationship between the antipsychotic effect of neuroleptics and the associated elevation of PRL secretion has been demostrated (Meltzer & Fang, 1976; Langer *et al.,* 1977; Cotes, Crow, Johnstone, Bartlett & Bourne, 1978; Siris, van Kamman & de Fraites, 1978) but the relationship is not strong and the effect is only obvious at low doses of neuroleptics as a ceiling effect develops (Gruen *et al.,* 1978a). There is a time lag (Cotes *et al.,* 1978) between the rapid elevation of PRL and the slower anti-psychotic effects associated with neuroleptics and this may point to processes of importance in clinical response other than straightforward dopamine blockade. Relationships have also been demonstrated between

(a) extra pyramidal symptoms, neuroleptic serum levels and PRL level after neuroleptic administration (Kolakowska, Wiles, McNeilly & Gelder, 1975) and (b) the rate of fall in PRL after cessation of neuroleptic therapy and extrapyramidal symptoms (Brown, Laughren & Robzyk, 1979) but these studies require confirmation.

It has been suggested (Beumont, 1979) that monitoring PRL levels is a possible method of assessing drug compliance in psychotic patients and that for this purpose it may be superior to the assessment of serum levels of neuroleptics or their metabolites. To some extent, this is so, but there are limitations to the value of this estimation in routine clinical use. It has been shown that many elderly men maintained on oral neuroleptics have normal PRL levels and this applies to a smaller percentage of female patients (de Rivera, Lal, Ettigi, Mantella, Miller & Freisen, 1976). This finding is not due to non-compliance because normal PRL levels have been found in men on depot neuroleptics (Huws & Groom, 1977) in whom significant serum levels of neuroleptics were measured (Ferrier *et al.,* unpublished observations). Drug interaction may be a relevant factor in studies of PRL levels. For example, concurrent medication with anticholinergics is said by some authors (de Rivera *et al.,* 1976) but not by others (Lawson & Gala, 1975) to be associated with higher prolactin levels.

There are much conflicting data on the effect of neuroleptics on growth hormone secretion. The basis of these differences appears firstly to be a significant species difference between primate and sub-primate species (Weiner & Ganong, 1978) and secondly the varying α-receptor blocking activity of different neuroleptics (Willoughby, Brazeau & Martin, 1977). Markedly fluctuating values, which may be due to sampling during spontaneous GH secretory episodes, are a problem in some patients (Rubin, 1977). The administration of pimozide, the most specific dopamine blocking agent among neuroleptics, is associated with a reduction in growth hormone both basally and in response to certain physiological stimuli (Martin, 1973; Liuzzi, Panerai, Chiodini, Secchi, Cocchi, Botalla, Silvestrini & Muller, 1976; Schwimm, Schwark, McIntosh, Milstrey, Wills & Kobberling, 1976). A summary of the relevant available findings is given in Table 2.

The role of dopamine in the control of LH secretion is uncertain. Direct pharmacological studies (McCann, Fawcett & Krulich, 1974) have indicated an excitatory role but this has been contradicted by histofluorescence studies (Fuxe & Hokfelt, 1969). Dopamine appears to release luteinising hormone releasing hormone (LHRH) from hypothalamic fragments *in vitro* (Bennett, Edwardson, Holland, Jeffcoate & White, 1975), but has also been shown to have a role in the degradation of LHRH (Marcano de

Cotte, Menezes, Bennett & Edwardson, 1980). Most studies show no effect of neuropleptics on LH or FSH in patients (Table 3) but there is some evidence that when LH levels are low neuroleptic treatment is associated with a return to the normal range (Brambilla *et al.*, 1975). This has also been demonstrated for FSH (Brambilla *et al.*, 1975). A summary of relevant available findings is given in Table 3.

Testosterone levels were unchanged by neuroleptic medication in a study where these were given for sexual deviance (Murray, Bancroft, Anderson, Tennant & Carr, 1975). Brambilla *et al.* (1975) found that testosterone levels rose in chronic schizophrenic patients after the introduction of a neuoleptic drug but Cotes *et al.* (1978) found that levels of testosterone in acute schizophrenic patients were unrelated to clinical state or neuroleptic medication and Beumont *et al.* (1974) found a rise in testosterone levels after withdrawal of long term neuroleptics in eight schizophrenic males.

Neuroleptics cause variable effects, predominantly excitatory on ACTH secretion in sub-primate species probably via a noradrenergic action (de Wied, 1967). There is no conclusive evidence in man for a consistent effect of neuroleptics on ACTH secretion.

Recent studies (Healy & Burger, 1977; Scanlon, Rees-Smith & Hall, 1978) have shown small but clear-cut elevations in TSH after acute challenge with metoclopramide, a dopamine receptor blocking agent which has probable anti-psychotic effects (Stanley, Lautin, Rotrosen & Gershon, 1979) although it is not clinically used for this purpose. No longer term changes in TSH/thyroid secretion have been noted (Shader & Dimascio, 1970) and otherwise effects of neuroleptics on this system are not described.

Lithium

The therapeutic efficacy of lithium in manic depressive illness both as an acute treatment (Cade, 1949; Mendels, 1976) and as a prophylactic agent (Baastrup & Schou, 1967) has been clearly established. The mechanism of action of this drug is poorly understood and many inconsistent neurotransmitter changes have been reported. Although an effect on post-synaptic dopamine receptors has recently been demonstrated (Gallager, Pert & Bunney, 1978) another study (Lal, 1978) found that lithium had no

Table 2   Effect of neuroleptics on growth hormone secretion

Type of patient and nature of study	Result	Authors
Normal subjects given haloperidol	Basal GH reduced GH response to hypoglycaemia reduced	Kim *et al.* (1971)
Normal subjects given chlorpromazine	Basal GH reduced GH response to hypoglycaemia reduced	Sherman *et al.* (1971)
Psychiatric patients of mixed sex, age and diagnosis chronically taking phenothiazines	Basal GH normal GH response to hypoglycaemia adequate	Beumont *et al.* (1974)
Patients with chronic schizophrenia given haloperidol	GH secretion unchanged	Brambilla *et al.* (1975)
Patients with acute schizophrenia treated with α-flupenthixol β-flupenthixol or placebo	No relationship between GH levels and neuroleptic medication or anti-psychotic effect	Cotes *et al.* (1978)
Three groups of subjects untreated schizophrenics, schizophrenics on chlorpromazine, normals	No differences between groups in basal GH or in GH response to hypoglycaemia	Beg *et al.* (1979)

effect upon the GH response to the dopamine agonist apomorphine or the PRL response to the dopamine receptor blocker haloperidol and that there was no alteration in the basal levels of these hormones. Long term administration of lithium has effects on thyroid functioning causing, in up to 20% of cases, hypothyroidism associated with raised TSH (Lindstedt, Nilssen, Walinder, Skott & Ohman, 1977). Long term lithium treatment may also be associated with a raised secretion of antidiuretic hormone (Padfield, Park, Morton & Braidwood, 1977) and indeed may produce a clinical picture of diabetes insipidus (Singer, Rotenberg & Puschett, 1972). These hormonal changes are thought to be due to peripheral effects on cyclic AMP (Forrest, Cohen, Torretti, Himmelhoch & Epstein, 1974) and to bear no relationship to central effects or clinical efficacy.

Antidepressants

Drugs with antidepressant properties cover a wide spectrum of neuropharmacological agents with a wide spectrum of differential effects on monoamines (Iversen & Mackay, 1979). In general, the administration of antidepressants does not lead to consistent hormonal change nor to endocrinological side effects. Although Turkington (1972) found elevated prolactin in patients treated with tricyclic antidepressants this has not been replicated by other workers (Meltzer, Piyakalmala, Schyre & Fang, 1977; Gruen et al., 1978b; Widerlov, 1978). An exception to this is clomipramine which has a strong action in inhibiting uptake of 5-hydroxytryptamine. The administration of this drug on an acute and a chronic basis causes increased prolactin secretion (Jones et al., 1977). The administration of L-dopa, L-tryptophan and 5-hydroxytryptophan, the precursors of dopamine, noradrenaline and 5-hydroxytryptamine is associated with increased PRL secretion in man and in animals (Checkley, 1980). These drugs have been used as antidepressants but their efficacy is uncertain (Johnstone, 1980). Nomifensine is an inhibitor of endogenous catecholamine uptake and a weak dopamine agonist. It has been shown to reduce

Table 3 Effects of neuroleptics upon secretion of luteinizing hormone

Type of patient and nature of study	Result	Authors
Normal males given sulpiride	Prolactin raised LH unchanged	Thorner et al. (1971)
Males and post-menopausal females on neuroleptics and after withdrawal or neuroleptics	Normal levels unaffected by drugs	Beumont et al. (1974)
Premenopausal females with and without normal menstrual cycles on neuroleptics. Neuroleptics withdrawn in 4 cases.	Normal levels in subjects with normal cycles Absent midcycle LH peak in amenorrhoeic subjects restored on withdrawal of neuroleptics.	Beumont et al. (1974)
Chronic schizophrenic patients initially untreated and then given haloperidol	Initially low levels rose following haloperidol administration	Brambilla et al. (1975).
Normal females aged 20–25 years given pimozide at mid-cycle	LH levels reduced compared with previous cycles	Leppaluoto et al. (1976)
38 acute schizophrenic patients treated with α-flupenthixol, β-flupenthixol and placebo	LH levels unrelated to clinical state or drug treatment	Cotes et al. (1978)

prolactin following the administration of a single 200 mg dose (Muller, Genazzi & Murru, 1978; Masala, Magna, Devella, Delitala & Novasio, 1980) although results of another study do not support this (Dunne, Walker, Cowden & Ratcliffe, 1979). Antidepressants show few consistent effects upon growth hormone secretion. 5-hydroxy-tryptophan increases GH secretion (Imura, Natakai & Yoshimi, 1973) but its antidepressant activity has been very little studied (Persson & Roos, 1967).

The TSH response to TRH is blunted in some cases of depression (Prange, Wilson, Lara, Alltop & Breese, 1972; Coppen, Peet, Montgomery & Bailey, 1974). This response has been postulated as a means of classification (Gold, Pottash, Davies, Ryan, Sweeeney & Martin, 1979) and a predictor of response to antidepressants (Langer et al., 1980) but as it may persist after recovery (Kirkegaard, Nørlem, Laundsen, Bjørun & Christiansen, 1975), it cannot be used as a marker of clinical effect. In general most studies have failed to show consistent relationships between TSH response to TRH and clinical features (Paykel & Rowan, 1979).

No consistent effects of antidepressants upon the secretion of other anterior pituitary hormones have been found.

Anxiolytics

These drugs are generally considered to be free of neuroendocrine effects (Beumont, 1979). Two recent studies of benzodiazepines which are the most commonly used anxiolytics (Blackwell, 1973) have shown results of theoretical interest to the general topic of neuroendocrine markers of central nervous system drug effects. In the first of these studies it was found that the administration of diazepam 10 mg gave a consistent rise in GH (Syvalahti & Kanto, 1975) and that this effect was blocked by pimozide and sodium valproate but not methysergide (Koulu, Lammentausta, Kangas & Dahlstrom, 1979). Since GABA is thought to be inhibitory to GH release this does not accord with diazepam's putative GABA agonist activity (Snyder, Enna & Young, 1977).

The second of the studies concerned the effects of benzodiazepines upon basal and stress related ACTH secretion. Diazepam has been shown to reduce ACTH output in man (Rees, 1970) and to reduce basal cortisol secretion in animals at low doses although in high doses cortisol secretion in animals is increased (Barlow, Knight & Sullivan, 1979). In neurotic male subjects a high correlation was found between ACTH and cortisol secretion and arousal as measured by galvanic skin response. In these patients there was an ACTH and cortisol response to acute stress. After 4 weeks treatment with diazepam the initial high correlation was lost, the ACTH responses were reduced and more variable and the cortisol

response was abolished (Ferrier *et al.*, unpublished observations).

Cyproheptadine

This drug is an antagonist of histamine and 5-hydroxytryptamine. Its properties in increasing weight were found fortuitously when its anti-histaminic actions were being utilized in the treatment of hay fever and asthma in children (Lavenstein, Dacanay, Horvath, Lasagna & van Metre, 1961). This finding has been replicated in patients with many diagnoses (General Practitioner Clinical Trials, 1970) and although the drug has been used in the treatment of anorexia nervosa systematic studies of its value in that condition have been few (Halmi & Goldberg, 1978). Endocrinological effects of cyproheptadine in man have been little studied but it has been found to reduce the growth hormone response to hypo-glycaemia in normal volunteers (Bivens, Lebovitz & Feldman, 1973) and to suppress sleep related GH and cortisol release (Chihara, Kato, Maeda, Matsukara & Imura, 1976).

Endocrine effects of drugs used to investigate psychiatric disorders

Neuroendocrine tests are increasingly being used as a means of investigating neurotransmission in psychiatric conditions and in other disorders of the CNS. The considerable body of information concerning this topic has been reviewed by Checkley (1980), Rotrosen, Angrist, Gershon, Parquin, Branchley, Oleshansky, Halpern & Sachar (1979), Langer, Sachar, Nathan, Tabriezi, Perez & Halpern, (1979) and Annunziato (1979). Studies confined to particular disorders concern acromegaly (Thorner, Chait, Aitken, Bender, Bloom, Mortimer, Sanders, Stuart-Mason & Besser, 1975), Huntington's chorea (Caraceni *et al.*, 1977) and Parkinsonism (Parkes, Debono & Marsden, 1976). A summary of the more consistent findings in normals and patient groups employing the drugs described below is given in Table 4.

(a) *Dopamine agonists*

There are several drugs in this category used in endocrinological research and the details of their modes of action are shown in Table 5. In addition to these drugs dopamine infusions are increasingly being employed. Apomorphine and bromocriptine both lower prolactin in cell culture lines, animals, normal subjects and hyperprolactinaemic patients (Besser, Parke, Edwards, Forsyth & McNeilly, 1972; McLeod & Lehemeyer, 1974; Martin, Lal, Tolis & Friesen, 1974; Lawson & Gala, 1975). Lisuride (Delitala, Wass, Stubbs, Jones, Williams & Besser, 1979) and

Table 4 Endocrine responses to centrally acting drugs used in the investigation of psychiatric and other conditions

Condition	Authors	Dopamine agonists Bromocriptine (**Bromo**), levodopa (L-D) Apomorphine (Apo)	x-noradrenergic receptor agonists Clonidine	Amphetamines
Normal	See text	PRL↓GH↑ ? LH ACTH→	GH↑ PRL→ ACTH→LH→	GH↑ PRL? ACTH↑ LH→
Schizophrenia	Pandey et al. (1977) Ettigi et al. (1976) Langer et al. (1976)	? enhanced GH↑ and reduced PRL↓ to Apo in some acute patients Blunted GH↑ and PRL↓ to Apo in many chronic patients	—	Normal GH responses
Huntington's chorea	Caraceni et al. (1977) Chalmers et al. (1978)	Enhanced GH↑ to Bromo but reduced PRL↓ Normal responses	—	—
Parkinson's disease	Hyppa (1978) Shaw et al. (1976) Parkes et al. (1976) Malarkey et al. (1974)	Enhanced PRL↓ and GH↓ to Bromo Reduced GH↑ to Bromo Reduced GH↑ to Bromo Normal to L-D Reduced GH↑ to L-D	—	—
Acromegaly	Thorner et al. (1975)	GH↓ PRL↓	—	—
Affective illness	Coppen & Ghose (1978) Gold et al. (1976) Mendels et al. (1974) Checkley (1980) Checkley (1979) Langer et al. (1976)	Normal PRL↓ Normal PRL↓ Normal GH↑	? Reduced GH↑ in depression	Reduced cortisol↑ in depression Reduced GH↑ in depression

2

lergotrile (Thorner, Ryan, Wass, Jones, Bouloux, Williams & Besser, 1978) inhibit basal prolactin. L-dopa has also been found to lower prolactin although this effect is less consistent (Lal, Martin, de la Vega & Friesen, 1975). Amphetamines, however, have weak and inconsistent effects upon PRL in both animal (Ravitz & Moore, 1977) and human studies (Wells, Silverstone & Rees, 1978; Slater, de la Vega, Shyler & Murphy, 1978). Dopamine infusions reduce PRL secretion from pituitary cell cultures (Birge, Jacobs, Hammer & Daughaday, 1970) animals, including stalk-sectioned monkeys (Diefenbach, Carmel, Frantz & Ferin, 1976) and from human subjects (Leblanc, Lachein, Abu-Fadel & Yen, 1976; Leebaw, Lee & Woolf, 1978). All dopamine agonists block the prolactin response to TRH *in vitro* (Dibbett, Bondreau, Bruni & Meites, 1974) and *in vivo* (Besses, Burrow, Spaulding & Donabedian, 1975).

It seems probable that these agents act directly on the pituitary dopamine receptor although additional effects on the hypothalamus cannot be ruled out and are supported by some evidence (Kamberi, Mical & Porter, 1971). It is possible that dopamine metabolism in the median eminence (Gudelsky & Moore, 1976) and dopamine receptors of the pituitary (Friend *et al.*, 1978) differ in pharmacological responses from central dopamine synapses. Functionally, however, many of the responses of this 'hypothalamic-pituitary dopamine system' resemble those more centrally (Lal, Harvey & Bikadoroff, 1977). One of the problems of using PRL reduction after dopamine agonists as a way of assessing

dopamine receptor function is that there is a very narrow range between normal levels and both the lower limit of detection of the assay system and the level below which even massive doses of the drug do not produce any further depression of PRL level. Langer *et al.* (1979) have suggested studying the suppressive effects of dopamine agonists after a dose of neuroleptic to raise PRL to half maximum but this method raises interpretative difficulties of its own. Another problem is that the nausea and emesis which dopamine agonists may produce is stressful. The abolition of these problems by the administration of the peripherally acting dopamine receptor blocker domperidone itself produces marked endocrine effects.

GH secretion is stimulated in man by the administration of dopamine agonists (Lal, de la Vega, Sourkes & Friesen, 1973; Camanni, Massara, Belforte & Molinatti, 1975; Thorner *et al.*, 1978; Delitala *et al.*, 1979) and this effect is blocked by dopamine receptor blockers (Lal, Martin, *et al.*, 1975; Thorner *et al.*, 1978; Delitala *et al.*, 1979) except in the case of L-dopa where the GH response is blocked by 5-HT antagonists (Smythe, Compton & Lazarus, 1976). The rise in GH produced by amphetamine does not differ between the ($+$) and ($-$) isomers (Langer & Matussek, 1977) and this, together with the fact that the effect is not blocked by pimozide suggests that this response is noradrenergic (Sachar, Gruen, Altman, Halpern & Frantz, 1976). Dopamine infusion has been reported to increase the secretion of GH in some studies (Burrow, May, Spaulding & Donabedian, 1977, Leebaw *et al.*, 1978)

Table 5 Actions of dopamine agonists used in endocrinological research

Drug	
1. Apomorphine	Potent dopamine receptor agonist, effective on dopamine sensitive adenylate cyclase system, ? selectively labels presynaptic dopamine receptors, decrease in dopamine turnover, ? increases 5-HT turnover.
2. Ergot derivatives	
a) bromocriptine	High affinity for dopamine receptor sites, no stimulation of dopamine sensitive
b) lisuride	adenylate cyclase system *in vitro*, reduce dopamine turnover. Probable effect on 5-HT
c) lergotrile	receptors but ? effect on 5-HT turnover.
3. Levodopa	Increases synthesis of dopamine and noradrenaline and 5-HT
4. Amphetamines	Indirect presynaptic agent—releases biogenic amines,—noradrenaline and dopamine and blocks re-uptake—increase in turnover of dopamine, noradrenaline and ? 5-HT.

References: Muller *et al.* (1977), Fuxe, (1979).

but not in others (Leblanc *et al.*, 1976; Camanni, Massara, Belforte, Rosatello & Molinatti, 1977). Direct acting dopamine agonists and dopamine infusion have no effect on ACTH secretion (Lal *et al.*, 1973). Methylamphetamine induces ACTH secretion but this effect is blocked by α-adrenoceptor blockers and enhanced by β-adrenoceptor blockers suggesting that the effects of amphetamine are mediated by noradrenergic synapses (Rees *et al.*, 1970).

In animal studies systemic dopamine agonists have been shown to reduce LH and LH pulsatile release (Arendash & Gallo, 1978; Drouva & Gallo, 1977), but the effects are small and there is much dispute in this area. It is established that apomorphine (Lal *et al.*, 1973) lergotrile (Thorner *et al.*, 1978) and lisuride (Delitala *et al.*, 1979) have little effect on LH but there are disputes regarding the effects of L-dopa and bromocriptine (Hayek & Crawford, 1971; Lachelin, Leblanc & Yen, 1977; Strauch, Valche, Mahoudeau & Bricair, 1977). However, some workers have found that dopamine infusions lower LH in humans although their results on male subjects differ (Leblanc *et al.*, 1976; Leebaw *et al.*, 1978).

No consistent data on FSH and TSH have been noted.

(b) *Drugs acting at noradrenergic synapses*

(1) *α-adrenoceptor agonists* It appears that drugs of this type e.g. clonidine stimulate the release of GH but have little effect on PRL secretion (Lal, Tollis, Martin, Brown & Guyda, 1975; Gil-Ad, Topper & Laron, 1979). There is some evidence that amphetamine acting through an α-adrenergic mechanism elevates ACTH secretion (Rees *et al.*, 1970) as does the specific α-agonist methoxamine (Nakai, Imura, Yoshumi & Matsukura, 1973). However clonidine which is more specific appears to have no such action (Lal, Tollis *et al.*, 1975). No consistent effects on LH, TSH or FSH are noted.

(2) *α-adrenoceptor blockers* This group of drugs appears to block the GH response to most physiological stimuli (Checkley, 1980) but not to sleep (Lucke & Gilke, 1971). No consistent effects on PRL are noted. The ACTH response to amphetamine and to hypoglycaemia is blocked by α-receptor blocking drugs (Rees *et al.*, 1970; Nakai *et al.*, 1973). In animals, α-adrenoceptor blockade produces lower LH levels and a reduction in LH episodic secretion (Weich, 1978; Plant, Nakai, Belchetz, Keogh & Knobil, 1978) but this effect is not noted in man.

(3) *β-adrenoceptor blockers* There is uncertainty about the effect of these drugs on PRL but stress effects particularly associated with hypotension may be paramount here. β-adrenoceptor blockage appears to enhance the GH response to most physiological

stimuli, (Checkley, 1980) and also the ACTH response to amphetamine and hypoglycaemia (Rees *et al.*, 1970; Nakai *et al.*, 1973) suggesting that β-receptors have an inhibitory role in these responses. Of itself, β-adrenoceptor blockade appears to be associated with little endocrinological effect.

(c) *Drugs acting on opiate receptors*

In both rats and primates clearcut effects with morphine and enkephalin analogues have been seen after intravenous, intraventricular and intrahypothalamic administration with elevations of PRL and GH and reductions in LH, TSH and ACTH (Lien, Feruchel, Garsby, Sarantako & Grant, 1976; Shaar, Frederickson, Doninger & Jackson, 1977). These effects were blocked by naloxone (Shaar *et al.*, 1977) and indeed reverse by naloxone administration alone (Bruni, van Vogt, Marshall & Meites, 1977; Gold, Redmond & Donabedian, 1978). In man morphine causes an elevation of PRL and GH but there appears to be an interaction with dopamine receptors (Tollis, Hickey & Guyda, 1975). Long acting enkephalin analogues produced the same picture with a reduction in LH and cortisol and in this case the effect was reversed by naloxone (Stubbs, Delitala, Jones, Jeffcoate, Edwards, Ratter, Besser, Bloom & Alberti, 1978). Naloxone administration *per se* has disputed actions on PRL and GH (Janowsky, Judd, Huey, Portman & Parker, 1979; Rubin, Swezy & Bluschke, 1979) although it is likely that pharmacodynamic and dose effects are important causes of these contradictions. Recently, it has been shown that intravenous heroin produces an acute fall in LH levels with a loss of the normal episodic LH pattern (Mirin, Mendelson, Ellingboe & Myer, 1976). This effect was blocked by pre-treatment with the specific opiate antagonist naltrexone. Naltrexone administration alone caused increased LH levels with an increased number of secretory LH bursts in normal subjects (Mendelson, Ellingboe, Keuhnle & Mello, 1978).

Endocrine effects of drugs of abuse

The difficulties of using endocrinological effects as an index of drug actions described in the introduction apply to drugs coming under this heading as they do to the other groups but there are additional difficulties peculiar to this group. Persons who abuse drugs are inclined to be unreliable, may give misleading information about their drug intake and if they abuse one drug may well abuse others (Brambilla, Resele, de Maio & Nobile, 1979). Furthermore, the drug in question, and alcohol is the best example of this, may have other effects such as the production of liver damage which may have endocrinological effects. The marked anxiety and other physiological changes which may be associated with withdrawal of some drugs have to be taken into account in designing studies in this area.

(a) *Alcohol*

Alcohol is widely abused in western society. Various studies of its endocrine effects have been conducted but their results tend to be conflicting (Table 6).

(b) *Amphetamine*

The acute effects of amphetamine have been discussed in the previous section. Although amphetamine is chronically abused and is sometimes taken on a long term basis for therapeutic purposes, abuse is not now common and therapeutic use is rare.

Thus, its endocrinological effects other than as an investigative tool have been little studied. Its effects on GH have been studied in a group of narcoleptic subjects, some of whom had been on amphetamine for up to 20 years .(Parkes, De Bono, Jenner & Walters, 1977). Although GH responses to amphetamine were reduced in the narcoleptic subjects this reduction did not appear to be due to previous amphetamine treatment.

(c) *Cocaine*

Cocaine has a multiplicity of effects on neuro-transmitters including the blocking of re-uptake of dopamine, 5-hydroxytryptamine and nor-adrenaline although it has other effects (Post, 1975). Although it is abused widely in South America its use is not widespread in Europe and its endocrinological effects in man have not been established. It is known

Table 6 Endocrinological effects of alcohol

Subjects	Hormonal effect	Reference
13 male alcoholics	Basal LH increased. LH response to LHRH raised in those with LH outside normal range. 17 OHA normal.	Wright *et al.* (*1976*)
7 male alcoholics (2–7 days off alcohol) *v* 5 or 6 male controls	Basal GH reduced and GH and cortisol responses reduced in alcoholics	Chalmers *et al.* (1977)
16 normal males given alcohol	Acute rise in LH and fall in testosterone following alcohol administration.	Mendelson *et al.* (1977)
174 abstinent alcoholics of whom half resumed intake during study	Testosterone reduced during alcohol administration	Persky *et al.* (1977)
22 chronic alcoholic males. 14 normal males all given LHRH (in normals before and after 3 days acute alcohol ingestion)	In alcoholics basal testosterone reduced LH and FSH raised and prolactin normal. LHRH response reduced in alcoholics: administration of alcohol to normals produced rise in LH, fall in testosterone.	Van Thiel (1978)
33 male alcoholics in withdrawal tested 2 and 9 days of alcohol	Basal GH raised, PRL low blunted response to TRH basal testosterone and cortisol normal. At second testing GH normal PRL normal TRH response more nearly normal	Loosen *et al.* (1979)

to produce a slight reduction in serum prolactin in rats (Ravitz & Moore, 1977).

(d) Heroin

The effects of heroin have been studied in patients currently abusing the drug, patients maintained on methadone and in abstinent former addicts. The results are shown in Table 7.

Thus, there may be dysfunction of pituitary gonadal axis in heroin/methadone users but the results are not consistent.

(e) Marihuana

A reduction in plasma testosterone was found to occur following chronic intensive marihuana use (Kolodny, Masters, Kolodner & Toro, 1974) and these authors also found that very heavy use of marihuana was associated with reduced FSH secretion. Both Mendelson, Kuehnle, Ellingboe & Babor (1974) and Schaefer, Gunn & Dubowski (1975) found normal testosterone levels in abusers of marihuana. Benowitz, Jones & Lerner (1976) studying normal volunteers found a reduced GH response to hypoglycaemia following 14 days administration of delta-9-tetrahydro-cannabinol.

Again there is a suggestion of dysfunction in the pituitary gonadal axis but the results are not consistent. Apart from the lack of consistency of these results the abnormalities which are found tend to represent a change within a wide normal range and even if they were replicable could not be used as an endocrine maker of the drug effect.

Conclusion

The fact that it has been established that the neurotransmitters which are thought to be involved in the cause of serious psychiatric and other disorders, and are known to be affected by the treatments used for these disorders, are important in the control of the secretion of anterior pituitary hormones which can now be accurately measured in small samples, is obviously of great interest. The possibility is raised that endocrine changes could be used as a readily measurable index of effects upon neurotransmission of centrally acting drugs. As yet, this is a future hope rather than a present reality. The exact nature of the neuronal control of some hormones is unclear, their secretion may be influenced by non-specific factors which are difficult to control, and some of the drugs have a variety of actions. Even where these problems apply only to a very limited extent as is the case with regard to the rise in prolactin produced by the dopamine blocking agents used to treat schizophrenia, the practical value of this 'endocrinological marker' is doubtful. As noted, some patients taking these drugs on a chronic basis no longer have elevated prolactin levels (de Rivera et al., 1976; Huws & Groom, 1977) but even if the acute situation only. is considered, although a correlation between clinical effect and the rise in prolactin can be found, some patients with very high levels show no clinical response and some improve without active medication (Cotes et al., 1978). Thus, despite the considerable theoretical interest of the topic, these techniques do not yet have a place in routine clinical practice.

Table 7 Endocrinological effects of heroin

Subjects	Hormonal effect	Reference
Heroin addicts; methadone maintained; former methadone maintained abstinent addicts; normal controls (all male)	Testosterone within normal range	Cushman (1973)
Heorin addicts; methadone users; controls (all male)	Testosterone reduced in methadone users but not in heroin addicts	Cicero et al. (1975)
Heroin addicts; high dose methadone users; low dose methadone users; normal controls (all male)	Testosterone reduced in heroin addicts and high dose methadone users but not in low dose methadone users.	Mendelson et al. (1975)
Heroin addicts (all male)	Reduced basal FSH, LH & testosterone	Brambilla et al. (1977)
Heroin addicts and controls both given GnRH (all male)	Basal LH and FSH low in addicts response to GnRH reduced in addicts	Brambilla et al. (1979)

References

ANNUNZIATO, L. (1979). Regulation of the tuberoinfundibular and nigrostriatal systems. *Neuroendocrinology*, **29**, 66–76.

ARENDASH, G.W. & GALLO, R.V. (1978). Apomorphine induced inhibition of episodic LH release on ovariectomized rats with complete hypothalamic de-afferentation. *Proc. Soc. exp. Biol. Med.*, **159**, 121–125.

BAASTRUP, P.C. & SCHOU, M. (1967). Lithium as a prophylactic agent. *Arch. Gen. Psychiat.*, **16**, 163–172.

BARLOW, S.M., KNIGHT, A.F. & SULLIVAN, F.M. (1979). Plasma corticosterone responses to stress following chronic oral administration of diazepam in the rat. *J. Pharm. Pharmac.*, **31**, 23–26.

BEG, A.A., VARMA, V.K. & DASH, R.J. (1979). Effect of chlorpromazine on human growth hormone. *Am. J. Psychiat.*, **136**, 914–917.

BEN-JONATHAN, N., OLIVER, C., WEINER, H.J., MICAL, R.S. & PORTER, J.C. (1977). Dopamine in hypophysial portal plasma of the rat during the oestrous cycle and throughout pregnancy. *Endocrinology*, **100**, 452–458.

BENNETT, G.W., EDWARDSON, J.A., HOLLAND, O., JEFFCOATE, S.L. & WHITE, N. (1975). Release of immunoreactive luteinizing hormone-releasing hormone and thyrotrophin-releasing hormone from hypothalamic synaptosomes. *Nature*, **257**, 323–325.

BENOWITZ, N.L., JONES, R.T. & LERNER, C.B. (1976). Depression of growth hormone and cortisol response to insulin-induced hypoglycaemia after prolonged oral delta-9-tetra hydrocannabinol administration in man. *J. clin. Endocrinol. Metab.*, **42**, 938–941.

BERNHEIMER, H., BIRKMAYER, W., HORNYKIEWICZ, O., JELLINGER, K. & SEITELBERGER, F. (1973). Brain dopamine and the syndromes of Parkinson and Huntington. *J. Neurol. Sci.*, **20**, 415–455.

BERSON, S.A. & YALOW, R.S. (1968). General Principle of radioimmunoassay. *Clin. Chem. Acta*, **22**, 51–69.

BESSER, G.M., PARKE, L., EDWARDS, C.R.W., FORSYTH, I.A. & McNEILLY, A.S. (1972). Galactorrhoea; successful treatment with reduction of plasma prolactin levels by bromergocryptine (1972). *Br. med. J.*, **3**, 669–672.

BESSES, G.S., BURROW, G.N. SPAULDING, S.W. & DONABEDIAN, R.K. (1975). Dopamine infusion acutely inhibits the TSH and prolactin response to TRH. *J. clin. Endocrinol. Metab.*, **41**, 985–988.

BEUMONT, P.J.V. (1979). The endocrinology of psychiatry. In *Recent Advances in Clinical Psychiatry*, ed. Granville-Grossman, K. London: Churchill-Livingstone.

BEUMONT, P.J.V., CORKER, C.S., FRIESEN, H.G., GELDER, M.G., HARRIS, G.W., KOLAKOWSKA, T., MACKINNON, P.C.B., MANDELBROTE, B.M., MARSHALL, J., MURRAY, M.A.F., & WILES, D.H. (1974). The effects of phenothiazines on endocrine function I. Patients with inappropriate lactation and amenorrhoea II. Effects in men and post-menopausal women. *Br. J. Psychiat.*, **124**, 413–430.

BIRD, E.D. & IVERSEN L.L. (1974). Huntington's chorea. Post-mortem measurement of glutamine acid decarboxylase, choline acetyltransferase and dopamine in basal ganglia. *Brain*, **97**, 457–472.

BIRGE, C.A., JACOBS, L.S., HAMMER, C.J. & DAUGHADAY, W.H. (1970). Catecholamine inhibition of prolactin secretion by isolated rat adenohypophyses. *Endocrinology*, **86**, 120–130.

BIVENS, C.H., LEBOVITZ, H.E. & FELDMAN, L.M. (1973). Inhibition of hypoglycaemia-induced growth hormone secretion by the serotonin antagonists cyproheptadine and methysergide. *New Engl. J. Med.*, **289**, 236–239.

BLACKWELL, B., (1973). Psychotropic drugs in use today. *J. Am. Med. Ass.*, **225**, 1637–1641.

BRAMBILLA, F., GUERRINI, A., GUASTALLA, A., ROVERE, C. & RIGGI, F. (1975). Neuroendocrine effects of haloperidol therapy in chronic schizophrenia. *Psychopharmacology*, **44**, 17–22.

BRAMBILLA, F., RESELE, L. & DE MAIO, D. NOBILE P. (1979). Gonadotrophin response to synthetic gonadotrophin hormone releasing hormone (GnRH) in heroin addicts. *Am. J. Psychiat.*, **136**, 314–317.

BRAMBILLA, F., SACCHETTI, E. & BRUNETTA, M. (1977). Pituitary-gonadal function in heroin addicts. *Neuropsychobiology*, **3**, 65–74.

BROWN, G.M., SEEMAN, P. & LEE, T. (1976). Dopamine/neuroleptic receptors in basal hypothalamus and pituitary. *Endocrinology*, **99**, 1407–1410.

BROWN, W.A. LAUGHREN, T.P. & ROBZYK, P.H. (1979). Serum prolactin in humans parallels neuroleptic induced changes in dopamine receptor sensitivity. *Society for Neurosciences*, 9th Annual Meeting, Atlanta, Georgia. Extract No. 1482.

BRUNI, J.F., van VOGT, D., MARSHALL, S. & MEITES, J. (1977). Effects of naloxone, morphine and methionine encephalin on serum prolactin, luteinizing hormone, thyroid stimulating hormone and growth hormone. *Life Sci.*, **21**, 461–466.

BURROW, G.N., MAY, P.B., SPAULDING, S.W. & DONABEDIAN, N.K. (1977). TRH and dopamine interactions affecting pituitary hormone secretion. *J. clin. Endocrinol. Metab.*, **45**, 65–72.

CADE, J.F.J. (1949). Lithium salts in the treatment of psychotic excitement. *Med. J. Aust.*, **2**, 349–352.

CAMANNI, F., MASSARA, F., BELFORTE, L. & MOLINATTI, G.M. (1975). Changes in plasma growth hormone levels in normal and acromegalic subjects, following 2-br-α ergocryptine. *J. clin. Endocrinol. Metab.*, **40**, 363–366.

CAMANNI, F., MASSARA, F., BELFORTE, L., ROSATELLO, N. & MOLINATTI, G.M. (1977). Effects of dopamine on growth hormone and prolactin levels in normals and acromegalic subjects. *J. clin. Endocrinol. Metab.*, **44**, 465–473.

CARACENI, T.A., PARATE, E.A., COCCHI, D., PANERAI, A.E. & MULLER, E.E. (1977). Altered growth hormone and prolactin responses to dopaminergic stimulation in Huntington's chorea. *J. clin. Endocrinol. Metab.* **44**, 870–875.

CHALMERS, R.J., BENNIE, E.H., JOHNSON, R.H. & KINNELL, H.G. (1977). The growth hormone response to insulin induced hypoglycaemia in alcoholics. *Psychol. Med.*, **7**, 607–611.

CHALMERS, R.J., JOHNSON, R.H., KEOGH, H.J. & NANDA, R.N. (1978). Growth hormone and prolactin response to bromocriptine in patients with Huntington's chorea. *J. Neurol. Neurosurg. Psychiat.*, **41**, 135–139.

CHECKLEY, S.A. (1979). Corticosteroid and growth hormones response to methylamphetamine in depressive illness. *Psychol. Med.*, **9**, 107–116.

CHECKLEY, S.A. (1980). Neuroendocrine tests of monoamine function in man: a review of basic theory and the application to the study of depressive illness. *Psychol. Med.,* 10, 35–53.

CHIHARA, K., KATO, Y., MAEDA, K., MATSUKARA, S., IMURA, (1976). Suppression by cyproheptadine of human growth hormone and cortisol secretion during sleep. *J. clin. Invest.,* 57, 1393–1402.

CHRISTY, N.P., LONGSON, D.S., HOROWITZ, W.A. & KNIGHT, M.M. (1957). Inhibitory effect of chlorpromazine upon the adrenal cortical response to insulin hypoglycaemia in man. *J. clin. Invest.,* 36, 543–549.

CICERO, T.J., BELL, R.D., WEST, W.G., ALLISON, L.H., POLAKOSKI, K. & ROBINS, E. (1975). Function of the male sex organs in heroin and methadone users. *New Engl. J. Med.,* 292, 882–887.

COCCHI, D., GIL-AD, I., PARENTI, M., STEFANINI, E., LOCATELLI, V. & MULLER, E.E. (1980). Prolactin-releasing effect of a novel anti-dopaminergic drug, domperidone, in the rat. *Neuroendocrinology,* 30, 65–69.

COPPEN, A. & GHOSE, K. (1978). Peripheral α-adrenoceptor and central dopamine receptor activity in depressed patients. *Psychopharmacology,* 59, 171–177.

COPPEN, A., PEET, M., MONTGOMERY, S. & BAILEY, J. (1974). Thyrotrophin-releasing hormone in the treatment of depression. *Lancet,* ii, 433–435.

COTES, P.M., CROW, T.J., JOHNSTONE, E.C., BARTLETT, W. & BOURNE, R.C. (1978). Neuroendocrine changes in acute schizophrenia as a function of clinical state and neuroleptic medication. *Psychol. Med.,* 8, 657–665.

CREESE, I., BURT, D.R. & SNYDER, S.H. (1976). Dopamine receptor binding predicts clinical and pharmacological potencies of antischizophrenic drugs. *Science,* 192, 481–483.

CUSHMAN, P. (1973). Plasma testosterone in narcotic addiction. *Am. J. Med.,* 55, 452–458.

DELITALA, G., WASS, J.A.H., STUBBS, W.A., JONES, A., WILLIAMS, S. & BESSER, G.M. (1979). The effect of lisuride hydrogen maleate, an ergot derivative on anterior pituitary secretion in man. *Clin. Endocrinol.,* 11, 1–9.

DE RIVERA, J.L., LAL, S., ETTIGI, P., MANTELLA, S., MILLER, H.F. & FREISEN, H.G. (1976). Effect of acute and chronic neuroleptic therapy on serum prolactin levels in men and women of different age groups. *Clin. Endocrinol.,* 5, 273–282.

DE WIED, (1967). Chlorpromazine and endocrine function. *Pharmac. Rev.,* 19, 251–298.

DIBBETT, S.A., BONDREAU, M.J., BRUNI, J.F. & MEITES, J. (1974). Possible role of dopamine in modifying prolactin (PRL) response to TRH. Proc. 56th Annual Meeting. *Am. Endocrinol. Soc.,* Atlanta, p. 186.

DIEFENBACH, W.M. P., CARMEL, P.W., FRANTZ, A.G. & FERIN, M. (1976). Suppression of prolactin secretion by L-DOPA in the stalk sectional rhesus monkey. *J. clin. Endocrinol. Metab.,* 43, 638–642.

DROUVA, S.V. & GALLO, R.V. (1977). Further evidence for inhibition of episodic luteinizing hormone release in ovariectomized rats by stimulation of dopamine receptors. *Endocrinology,* 100, 792–798.

DUNNE, M.J., WALKER, J., COWDEN, E.A., & RATCLIFFE, J.G. (1979). Nomifensine test for investigation of hyperprolactinaemia. *Lancet,* ii, 1243.

ETTIGI, P.G. & BROWN, G.M. (1977). Psychoneuro-endocrinology of affective disorder: an overview. *Am. J. Psychiat.* 134, 493–501.

ETTIGI, P.G., NAIR, N.P.W., LAL, S., CERVANTES, P. & GUYDA, H. (1976). Effect of apomorphine on growth hormone and prolactin secretion in schizophrenic patients with or without oral dyskinisia, withdrawn from chronic neuroleptic therapy. *J. Neurol. Neurosurg. Psychiat.,* 39, 870–876.

FORREST, J.N., COHEN, A.D., TORRETTI, J., HIMMELHOCH, J. & EPSTEIN, F.H. (1974). On the mechanism of lithium-induced diabetes insipidus in man and the rat. *J. clin. Invest.,* 53, 1115–1123.

FRIEND, W.C., BROWN, G.M., JAWAHIR, G., LEE, T. & SEEMAN, P. (1978). Effect of haloperidol and apomorphine treatment on dopamine receptors in pituitary and striatum. *Am. J. Psychiat.* 135, 839–841.

FRIESEN, H.G., GUYDA, H., HWANG, P., TYSON, J.E. & BARBEAU, A. (1972). Functional evaluation of prolactin secretion: a guide to therapy. *J. clin. Invest.,* 51, 706–709.

FUXE, K. (1979). Dopamine receptor agonists in brain research and therapeutic agents. *Trends in Neurosciences,* 2, 1–5.

FUXE, K. & HOKFELT, T. (1969). Catecholamines in the hypothalamus and the pituitary gland. In eds Ganong, W.F. & Martini, L. *Frontiers in Neuroendocrinology,* New York: Oxford University Press.

GALLAGER, D.W., PERT, A. & BUNNEY, W.E. (1978). Haloperidol-induced presynaptic dopamine supersensitivity is blocked by chronic lithium. *Nature,* 273, 309–312.

GENERAL PRACTITIONER CLINICAL TRIALS (1970). A weight-promoting drug. *Practitioner,* 205, 101–105.

GIL-AD, I., TOPPER, E. & LARON, Z. (1979). Oral clonidine as a growth hormone stimulation test. *Lancet,* ii, 278–279.

GOLD, P.W., GOODWIN, F.K., WEHR, T. & REBAR, R. & SACK, R. (1976). Growth hormone and prolactin response to L-DOPA in affective illness *Lancet,* ii, 1308–1309.

GOLD, M.S. POTTASH, A.L.C., DAVIES, R.K., RYAN, N., SWEENEY, D.R. & MARTIN, D.M. (1979). Distinguishing unipolar and bipolar depression by thyrotropin release test. *Lancet,* ii, 411–412.

GOLD, M.S., REDMOND, D.E. & DONABEDIAN, R.K. (1978). Prolactin secretion: A measurable central effect of opiate receptor antagonists. *Lancet,* i, 323–324.

GRAHAME-SMITH, D. (1976). cit. by Crow, T.J., Deakin, J.F.W., Johnstone, E.C. & Longden, A. Dopamine and schizophrenia. *Lancet,* ii, 563–566.

GRUEN, P.H., SACHAR, E.J., ALTMAN, N., LEIFER, M., FRANTZ, A.G. & HALPERN, F.S. (1978a). Prolactin responses to neuroleptics in normal and schizophrenic subjects. *Arch. Gen. Psychiat.* 35, 108–116.

GRUEN, P.H., SACHAR, E.J., ALTMAN, N., LANGER, G., TABRIZI, M.A. & HALPERN, F.S. (1978b). Relation of plasma prolactin to clinical response in schizophrenic patients. *Arch. Gen. Psychiat.,* 35, 1222–12227.

GRUEN, P.H., SACHAR, E.J., ALTMAN, N. & SASSIN, H. (1975). Growth hormone response to hypoglycaemia in post-menopausal depressed women. *Arch. Gen. Psychiat.,* 32, 31–33.

GUDELSKY, G.A. & MOORE, K.F. (1976). Differential drug effects on dopamine concentrations and rates of turnover in the median eminence, olfactory tubercle and corpus striatum. *J. Neurol. Transmission,* 38, 96–105.

HALMI, K.A. & GOLDBERG, S.C., (1978). Cyproheptadine in anorexia nervosa. *Psychopharmac. Bull.*, **14**, 31–33.

HANSSEN, T., HEYDEN, T., SUNDBERG, I., WETTERBERG, L. & ENROTH, P. (1978). Decrease in propranolol in schizophrenia. *Lancet*, **i**, 101–102.

HAYEK, A. & CRAWFORD, J.D. (1972). L-Dopa and pituitary hormone secretion. *J. clin. Endocrinol. Metab.*, **34**, 764–766.

HEALEY, D.L. & BURGER, H.G. (1977). Increased prolactin and thyrotrophin secretion following oral metoclopramide: dose-response relationships. *Clin. Endocrinol.*, **7**, 195–201.

HIMSWORTH, R.L., CARMEL, P.W. & FRANTZ, A.G. (1972). The location of the chemoreceptor controlling growth hormone secretion during hypoglycaemia in primates. *Endocrinology*, **91**, 217–226.

HOLLISTER, L.E., DAVIS, K.L. & BERGER, P.A. (1976). Pituitary response to thyrotropin releasing hormone in depression. *Arch. Gen. Psychiat.*, **33**, 1393–1396.

HUWS, D. & GROOM, G.V. (1977). Luteinizing hormone releasing hormone and thyrotrophin releasing hormone stimulation studies in patients given clomipramine or 'depot' neuroleptics. *Postgrad. med. J.*, **53**, (Suppl. 4), 175–181.

HYYPPA, M.T. (1978). Plasma pituitary hormones in patients with Parkinson's disease treated with bromocriptine. *J. Neurol. Transmission*, **42**, 151–7.

IDANPAAN-HAKKILA, J., ALHAVA, E. & OLKINVORA, M. (1977). Agranulocytosis during treatment with clozapine. *Eur. J. clin. Pharmac.*, 11, 193–198.

IMURA, H., NAKAI, Y. & YOSHIMI, T. (1973). Effect of 5-hydroxytryptophan (5-HTP) on growth hormone and ACTH release in man. *J. clin. Endocrinol. Metab.*, **36**, 204–206.

IVERSEN, L.L. & MacKAY, A.V.P. (1979). Pharmacodynamics of antidepressants and antimanic drugs. In *Psychopharmacology of Affective Disorders*, eds. Paykel, E.S. & Coppen, A. Oxford: Oxford University Press.

JANOWSKY, D., JUDD, L., HUEY, L., PORTMAN, L. & PARKER, D. (1979). Naloxone effects on serum growth hormone and prolactin in man. *Psychopharmacology*, **65**, 95–97.

JOHNSTONE, E.C. (1980). Affective Disorders In *Disorders of Neurotransmission*, ed. Crow, T.J. New York: Academic Press (in press).

JOHNSTONE, E.C., CROW, T.J. & MASHITER, K. (1977). Anterior putuitary hormone secretion in chronic schizophrenia—an approach to neurohumeral mechanisms. *Psychol. Med.* **7**, 223–228.

JONES, R.B., LUSCOMBE D.K. & GROOM G.V. (1977). Plasma prolactin concentrations in normal subjects and depressive patients following oral clomipramine. *Post grad. med. J.*, **53**, (Suppl. 4), 166–171.

KAMBERI, I.A., MICAL, R.S. & PORTER, J.C. (1971). Effect of anterior pituitary perfusion and intraventricular injection of catecholamines on prolactin release. *Endocrinology*, **88**, 1012–1020.

KIM, S., SHERMAN, L., KOLODNY, H.D., BENJAMIN, F. & SINGH, A. (1971). Attenuation by haloperidol of human serum growth hormone (HGH) by response to insulin. *Clin. Res.*, **19**, 718.

KIRKEGAARD, C., NØRLEM, N., LAUNDSEN, U.B., BJØRUN, N. & CHRISTIANSEN, C. (1975). Protirelin stimulation test and thyroid function during treatment of depression. *Arch. Gen. Psychiat.*, **32**, 1115–1118.

KLEINBERG, D.L., WHARTON, R.N. & FRANTZ, A.G. (1971). Rapid release of prolactin in normal adults following chlorpromazine stimulation. 53rd Programme of *Endocrine Society* Meetings, San Francisco, 126.

KOLAKOWSKA, T., WILES, D.H., McNEILLY, A.S. & GELDER, M.G. (1975). Correlation between plasma levels of prolactin and chlorpromazine in psychiatric patients. *Psychol. Med.*, **5**, 214–216.

KOLODNY, R.C., MASTERS, W.H., KOLODNER, R.M. & TORO, G. (1974). Depression of plasma testosterone levels after chronic intensive marihuana use. *New Engl. J. Med.*, **290**, 872–874.

KOULU, M., LAMMENTAUSTA, R. KANGAS, L. & DAHLSTROM, S. (1979). The effect of methysergide, pimozide and sodium valproate on the diazepam-stimulated growth hormone secretion in man. *J. clin. Endocrinol. Metab.*, **48**, 119–122.

LACHELIN, G.C.L., LEBLANC, H. & YEN, S.S.C. (1977). The inhibitory effects of dopamine agonists on LH release in women. *J. clin. Endocrinol. Metab.*, **44**, 728–732.

LAL, H., BROWN, W., DRAWBURGH, R., HYNES, M., & BROWN G. (1977). Enhanced prolactin inhibition following chronic treatment with haloperidol and morphine. *Life Sci.*, **20**, 101–106.

LAL, S., DE LA VEGA, C.E., SOURKES, T.L. & FRIESEN, H.G. (1973). Effect of apomorphine on growth hormone, prolactin, luteinizing hormone, follicle stimulating hormone in human serum. *J. clin. Endocrinol. Metab.*, **37**, 719–724.

LAL, S., HARVEY, G. & BIKADOROFF, S. (1977). Effect of methysergide and pimozide on apomorphine induced growth hormone secretion in man. *J. clin. Endocrinol. Metab.*, **44**, 766–770.

LAL, S., MARTIN, J.B., DE LA VEGA, C., & FRIESEN, H. (1975). Comparison of the effect of apomorphine and levodopa on the serum hormone levels in normal men. *Clin. Endocrinol.*, **4**, 277–285.

LAL, S., TOLLIS, G., MARTIN, J.B., BROWN, G.M. & GUYDA, M. (1975). Effect of clonidine on growth hormone, prolactin, luteinizing, hormone folicle stimulating hormone and thyroid stimulating hormone in the serum of normal men. *J. clin. Endocrinol. Metab.*, **41**, 823–832.

LAL, S. (1978). Effect of lithium on hypothalamic-pituitary dopaminergic function. *Acta Psychiat. Scand.*, **57**, 91–6.

LANGER, G., HEINZE, G., REIM, B. & MATUSSEK, N. (1976). Reduced growth hormone responses to amphetamine in 'endogenous' depressive patients. *Arch. Gen. Psychiat.*, **33**, 1471–1475.

LANGER, G. & MATUSSEK, N. (1977). D and L-amphetamine are equivalent in releasing human growth hormone. *Psychoneuroendocrinology*, **2**, 379–382.

LANGER, G., SACHAR, E.J., NATHAN, R.S., TABRIEZI, M.A., PEREZ, J.M. & HALPERN, F.S. (1979). Dopaminergic factors in human prolactin regulators a pituitary model for the study of a neuroendocrine system in man. *Psychopharmacology*, **65**, 161–164.

LANGER, G., SACHAR, E.J., GRUEN, P.H. & HALPERN, F.S. (1977). Human prolactin responses to neuroleptic drugs correlate with antischizophrenic potency. *Nature*, **266**, 639–640.

LANGER, G., SCHONBECK, G., KORNIG, G., KESCH, O., SCHUSSLER, M. & WALDHAUSL, W. (1980). Antidepressant drugs and the hypothalamic pituitary thyroid axis. *Lancet*, **i**, 100.

LAPIN, I.P. & OXENKRUG, G.F. (1969). Intensification of the

central serotoninergic processes as a possible determinant of the thymoleptic effect. *Lancet*, i, 132–136.

LAVENSTEIN, A.F., DACANAY, E.P., HORVATH, J., LASAGNA, L.C. & VAN METRE, T.E. (1961). The effect of cyproheptadine on appetite and body weight. *Am. J. Dis. Child.*, **102**, 537.

LAWSON, D.M. & GALA, R.R. (1975). The influence of adrenergic, dopaminergic, cholinergic and serotonergic drugs on plasma prolactin levels in ovarictomized, oestrogen treated rats. *Endocrinology*, **96**, 313–318.

LEBLANC, H., LACHELIN, G.C.L., ABU-FADIL, S. & YEN, S.S.C. (1976). Effect of dopamine infusion on pituitary hormone secretion in humans. *J. clin. Endocrinol. Metab.*, **43**, 668–674.

LEEBAW, W.F., LEE, L.A. & WOOLF, P.O. (1978). Dopamine effect level and augmented pituitary hormone secretion. *J. clin. Endocrinol. Metab.*, **47**, 480–487.

LEPPALUOTO, J., MANNISTO, P. RANTA, T. & LINNOILA, M. (1976). Inhibition of mid-cycle gonadotrophin release in healthy women by pimozide and fusaric acid. *Acta Endocrinol.*, **81**, 455–460.

LIEN, E., FERUCHEL, R.L., GARSBY, D., SARANTAKO, D. & GRANT, N. (1976). Enkephalin—stimulated prolactin release. *Life Sci.*, **19**, 37–40.

LINDSTEDT, G., NILSSEN, L., WALINDER, J., SKOTT, A. & OHMAN, R. (1977). On the prevalence, diagnosis and management of lithium induced hypothyroidism in psychiatric patients. *Br. J. Psychiat.*, **130**, 452–458.

LIUZZI, A., PANERAI, A.E., CHIODINE, P.G., SECCHI, C., COCCHI, O., BOTALLA, L., SILVESTRINI, F. & MULLER, E.E. (1976). In *Growth hormone and related peptides*. eds Pecile, A. & Muller, E.E., pp. 236–251. Amsterdam: Excerpta Medica.

LOOSEN, P.T., PRANGE, A.J. & WILSON, I.C. (1979). TRH (Protirelin) in depressed alcoholic men. *Arch. Gen. Psychiat.*, **36**, 540–547.

LUCKE, C. & GILKE, S. (1971). Experimental modification of the sleep-induced peak of growth hormone secretion. *J. clin. Endocrinol. Metab*, **32**, 729–736.

McCANN, S.M., FAWCETT, C.P. & KRULICH, L. (1974). *Endocrine Physiology* ed. McCann, S.M., pp. 31–65. London: Butterworth.

McLEOD, R.M. & LEHEMEYER, J.E. (1974). Studies on the mechanism of dopamine mediated inhibition of prolactin secretion. *Endocrinology*, **94**, 1077–1085.

McNEILL, T.H. & SLADEK, J.R. (1978). Fluorescence—immunocytochemistry: simultaneous localization of catecholamines and gonadotrophin-releasing hormone. *Science*, **200**, 72–74.

MALARKEY, W.B., CYRUS, J. & PAULSON, G.W. (1974). Dissociation of growth hormone and prolactin secretion in Parkinson's disease following chronic L-dopa therapy. *J. clin. Endocrinol. Metab.* **39**, 229–235.

MARCANO DE COTTE, D., MENEZES, C.E.L., BENNETT, G.W. & EDWARDSON, J.A. (1980). Dopamine stimulates the degradation of gonadotrophin releasing hormone by rat synaptosomes. *Nature*, **283**, 487–489.

MARTIN, J.B. (1973). Neural regulation of growth hormone secretion. *New Engl. J. Med.*, **288**, 1384–1393.

MARTIN, J.B., LAL, S., TOLIS, G. & FRIESEN, H.G. (1974). Inhibition by apomorphine of prolactin secretion in patients with elevated serum prolactin. *J. clin. Endocrinol. Metab.*, **39**, 180–182.

MARTIN, J.B., REICHLIN, S. & BROWN, G.M. (1977). In *Clinical Neuroendocrinology, Contemporary Neurology*. Philadelphia: G.A. Davis Co.

MARTINI, L. & BESSER, G.M. (1977). *Clinical Neuroendocrinology*. New York: Academic Press.

MASALA, A., MAGNA, A., DEVELLA, L., DELITALA, G. & NOVASIO, P.P. (1980). Inhibition of prolactin secretion by nomifensine in man. *Clin. Endocrinol.*, **12**, 237–241.

MELTZER, H.Y. & FANG, V.S. (1976). The effect of neuroleptics on serum prolactin in schizophrenic patients. *Arch. Gen. Psychiat.*, **33**, 279–284.

MELTZER, J.Y., GOODE, D.J., SCHYRE, P.M., YOUNG, M. & FANG, V.S. (1979). Effects of clozapine on human serum prolactin levels. *Am. J. Psychiat.*, **136**, 1550–1554.

MELTZER, H.Y., PIYAKALMALA, S., SCHYRE, P. & FANG, V.S. (1977). Lack of effect of tricyclic antidepressants on serum prolactin levels. *Psychopharmacology*, **51**, 185–187.

MENDELS, J. (1976). Lithium in the treatment of depression. *Am. J. Psychiat.*, **133**, 373–378.

MENDELS, J., FRAZER, A. & CARROL, B. (1974). Growth hormone responses in depression. *Am. J. Psychiat.*, **131**, 1154–1155.

MENDELSON, J.H., ELLINGBOE, J., KEUHNLE, J.C. & MELLO, N.Y. (1978). Effects of naltrexone on mood and neuroendocrine function in normal adult males. *Psychoneuroendocrinology*, **3**, 231–236.

MENDELSON, J.H., KUEHNLE, J., ELLINGBOE, J. & BABOR, T.F. (1974). Plasma testosterone levels, before, during and after chronic marihuana smoking. *New Engl. J. Med.*, **292**, 1051–1055.

MENDELSON, J.H., MELLO, N.K. & ELLINGBOE, J. (1977). Effects of acute alcohol intake on pituitary-gonadal hormones in normal human males. *J. Pharmac. exp. Ther.*, **202**, 676–682.

MENDELSON, J.H., MENDELSON, J.E. & PATCH, V.D. (1975). Plasma testosterone levels in heroin addiction and during methadone maintenance. *J. Pharmac. exp. Ther.*, **192**, 211–217.

MIRIN, S.M., MENDELSON, J.H., ELLINGBOE, J. & MYER, R.E. (1976). Acute effects of heroin and naltrexone on testosterone and gonadotrophin secretion in pilot study. *Psychoneuroendocrinology*, **1**, 359–369.

MULLER, E.E., NISTICO, G. & SCAPAGINI, E. (1977). In *Neurotransmitters and anterior pituitary function*. New York: Academic Press.

MULLER, E.E., GENAZZI, A.R. & MURU, S. (1978). Nomifensine: diagnostic test in hyperprolactinaemic states. *J. clin. Endocrinol. Metab.*, **47**, 1352–1357.

MURRAY, M.A.F., BANCROFT, J.H.J., ANDERSON, D.C., TENNENT, T.C. & CARR, P.J. (1975). Endocrine changes in male sexual deviants after treatment with anti-androgens, oestrogens or tranquillisers. *J. Endocrinol.*, **67**, 179–188.

NAKAI, Y., IMURA, H., YOSHUMI, T. & MATSUKURA, S. (1973). Adrenergic control mechanism for ACTH secretion in man. *Acta Endocrinol.*, **74**, 263–270.

NASRALLAH, H.A., FREED, W.J., ROGOL, A. & WYATT, R.J. (1977). Propranolol and prolactin. *Lancet* ii, 1175–1176.

NOEL, G.L., SUK, H.K., STONE, G.J. & FRANTZ, A.G. (1972). Human prolactin and growth hormone release during surgery and other conditions of stress. *J. clin. Endocrinol. Metab*, **35**, 840–851.

PADFIELD, P.L., PARK, S.J., MORTON, J.J. & BRAIDWOOD, A.E. (1977). Plasma levels of antidiuretic hormone in patients receiving prolonged lithium therapy. *Br. J. Psychiat.*, **130**, 144–147.

PANDEY, G.N., GARVER, D.L., TAMMINGA, C., ERICKSON, S., SYAD, I.A. & DAVIS, J.M. (1977). Post-synaptic supersensitivity in schizophrenia. *Am. J. Psychiat.*, **134**, 518–522.

PARKES, J.D., DEBONO, A.G., JENNER, P. & WALTERS, J. (1977). Amphetamines, growth hormone and narcolepsy. *Br. J. clin. Pharmac.*, **4**, 343–349.

PARKES, J.D., DEBONO, A.G. & MARSDEN, C.D. (1976). Growth—hormone response in Parkinson's disease. *Lancet*, **i**, 483.

PAYKEL, E.S. & ROWAN, P.R. (1979). Affective disorders. In *Recent Advances in Clinical Psychiatry*, ed. Granville-Grossman, K. pp. 37–90. London: Churchill-Livingstone.

PERSKY, H., O'BRIEN, C.P., FINE, E., HOWARD, W.J., KHAN, M.A. & BECK, R.W. (1977). The effect of alcohol and smoking on testosterone function and aggression in chronic alcoholics. *Am. J. Psychiat.*, **134**, 621–625.

PERSSON, T. & ROOS, B.E. (1967). 5-hydroxytryptophan for depression. *Lancet*, **ii**, 987–988.

PLANT, T.M., NAKAI, Y., BELCHETZ, P., KEOGH, E. & KNOBIL, E. (1978). The sites of action of estradiol and phentolamine in the inhibition of the pulsatile circhoral discharges of LH in the rhesus monkey. *Endocrinology*, **102**, 1015–1018.

POST, R.M. (1975). Cocaine psychoses: A continuum model. *Am. J. Psychiat.*, **132**, 225–231.

PRANGE, A.J., WILSON, I.C., LARA, P.P., ALLTOP, L.B. & BREESE, G.R. (1972). Effects of thyrotropin-releasing hormone in depression. *Lancet*, **ii**, 999–1002.

RANDRUP, A. & MUNKVAD (1972). Evidence indicating an association between schizophrenia and dopaminergic hyperactivity in the brain. *Orthomolec. Psychiat.*, **1**, 2–7.

RAVITZ, A.J. & MOORE, K.E. (1977). Effects of amphetamine, methylphenidate and cocaine on serum prolactin concentrations in the male rat. *Life Sci.*, **21**, 267–272.

REES, L. (1970). *M.D. thesis.* University of London.

REES, L., BULLER, P.W.P., GOSLING, C. & BESSER, G.M. (1970). Adrenergic blockade and the corticosteroid and growth hormone response to methylamphetamine. *Nature*, **228**, 565–566.

RIDGES, A.P., LAWTON, K., HARPER, P., GHOSH, C. & HINDSON, N. (1977). Propranolol in schizophrenia. *Lancet*, **ii**, 986.

ROTROSEN, J., ANGRIST, O., GERSHON, S., PARQUIN, T., BRANCHEY, L., OLESHANSKY, M., HALPERN, F. & SACHAR, E.J. (1979). Neuroendocrine effects of apomorphine, Characterization of response patterns and application to schizophrenia research. *Br. J. Psychiat.*, **135**, 444–456.

RUBIN, R.T. (1977). Strategies of neuroendocrine research in psychiatry. In *Neuroregulators and Psychic Disorders*, eds. Usdin, E., Hamburg, D.A. & Barches, J.D., pp. 233–241, New York: Oxford University Press.

RUBIN, P., SWEZEY, S. & BLUSCHKE, T. (1979). Naloxone lowers plasma prolactin in man. *Lancet*, **i**, 1293.

SACHAR, E.J., GRUEN, P.H., ALTMAN, N., HALPERN, F.S. & FRANTZ, A.G. (1976). Use of neuroendocrine techniques in psychopharmacological research. In *Hormones, Behaviour and Psychopathology*, Sachar, E.J., pp. 161–176. New York: Raven Press.

SALDANHA, V.F., HARVARD, C.W.H., BIRD, R. & GARDNER, A. (1972). The effect of chlorpromazine on pituitary function. *Clin. Endocrinol.*, **1**, 173–180.

SCANLON, M.F., GOMEZ-PAIN, A., MORA, B., COOK, D.B., DEWAR, J.H., HILDYARD, A. WEIGHTMAN, D.R., EVERED, D.C. & HALL, R. (1977). Effects of nomifensine, an inhibitor of endogenous catecholamine re-uptake in acromegaly, in hyperprolactinaemia and against stimulated prolactin release in man. *Br. J. clin. Pharmac.*, **4**, 191S–197S.

SCANLON, M.F., REES SMITH, B. & HALL, R. (1978). Thyroid-stimulating hormone: neuroregulation and clinical applications. *Chem. Sci. Med.*, **55**, 129–138.

SCHAEFER, C.F., GUNN, C.G. & DUBOWSKI, K.M. (1975). Normal plasma testosterone concentrations after marihuana smoking. *New Eng. J. Med.*, **292**, 867–868.

SCHILDKRAUT, J.J. (1965). The catecholamine hypothesis—a review of the supporting evidence. *Am. J. Psychiat.* **122**, 509–522.

SCHWIMM, C., SCHWARK, H. McINTOSH, C., MILSTREY, H.R., WILLS, B. & KOBBERLING, J. (1976). Effect of dopamine receptor blocking agent pimozide on the growth hormone response to arginine and exercise and the spontaneous growth hormone fluctuations. *J. clin. Endocrinol. Metab.*, **43**, 1183–1185.

SHAAR, C.J., FREDERICKSON, R.C.A., DONINGER, M.B. & JACKSON, L. (1977). Enkephalin analogues and naloxone modulate the release of growth hormone and prolactin. Evidence for regulation by an endogenous opioid peptide in brain. *Life Sci.*, **21**, 853–860.

SHADER, R.I. & Di MASCIO R. (1970). *Psychotropic drug side-effects* Baltimore: Williams and Wilkins.

SHAW, K.M., LEES, A.J., HAYES, S., ROSS, E.J., STERN, G.M. & THOMSON B.D. (1976). Growth hormone response to bromocriptine in Parkinsonism. *Lancet*, **i**, 194.

SHERMAN, L., KIM, S., BENJAMIN, F. & KOLODNY, H. (1971). Effect of chlorpromazine on serum growth hormone concentration in man. *New Engl. J. Med.*, **284**, 72–74.

SINGER, I., ROTENBERG, D. & PUSCHETT, J.B. (1972). Lithium induced nephrogenic diabetes insipidus *in vivo* and *in vitro* studies. *J. clin. Invest.*, **51**, 108–1091.

SIRIS, S.S., van KAMMAN, D.P. & de FRAITES, E.G. (1978). Serum prolactin and antipsychotic responses to pimozide in schizophrenia. *Psychopharmac. Bull.*, **14**, 8–9.

SLATER, S.,DE LA VEGA,C.E., SHYLER, J. & MURPHY, D.L. (1978). Plasma prolactin secretion by fenfluramine and amphetamine. *Psychopharmac. Bull.*, **12**, 26.

SMYTHE, G.A., COMPTON, P.J. & LAZARUS, L. (1976). Serotonergic control of human growth hormone secretion: the actions of L-dopa and 2-bromo-alpha-ergocryptine. In *Growth Hormone and Related Peptides*, eds. Pecile, A. & Muller, E.E. pp. 222–225. Amsterdam: Excerpta Medica.

SNYDER, S.H., ENNA, S.J. & YOUNG, A.B. (1977). Brain mechanisms associated with therapeutic actions of benzodiazepines: focus on neurotransmitters. *Am. J. Psychiat.* **134**, 662–664.

STANLEY, M., LAUTIN, A., ROTROSEN, J. & GERSHON, S. (1979). Antipsychotic efficacy of metoclopramide. Do DA/neuroleptic receptors mediate the action of anti-psychotic drugs? *IRCS Medical Science*, **7**, 322.

STRAIN, G.W. & STRAIN, J.J. (1978). Editorial: *Psychosom. Med.*, **40**, 2–4.

STRAUCH, G., VALCHE, J.C., MAHOUDEAU, J.A. & BRICAIR, H. (1977). Hormonal changes induced by bromocriptine (CB-154) at the early stage of treatment. *J. clin. Endocrinol. Metab.,* **44,** 588–590.

STUBBS, W.A., DELITALA, G., JONES, A., JEFFCOATE, W.J., EDWARDS, C.R.W., RATTER, S.J., BESSER, G.M., BLOOM, S.R. & ALBERTI, K.G.M.M. (1978). Hormonal and metabolic responses to an enkephalin analogue in normal man. *Lancet,* **ii,** 1225–1227.

SYLVALAHTI, E. & KANTO, J. (1975). Serum growth hormone, serum immunoreactive insulin and blood glucose responses to oral and intravenous diazepam in man. *Int. J. clin. Pharmac.,* **12,** 74.

THORNER, M.O., BESSER, G.M., HAGAN, C. & McNEILLY, A.S. (1971). Introduction of a new stimulation test for prolactin: the sulpiride test: a comparison with other dynamic function tests. *J. Endocrinol.,* **61,** 83.

THORNER, M.O., CHAIT, A., AITKEN, M., BENDER, G., BLOOM, S.M., MORTIMER, C.H., SANDERS, P., STUART-MASON, A. & BESSER, G.M. (1975). Bromocriptine treatment of acromegaly. *Br. med. J.,* **i,** 299–303.

THORNER, M.O., RYAN, S.M., WASS, J.A.H., JONES, A., BOULOUX, P., WILLIAMS, S. & BESSER, G.M. (1978). Effect of dopamine agonist, lergotrile mesylate, on circulating anterior pituitary hormones in man. *J. clin. Endocrinol. Metab.,* **47,** 372–378.

TOLLIS, G., HICKEY, J. & GUYDA, H. (1975). Effect of morphine on serum growth hormone, cortisol, prolactin and thyroid stimulating hormone in man. *J. clin. Endocrinol. Metab.,* **41,** 797–800.

TURKINGTON, R.W. (1972). The clinical endocrinology of prolactin. *Ad. int. Med.,* **18,** 363.

van THIEL, D.H., LESTER, R. & VAITUKAITIS, J. (1978). Evidence of a defect in pituitary secretion of luteinizing hormone in chronic alcoholic men. *J. clin. Endocrinol. Metab.,* **47,** 499–507.

WEICH, R.F. (1978). Acute effects of adrenergic blocking drugs and neuroleptic agents on pulsatile discharges of luteinizing hormone in the ovariectomized rat. *Neuroendocrinology,* **26,** 108–117.

WEINER, R.I. & GANONG, W.F. (1978). Role of monoamines and histamine in the regulation of anterior pituitary hormone secretion. *Physiol. Rev.,* **58,** 905–976.

WELLS, B., SILVERSTONE, T. & REES, L. (1978). The effect of oral dextroamphetamine on PRL secretion in man. *Neuropharmacology,* **17,** 1060–1061.

WIDERLOV, E. (1978). Effect of tricyclic antidepressants on human plasma levels of TSH/GH and PRL. *Acta Psychiat. Scand.,* **58,** 449–456.

WILLOUGHBY, J.O., BRAZEAU, P. & MARTIN, J.B. (1977). Effects of (+)-butaclamol on episodic GH and PRL release. *Endocrinology,* **101,** 1298–1303.

WRIGHT, J.W., FRY, D.E., MERRY, J. & MARKS, (1976). Abnormal hypothalamic—pituitary—gonadal function in chronic alcoholics. *Br. J. Addiction,* **71,** 211–215.

YEN, S.C. (1977). Neuroendocrine aspects of the regulation of cyclic gonadotrophin release in women. In *Clinical Neuroendocrinology,* eds Martin, L. & Besser, G.M. pp. 175–196. New York: Academic Press.

YORKSTON, N.J., GRUZELIER, J.H., ZAKI, S.A., HOLLANDER, D., PITCHER, D.R. & SERGEANT, H.G.S. (1977). Propranolol as an adjunct to the treatment of schizophrenia. *Lancet,* **ii,** 575–578.

TESTS OF AUTONOMIC FUNCTION IN ASSESSING CENTRALLY-ACTING DRUGS

PAUL TURNER

Department of Clinical Pharmacology, St. Bartholomew's Hospital, London EC1A 1BE

The major classes of centrally-acting drugs in psychotherapeutic use have marked peripheral autonomic actions in man, which may appear at therapeutic doses and not be related only to overdosage. Studies on the central nervous pharmacological effects of these drugs in man are severely limited methodologically, and it has been tempting, therefore, to extrapolate from their peripheral autonomic effects to possible central actions. It has to be admitted with disappointment, however, that no consistent spectra of such actions have been described which provide convincing bases for hypothetical central mechanisms of action. Nevertheless, studies of the peripheral autonomic actions of drugs of any therapeutic class are an important part of their early screening because they may be predictive of important adverse effects and drug interactions that may be encountered during their long-term therapeutic use.

The neurochemical basis of transmission in the autonomic nervous system continues to attract attention (Burnstock, 1979) and in recent years evidence has been produced for purinergic and peptidergic mechanisms. It is probable that many psychotropic drugs will be found to influence these systems, but this review will be limited to some of the methods available for studying their actions on the better known human cholinergic (ACh), noradrenergic (NA), dopaminergic (DA) and serotoninergic (5HT) systems.

Human isolated tissue

a) *Smooth muscle* The autonomic receptor population of different types of human smooth muscle have been characterized and used to study the postsynaptic agonist and antagonist actions of many drugs. The value of such studies was illustrated by the demonstration that the so-called 'false transmitter' α-methylnoradrenaline had α-adrenoceptor agonist activity similar to that of noradrenaline on human isolated smooth muscle (Coupar & Turner, 1970). The facilitatory effect of methysergide on cholinergic transmission (Katsuragi & Furukawa, 1979) was first demonstrated on human isolated intestinal muscle (Metcalfe & Turner, 1970). Human tissue, including vascular tissue, may also be used to study presynaptic effects of drugs (Moulds, Rittinghausen & Shaw, 1979). Many psychotropic drugs have cardiotoxic

properties, and the measurement of human intracellular action potentials, and their modification by drugs (Coltart & Meldrum, 1971) may prove of value in elucidating their action and predicting their effects.

b) *Platelets* The human platelet has two properties which have been used in the study of psychotropic drug action; 1) DA and 5-HT uptake, storage and release; 2) aggregation. These will be discussed in greater detail in later articles in this series.

Cardiovascular system

a) *Superficial hand vein* Sicuteri (1973) described a method for recording pressure changes in a human peripheral vein *in vivo* in which a small gauge needle inserted in the vein was used both to perfuse it with pharmacologically active agents and also to measure intraluminal pressure changes by means of a pressure transducer. Although sensitive enough to record the vascular effects of agonists such as 5-HT, it suffered from practical problems such as blockage of the needle which interfered with pressure recordings. Nachev, Collier & Robinson (1971) described a simple but elegant method for estimating changes in hand vein diameter in which a dissecting stereomicroscope was focussed on a cross drawn over the chosen vein after inflation of a sphygmomanometer cuff on the upper arm to 45 mmHg and refocussed as the vein dilated or constricted in response to pharmacological agents infused distal to the site under study. The distance through which the microscope moved to refocus the cross was a measure of the change in vein diameter. Limitations to this method are that continuous recording of vessel diameter is not possible, and observer bias is difficult to eliminate. These have been overcome by means of a light lever resting on the dorsal surface of the hand over the vein and connected to a displacement transducer with an appropriate amplifier and recorder (White & Udwadia, 1975). Aellig (1979) has recently devised a further modification of the method in which a light core mounted in a small tripod is placed over the summit of the vein under study. This core alters the voltage generated in surrounding coils, the changes being proportional to its displacement. This method has the advantage that the device can be exactly calibrated and therefore allows direct measurement of venous diameter at a chosen congestion pressure.

This *in vivo* preparation is sensitive to the effects of many agonists including NA, 5-HT, histamine and prostaglandins, and to the actions of specific and non-specific antagonists (Robinson & Collier, 1979). A limitation, however, is that the tone of a venous segment under study depends not only on local pharmacological treatments but also on reflex changes in vascular tone due to other events, both physiological and environmental. The success of the method therefore depends on strict control of experimental conditions and frequent repetition of control dose response curves to the agonist under investigation in order to confirm the stability and sensitivity of the preparation.

Other methods of studying the effects of drugs on the venous system in man have been reviewed by Robinson (1978).

b) *Skin temperature* Skin temperature depends primarily on arterial blood flow and acute changes following drug administration may reflect changes in flow. However, psychological changes such as anxiety can influence skin temperature as do metabolic events in underlying tissues. It is essential to control strictly experimental conditions, to record accurately ambient temperature with thermocouples and to allow adequate time for temperature equilibration. It is also necessary to ensure mental relaxation as far as possible, although in studies involving psychiatric patients this may be impossible and make difficult a true assessment of experimental results. Pharmacological responses of cutaneous vessels vary in different areas, vasoconstrictor α-adrenoceptors being present in hand and forearm but absent from the chest. Vasodilatation of the skin of the neck and upper chest is generally due to active dilatation, while in the hand it depends mainly on decreased vasoconstrictor tone. Despite the limitations of this procedure, the influence of adrenergic receptor agonists and antagonists have been investigated (for example Royds & Lockhart, 1974).

c) *Plethysmography* Arterial flow into a limb or part of a limb may be measured by a variety of methods (Roddie & Wallace, 1979) of which venous occlusion plethysmography appears to be the best. Reflex vascular changes following intravenous or oral drug administration may be avoided by infusing the drug into the brachial artery of one arm and using the other arm as a control (Collier, Large & Robinson, 1978). Although this method is only suitable for short-term studies of drug action, and the effects of long-term treatment may differ from those of acute administration, it has permitted assessment of the relative effects of drugs on the venous and arterial systems (Robinson & Collier, 1979).

d) *Heart rate* Resting heart rate is largely determined by the balance of cardiac para-sympathetic and sympathetic tone. A modest increase in heart rate is usually due to withdrawal of parasympathetic tone due either to an anticholinergic action of a drug, or to an α-adrenoceptor blocking or direct vasodilator action producing reflex withdrawal of cholinergic tone. Many psychotropic drugs have one or more of these actions, but the possession of anticholinergic properties is usually shown more easily by other more prominent atropine-like effects such as reduction in salivary volume. Some psychiatric conditions such as anxiety are associated with resting heart rates which differ significantly from normal controls, and this has to be considered in any study of drug action. This subject has been discussed in detail by Tyrer (1976).

Inhibition of exercise-induced tachycardia is used routinely for the assessment of a drug's β-adreno-ceptor blocking properties (McDevitt, 1977). A control tachycardia of greater than 150 beats/min is desirable if adequate dose response curves are to be obtained.

e) *Baroreflex activity* Uncertainty often exists as to whether drug-induced changes in heart rate and blood pressure are direct effects or mediated through an influence on baroreflex activity. A variety of methods have been described for assessing baroreflex function in man, but few unequivocal effects of drugs upon it have been demonstrated.

i) Increases in blood pressure are produced by intravenous injections of small boluses of phenylephrine. A stimulus response line is obtained from the regression of pulse interval on systolic arterial pressure during the rise in pressure produced by phenylephrine. The slope of the regression line is used as an index of baroreflex sensitivity, and is expressed as milliseconds of increase in pulse interval per mmHg rise in arterial pressure (Smyth, Sleight & Pickering, 1969). Clonidine appears to increase the gain of the baroreflex arc (Sleight & West, 1975). In one study short and long-term antihypertensive treatment with β-adrenoceptor antagonists did not appear to influence it, but no positive control drug was included in the study (Simon, Kiowski & Julius, 1977). In another study, however, baroreflex activity increased significantly in young hypertensive patients after treatment with β-adrenoceptor antagonists (Watson, Stallard & Littler, 1979). The sensitivity of this method to assess drug action on baroreflex activity must, therefore, be considered uncertain.

ii) Circulatory changes following a standard Valsalva manoeuvre in which subjects support a column of water for a given period of time by a forced expiration have been used to assess baroreflex activity (Korner, Tonkin & Uther, 1979). No unequivocal drug-induced changes appear to have been demonstrated by this method.

iii) A techique has been developed which involves the application to the neck of variable pressure by means of a sealed chamber applied around the neck, thus changing carotid sinus transmural pressure. This selectively tests carotid baroceptors and permits study of reflex responses of both heart and peripheral circulation (Ludbrook, Marcia, Ferrari & Zanchetti, 1977). Results of its use in the study of drug action are awaited with interest.

f) *Blood pressure* Methods available for measurement of blood pressure in clinical pharmacological studies have been reviewed by Raftery (1978).

i) Autonomic neuropathy, such as that found in some patients with diabetes mellitus, may be associated with changes in cardiovascular responses. For example, the increases in blood pressure and heart rate produced by static muscular exercise such as sustained hand grip are reduced in the presence of such a neuropathy (Ewing, Irving, Kerr, Wildsmith & Clarke, 1974). This autonomic response, which is reflex in nature, is thought to be initiated by stimuli from the exercising muscle. The pressor response is thought to be mediated partly by an increase in cardiac output and partly by peripheral α-adrenoceptor mediated vasoconstriction. In essence, therefore, it resembles other reflex responses such as the Valsalva manoeuvre. It has been argued (Harrison, 1964) that a similar test involving the maintenance of an outstretched leg against gravity for as long as possible is in reality a form of stress with important physiological effects, as it is accompanied by increased levels of plasma catecholamines and cortisol, and pupillary dilatation, as well as raised heart rate and blood pressure. There is no doubt that this task is unpleasant and painful, but the relative contribution of somatic and psychic distress to the physiological changes is open to question, as are the effects of anxiolytic agents upon these physiological variables (Farhoumand, Harrison, Pare, Turner & Wynn, 1979).

ii) Tyramine is an indirectly-acting sympathomimetic amine which releases NA from storage sites in adrenergic nerve endings. The released NA stimulates postsynaptic receptors leading to a rise in systolic blood pressure. Monoamine reuptake inhibiting antidepressives such as imipramine inhibit reuptake of NA released into the synaptic cleft, and also inhibit the uptake of tyramine, so reducing the pressor response to injected tyramine (Ghose, Gifford, Turner & Leighton, 1976). The pressor effect of noradrenaline, on the other hand, is potentiated (Ghose, 1977). Essentially, the tyramine pressor response test consists of administration of incremental doses of intravenous tyramine, beginning with 0.5 mg, in a relaxed supine subject. Following injection of each dose, the blood pressure rises rapidly

after a latent period of 1 min to reach a maximum within 3 min. The baseline is reached again within about five minutes. The dose is increased until the systolic pressure rises to 30 mmHg or more above baseline. From the dose response curve obtained, the tyramine dose required to elevate the systolic pressure by 30 mmHg after treatment with a drug is compared with that after placebo, to give a dose-ratio. Tyramine sensitivity is influenced by age, sex, hormonal status and psychiatric condition (Ghose, Turner & Coppen, 1975; Ghose & Turner, 1977), all of which must be considered when using it in clinical pharmacological studies. Nevertheless, when carried out under carefully controlled conditions, changes in tyramine sensitivity have been shown to correlate closely with plasma levels of monoamine uptake inhibiting drugs (Ghose et al., 1976).

g) *Systolic time intervals and high speed surface ECG* Many psychotropic drugs, particularly the monoamine reuptake inhibitors, possess cardiotoxic actions, the mechanism of which is not yet clear. Several experimental techniques have been used to study the cardiac effects of these drugs, including His bundle ECG (Burrows, Vohra, Hunt, Sloman, Scoggins & Davies, 1976), but noninvasive techniques such as systolic time intervals and high speed surface ECG (Burgess, Turner & Wadsworth, 1978) are more appropriate for routine screening procedures in patients and normal volunteers. The use of systolic time intervals in clinical pharmacology has been reviewed elsewhere (Gibson, 1979).

Salivary volume

The most sensitive and easily measurable anticholinergic effect of psychotropic drugs is a reduction in salivary flow rate and a variety of methods have been described for this purpose. Basal or stimulated flow rates may be measured, stimulation usually taking the form of chewing on a neutral insoluble material such as wax or parafilm, or sucking an acid-flavoured sweet. In all types of test, saliva flow per unit time is measured. The volume can be measured by (i) spitting all saliva secreted into a measuring cylinder through a funnel (Kingsley & Turner, 1974); (ii) a suction mechanism ensures that a saliva ejector applied orally collects all saliva on the floor of the mouth (Bertram, Kragh-Sorensen, Rafaelsen & Larsen, 1979); (iii) a suction cup applied over the orifice of the parotid duct collects all saliva produced from that gland during a given time (Speirs, 1977). The last method is particularly useful for studies of salivary drug concentration, but is difficult to apply to all subjects for most purposes.

Another approach is to measure salivary production by increase in weight of dental wool cylinders inserted into the cheeks and floor of the mouth for a given time period (Dollery, Davies, Draffan, Dargie, Dean, Reid, Clare & Murray, 1976). Although no formal comparison of these methods appears to have been carried out, personal experience suggests that the first method described is the most simple and convenient, and is adequate for screening psychotropic drugs for clinically significant anticholinergic activity.

Gastrointestinal function

The most important and frequent effect of psychotropic drugs on gastrointestinal function is to inhibit motility, generally through an anticholinergic action. This may result in clinical constipation, but may also produce important effects on gastric emptying and the absorption of other drugs.

a) *Gastric emptying* Although a variety of methods to measure gastric emptying rate have been described (Prescott, 1974; Bateman, Kahn, Mashiter & Davies, 1978), none are free from problems of interpretation, methodology or safety. The best available appears to be the comparison of the rate of absorption of an orally administered marker such as paracetamol or alcohol after treatment with the test drug compared with that after a standard anticholinergic drug and after a placebo.

b) *Colonic motility* A variety of psychotropic drugs with ACh, NA, DA and 5-HT agonist or antagonist activity may influence colonic motility. Changes in intraluminal pressure in the sigmoid colon and rectum may be measured through catheters introduced through a proctosigmoidoscope, connected to differential air pressure transducers and recorded on an appropriate polygraph (Lechin & Van der Dijs, 1979).

The eye

a) *Pupil diameter* Pupil diameter is determined by cholinergic tone on the constrictor pupillae and α-adrenoceptor tone on the dilator pupillae muscles, and a variety of psychotropic drugs influence it (Turner, 1975). The interpretation of many past studies is now recognized to be complicated by recent increased understanding of the importance of central mechanisms controlling parasympathetic outflow and it is often difficult to be certain that the pupillary actions of a drug are due to peripheral rather than central influences, even if the drug has been administered by local topical application to the eye. A variety of methods for recording pupil diameter are available ranging from simple subjective matching of the pupil with a series of holes of different known diameters, through photographic methods using ordinary light sources or infrared illumination, to sophisticated infrared and television pupillometers. The method used should depend on the information required. Changes in resting pupil diameter can probably adequately be recorded by photographic methods; for example comparison of the effects of desipramine and amitriptyline on pupillary responses to NA and methoxamine using a simple photographic method yielded results consistent with their known pre- and postsynaptic effects (Gaszner, Szabadi & Bradshaw, 1980). Changes in pupil reactivity to light and accommodation, however, require the ability to record rapid changes in pupil size in darkness and this is now best achieved by a television pupillometer (Bye, Clubley, Henson, Peck, Smith & Smith, 1979), although its cost puts this piece of equipment beyond the budget of most research departments.

b) *Accommodation* Although large changes in pupil diameter can be produced by both cholinergic and adrenergic influences, marked changes in accommodation are usually cholinergic in origin, as α-adrenoceptor agonism and antagonism produce only small albeit significant changes (Mayer, Stewart-Jones & Turner, 1977). For most purposes, determination of the near point by Scheiner's method (Taylor, 1950) is adequate, mean values of at least three recordings per eye being recorded at each time period.

c) *Intraocular pressure* Many psychotropic drugs possess atropine like effects which have the potential to raise intraocular pressure and precipitate glaucoma in patients at risk. Drug-induced changes in intraocular pressure may be measured by means of a contact tonometer which requires the production of local corneal anaesthesia before its application. This has been criticized as possibly leading to changes in corneal permeability to other drugs and more recently a non-contact tonometer has been described which was sensitive enough to demonstrate an ocular hypotensive action of a β-adrenoceptor antagonist in normal volunteers (Hill, Lewis, Stewart-Jones, Wadsworth & Turner, 1979). It depends upon the scattering of a collimated beam of light directed at the cornea when the corneal surface is indented by a pulsed column of compressed air. Its potential to detect intraocular pressure changes induced by psychotropic drugs is worthy of assessment in view of its non-invasive nature.

Critical flicker frequency

Although not a test of autonomic activity but of central nervous arousal, it is appropriate to consider critical flicker frequency (CFF) here, as it is markedly influenced by autonomic activity, particularly on pupil diameter. The CFF may be defined as the rate at which an intermittent light source appears to a subject to be flickering as opposed to steady. The threshold frequency is determined by a large number of factors such as the wavelength, waveform and light-dark ratio of the light source, and age, pupil size and states of light adaptation and accommodation to intermittency of the subject. When these variables are controlled, however, the CFF is a remarkably stable phenomenon which is sensitive to influence by central depressant and stimulant drugs in therapeutic doses and under different physiological conditions (Turner, 1968). It is particularly useful in studying the duration of action of centrally-acting drugs and in comparing their relative central effects in multidose studies.

This test of visual intermittency has its equivalent in the auditory system (Besser, 1967; Besser & Duncan, 1967), but the latter is more difficult to carry out as a routine procedure and is subject to considerable variation over long periods of time due to changes in auditory function associated, for example, with obstructions of the Eustachian tube and external auditory meatus.

Micturition

The importance of studying the effects of a drug on micturition is to predict a potential for producing urinary retention by an atropine-like action in patients at risk. A method has been described (Kopera, 1978) in which volunteers are given a measured quantity of fluid to drink, and then void their urine into a urodropspectrometer which uses the interruption of a light beam to record passage of urine drops, permitting accurate measurement of individual drop diameter, their temporal spacing and velocity.

Sweating

Sweating is increased in anxiety and emotional excitement and its measurement forms an important part of the investigation of potential anxiolytic drugs. Methods used include a variety which measure skin conductance under different conditions (Tyrer, 1976) and others which record the number of active sweat glands. A simple method recently described (Clubley, Bye, Henson, Peck & Riddington, 1978) involves painting an area of skin with a plastic impression paint. The plastic impression is then removed using 'sellotape', mounted on a 35 mm slide, projected and the glands counted. The anticholinergic activity of drugs can be studied by producing a sweat gland response by intradermal injections of increasing concentrations of ACh and determining the inhibitory effects of drugs on the ACh dose response

curve, under strictly controlled conditions of ambient temperature and physical activity.

Reductions of salivary volume and of sweat gland responses to ACh appear to be the most sensitive indices of anticholinergic activity, while changes in pupil diameter, accommodation and heart rate are less sensitive.

Tremor

Many drugs produce, exacerbate or inhibit tremor by central or peripheral mechanisms and tremor is a common symptom of psychiatric and neurological conditions. Its measurement is therefore an important part of clinical pharmacology and will be discussed in detail in a later paper in this series.

Experimental design

Although studies of autonomic pharmacology are popular in clinical pharmacology, they are beset by problems of methodology and interpretation. Chief among these is the marked variation within and between subjects in autonomic function, associated with a bewildering array of physiological, psychological and environmental factors. In any study of this type, therefore, the following should be considered:—

1) Experimental conditions should be strictly controlled, including ambient temperature, humidity, noise and other distractions.

2) The sensitivity of the method in the hands of the investigator should be established for each study, whenever possible, by the inclusion of an active standard preparation and a placebo. For example, if a new drug is being examined for potential anticholinergic activity on the eye, salivary volume and sweat gland activity, a standard anticholinergic drug should be included as well as a placebo, in the experimental design. Only if the standard drug can be differentiated from placebo in a particular test can the absence of an effect 'with the new drug be interpreted as freedom from such an action. It should not be necessary to add that each treatment should be administered under strictly randomized and double-blind conditions, if necessary using a double-dummy technique.

3) The time course of an experiment must be so designed to permit adequate time for acclimatization of subjects to the environmental conditions and, for example, for equilibration of thermocouples. If too much information is sought by means of a number of tests which cannot easily be accommodated within the experimental period, the inevitable haste and harrassment that ensue can produce their own

26

autonomic effects and prejudice the experimental results.

4) An attempt to combine pharmacokinetic with pharmacodynamic studies of this kind may lead to failure because the trauma of venesection may

produce a degree of arousal in the subject which interferes with tests of autonomic function. If a marker of drug absorption is required, it is probably better to use identification in saliva or urine at appropriate times.

References

AELLIG, W.H. (1979). Use of a linear variable differential transformer to measure compliance of human hand vein in situ. *Br. J. clin. Pharmac.*, **8**, 395P.

BATEMAN, D.N., KAHN, C., MASHITER, K. & DAVIES, D.S. (1978). Pharmacokinetics and concentration-effect studies with intravenous metoclopramide. *Br. J. clin. Pharmac.*, **6**, 401–407.

BERTRAM, U., KRAGH-SORENSEN, P., RAFAELSEN, O.J. & LARSEN, N. (1979). Saliva secretion following long-term antidepressant treatment with nortriptyline controlled by plasma levels. *Scand. J. dent. Res.*, **87**, 58–64.

BESSER, G.M. (1967). Auditory flutter fusion as a measure of the actions of centrally acting drugs. *Br. J. Pharmac.*, **30**, 329–340.

BESSER, G.M. & DUNCAN, C. (1967). The time course of action of single doses of diazepam, chlorpromazine and some barbiturates as measured by auditory flutter fusion and visual flicker fusion thresholds in man. *Br. J. Pharmac.*, **30**, 341–348.

BURGESS, C.D., TURNER, P. & WADSWORTH, J. (1978). Cardiovascular responses to mianserin hydrochloride; a comparison with tricyclic antidepressant drugs. *Br. J. clin. Pharmac.*, **5**, Suppl. 1. 21s–28s.

BURNSTOCK, G. (1979). Autonomic innervation and transmission. *Br. med. Bull.*, **35**, 255–262.

BURROWS, G.D., VOHRA, J., HUNT, D., SLOMAN, J.G., SCOGGINS, B.A. & DAVIES, B. (1976). Cardiac effects of different tricyclic antidepressant drugs. *Br. J. Psychiat.*, **129**, 335–341.

BYE, C.E., CLUBLEY, M., HENSON, T., PECK, A.W., SMITH, S.A. & SMITH, S.E. (1979). Changes in the human light reflex as a measure of the anticholinergic effects of drugs. A comparison with other measures. *Eur. J. clin. Pharmac.*, **15**, 21–25.

CLUBLEY, M., BYE, C.E., HENSON, T., PECK, A.W. & RIDDINGTON, C. (1978). A technique for studying the effects of drugs on human sweat gland activity. *Eur. J. clin. Pharmac.*, **14**, 221–226.

COLLIER, J.G., LARGE, R.E. & ROBINSON, B.F. (1978). Comparison of the effects of tolmesoxide, diazoxide, hydrallazine, prozosin, glyceryl trinitrate and sodium nitroprusside on forearm arteries and dorsal hand veins in man. *Br. J. clin. Pharmac.*, **5**, 35–44.

COLTART, D.J. & MELDRUM, S.J. (1971). The effects of racemic propranolol, dextropropranolol and racemic practolol on the human and canine transmembrane action potential. *Arch. int. Pharmacodyn.*, **192**, 188–193.

COUPAR, I.M. & TURNER, P. (1970). Relative potencies of some false transmitters on isolated human smooth muscle. *Br. J. Pharmac.*, **38**, 463P.

DOLLERY, C.T., DAVIES, D.S., DRAFFAN, G.H., DARGIE, H.J., DEAN, C.R., REID, J.L., CLARE, R.A. & MURRAY, S.

(1976). Clinical pharmacology and pharmacokinetics of clonidine. *Clin. Pharmac. Ther.*, **19**, 11–17.

EWING, D.J., IRVING, J.B., KERR, F., WILDSMITH, J.A.W. & CLARKE, B.F. (1974). Cardiovascular responses to sustained handgrip in normal subjects and in patients with diabetes mellitus: a test of autonomic function. *Clin. Sci.*, **46**, 295–306.

FARHOUMAND, N., HARRISON, J., PARE, C.M.B., TURNER, P. & WYNN, S. (1979). The effect of high dose oxprenolol on stress-induced physical and psychophysiological variables. *Psychopharmacology*, **64**, 365–369.

GASZNER, P., SZABADI, E. & BRADSHAW, C.M. (1980). Comparison of the effects of desipramine and amitriptyline on pupillary responses to noradrenaline and methoxamine in healthy volunteers. *Br. J. clin. Pharmac.*, **9**, 307P–309P.

GHOSE, K. (1977). Studies on the interaction between mianserin and noradrenaline in patients suffering from depressive illness. *Br. J. clin. Pharmac.*, **4**, 712–714.

GHOSE, K., TURNER, P. & COPPEN, A. (1975). Intravenous tyramine pressor response in depression. *Lancet*, **ii**, 1317–1318.

GHOSE, K., GIFFORD, L., TURNER, P. & LEIGHTON, M. (1976). Studies of the interactions of desmethylimipramine with tyramine in man and its correlation with the plasma concentrations. *Br. J. clin. Pharmac.*, **3**, 335–337.

GHOSE, K. & TURNER, P. (1977). The menstrual cycle and the tyramine pressor response test. *Br. J. clin. Pharmac.*, **4**, 500–502.

GIBSON, D.G. (1978). Use of systolic time intervals in clinical pharmacology. *Br. J. clin. Pharmac.*, **6**, 97–102.

HARRISON, J. (1964). The behaviour of the palmar sweat glands in stress. *J. Psychosom. Res.*, **8**, 187–191.

HILL, S.E.W., LEWIS, K., STEWART-JONES, J.H., WADSWORTH, J. & TURNER, P. (1979). Effect of local atenolol on intraocular pressure in normal subjects using a noninvasive method. *Pharmacotherapeutica*, **2**, 136–139.

KATSURAGI, T. & FURUKAWA, T. (1979). Methysergide induces selective potentiation in cholinergic contractions of the guinea-pig vas deferens by facilitating acetylcholine release. *J. Pharm. Pharmacol.*, **31**, 822–825.

KINGSLEY, P.J. & TURNER, P. (1974). Class experiment in clinical pharmacology with benzilonium bromide, an anticholinergic drug. *Eur. J. clin. Pharmac.*, **7**, 141–143.

KOPERA, H. (1978). Anticholinergic and blood pressure effects of mianserin, amitriptyline and placebo. *Br. J. clin. Pharmac.*, **5**, Suppl 1., 29s–4s.

KORNER, P.I., TONKIN, A.M. & UTHER, J.B. (1979). Valsalva constrictor and heart rate reflexes in subjects with essential hypertension and with normal blood pressure. *Clin. exp. Pharmac. Physiol.*, **6**, 97–110.

LECHIN, F., VAN DER DIJS, B. (1979). Effects of dopaminergic blocking agents on distal colon motility. *J. clin. Pharmac.*, **19**, 617–625.

LUDBROOK, J., MARCIA, G., FERRARI, A. & ZANCHETTI, A. (1977). The variable-pressure neck-chamber method for studying the carotid baroreflex in man. *Clin. Sci. mol. Med.*, **53**, 165–171.

MAYER, G.L., STEWART-JONES, J.H. & TURNER, P. (1977). Influence of α-adrenoceptor blockade with thymoxamine on changes in pupil diameter and accommodation produced by tropicamide and ephedrine. *Curr. med. Res. Opin.*, **4**, 660–664.

McDEVITT, D.G. (1977). The assessment of β-adrenoceptor blocking drugs in man. *Br. J. clin. Pharmac.*, **4**, 413–425.

METCALFE, H.L. & TURNER, P. (1970). A comparison of the effects of cinanserin and methysergide on responses of isolated human smooth muscle to acetylcholine. *Arch. int. Pharmacodyn.*, **183**, 148–158.

MOULDS, R.F.W., RITTINGHAUSEN, R. & SHAW, J. (1979). Prejunctional receptors in human digital arteries. *Proceedings 5th Triennial Conference of National Heart Foundation,* Canberra.

NACHEV, C., COLLIER, J. & ROBINSON, B. (1971). Simplified method for measuring compliance of superficial veins. *Cardiovascular Res.*, **5**, 147–156.

PRESCOTT, L.F. (1974). Gastric emptying and drug absorption. *Br. J. clin. Pharmac.*, **1**, 189–190.

RAFTERY, E.B. (1978). The methodology of blood pressure recording. *Br. J. clin. Pharmac.*, **6**, 193–202.

ROBINSON, B.F.(1978). Assessment of the effects of drugs on the venous system in man. *Br. J. clin. Pharmac.*, **6**, 381–386.

ROBINSON, B.F. & COLLIER, J.G. (1979). Human vascular muscle. *Br. med. Bull.*, **35**, 305–312.

RODDIE, I.C. & WALLACE, W.F.M. (1979). Methods for the assessment of the effects of drugs on the arterial system in man. *Br. J. clin. Pharmac.*, **7**, 317–324.

ROYDS, R.B. & LOCKHART, J.D.F. (1974). The effect of indoramin on peripheral blood flow. *Br. J. clin. Pharmac.*, **1**, 13–17.

SICUTERI, F. (1973). 5-Hydroxytryptamine supersensitivity as a new theory of essential headache. In *Background to Migraine.* Vol. 5, ed. Cummings, J.N. pp. 45–56. London: Heinemann Medical.

SIMON, G., KIOWSKI, W. & JULIUS, S. (1977). Effect of β-adrenoceptor antagonists on baroreceptor reflex sensitivity in hypertension. *Clin. Pharmac. Ther.*, **22**, 293–298.

SLEIGHT, P. & WEST, M.J. (1975). The effects of clonidine on the baroreflex arc in man. In *Central action of drugs in blood pressure regulation,* eds. Davies, D.S. & Reid, J.L. pp. 291–298. Tunbridge Wells: Pitman Medical.

SMYTH, H.S., SLEIGHT, P. & PICKERING, G. (1969). Reflex regulation of arterial pressure during sleep in man. *Circulation Res.*, **24**, 109–121.

SPEIRS, C.F. (1977). Oral absorption and secretion of drugs. *Br. J. clin. Pharmac.*, **4**, 97–99.

TAYLOR, N.B. (1950). The special senses. In *The Physiological Basis of Medical Practice,* eds. Best, C.H. & Taylor, N.B. p. 1139. London: Bailliere, Tindall and Cox.

TURNER, P. (1968). Critical flicker frequency and centrally acting drugs. *Br. J. Ophthal.*, **52**, 245–250.

TURNER, P. (1975). The human pupil as a model for clinical pharmacological investigations. *J. Roy. Coll. Phys. Lond.*, **9**, 165–173.

TYRER, P. (1976). *The role of bodily feelings in anxiety.* Oxford: Oxford University Press.

WATSON, R.D.S., STALLARD, T.J. & LITTLER, W.A. (1979). Effects of β-adrenoceptor antagonists on sino-aortic baroreflex sensitivity and blood pressure in hypertensive man. *Clin. Sci.,* **57**, 241–247.

WHITE, C. de B. & UDWADIA, B.P. (1975). β-adrenoceptors in the human dorsal hand vein, and the effects of propranolol and practolol on venous sensitivity to noradrenaline. *Br. J. clin. Pharmac.*, **2**, 99–105.

PSYCHOMOTOR FUNCTION AND PSYCHOACTIVE DRUGS

IAN HINDMARCH

Department of Psychology, University of Leeds, Leeds LS2 9JT

A cursory review of the literature reveals that the techniques used to assess psychomotor functions are diverse, often complex, frequently insensitive to drug induced changes and sometimes inconvenient to enact or replicate. Adams (1974) used proof reading ability; Croucher & Hindmarch (1974), the duration of the spiral after effect; Betts, Clayton & Mackay (1972), low speed car handling tasks; Malpas, Rowan, Joyce & Scott (1970), card sorting ability; Fargus & Hindmarch (1974), a cardriving simulator; Ashton, Hall, Savage, Telford & Thompson (1972), a pursuit rotor; File & Bond (1979), symbol copying; Van Houten & Zenhausern (1967), the absolute auditory threshold; Davis, Hollister, Overall, Johnson & Train (1976), short and long term memory; Ghoneim & Mewaldt (1977), verbal learning; Gendreau, Sherlock, Parsons, McLean, Scott & Suboske (1972), discrimination conditioning of the eyelid response; Gupta (1974), the kinaesthetic figural after effect; Adamson & Finlay (1966), muscular grip strength; Borland & Nicholson (1974), adaptive tracking; Wittenborn, Flaherty, McGough & Nash (1979), a beam balancing task; Bond & Lader (1972), the digit symbol substitution task; Bernstein, Hughes & Forney (1967), delayed auditory feedback; Veldkamp, Straw, Metzler & Demissianos (1974), ocular convergence; Lahtinen, Lahtinen & Pekkola (1978), the speed of putting caps on ball point pens; Ideström & Cadenius (1963) used tapping speed; Masuda & Bakker (1966), the galvanic skin response; Stitt, Latour & Frane (1977), a hidden word task; Bond & Lader (1973), auditory reaction time; Zimmermann-Tansella, Tansella & Lader (1976), the Gibson Spiral Maze; Hedges, Turner & Harry (1971), the critical flicker fusion frequency; Wittenborn, Flaherty, Hamilton, Schiffman & McGough (1976), a time estimation procedure; Church & Johnson (1979), electro-encephalographic changes; Peck, Adams, Bye & Wilkinson (1976), a digit span test; Landauer, Pococke & Prott (1974), a simple response timer; Holmberg & William-Ollson (1963), used body sway; Malpas & Joyce (1969), the duration of after images; Hindmarch & Parrott (1979), the serial subtraction of numbers; Roth, Kramer & Lutz (1977), the Purdue pegboard; Hindmarch (1979a), the stabilometer; Busch, Klapproth, Lücker & Schmitz (1979), concentration; Hindmarch & Parrott (1978), a concept identification task; Jones, Lewis & Spriggs (1978), a group vigilance task; Bond & Lader (1975), the cancellation of 4's; Jones, Jones, Lewis & Spriggs (1979), category clustering; Aschoff, Becker & Weinert (1975), saccadic eye movements; Gagné & Fleishman (1959), the rudder control test; Fleishman & Hempel (1956), multiple limb co-ordination; Jones (1958), an auditory discrimination test; Hindmarch (1975), the choice reaction time task; Hindmarch (1977a), simulated night time car driving performance; Biehl (1979), actual car driving ability; Wittenborn et al. (1979), spontaneous reversals of the Necker cube; Taeuber (1977), two handed cordination; Doongaji, Sheth, Apte, Lakdawala, Khare & Thatte (1979) used Whipple's tracing board and Hindmarch & Clyde (1980a, b), a trigram recognition task.

The foregoing examples of tests of psychomotor function are in no way exhaustive of the diversity of tests which have been used to measure the effects of psychoactive compounds on human behaviour. Each test has its own merits and defects but it can be questioned to what extent each researcher has viewed his approach within a theoretical framework. The major assumption of the psychopharmacologist is that the effects of a drug can be ultimately judged in behavioural terms. However, the range of behavioural activities presented above makes the choice of measure difficult to effect. If psychopharmacology is to be psychologically relevant, the study of the effect of drugs in the context of a well defined model of behaviour must be consistently pursued (Michon, 1973).

The complexity of the relationship between the overt behavioural activity of the organism and the stimulus impinging on the individual at a particular point in time makes the task of providing a reliable and parsimonious model of behaviour most difficult. However, it is possible to isolate the major variables of performance which go to make up the psychological reaction to the administration of a psychoactive substance (Figure 1).

It is obvious that the mode and level of activity of the brain and central nervous system will be

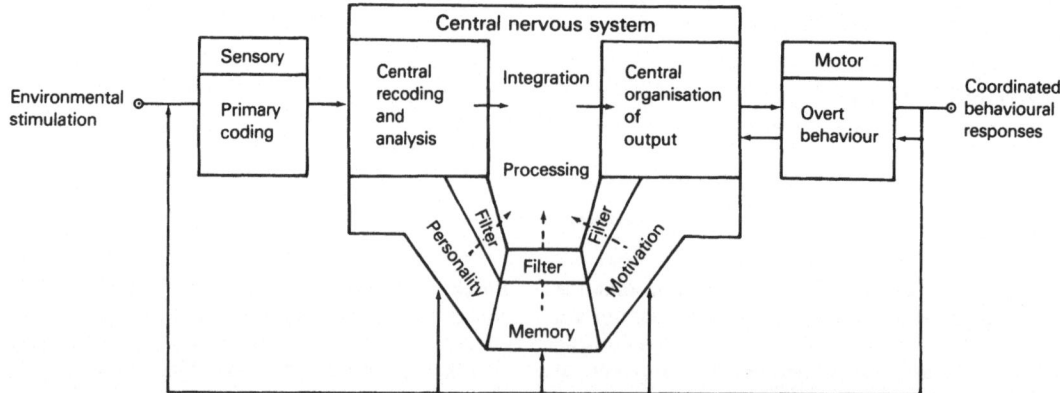

Figure 1 Psychomotor performance results from the co-ordination of sensory and motor systems through the integrative and organisational processes of the brain and central nervous system. The processing of sensory information is influenced by personality, memory and individual motivation, while the overall function of the integrative mechanism is governed by the state of arousal of the central nervous system. Complex feedback and adaptive systems complete the process by which environmental stimuli produce appropriate, co-ordinated behavioural responses.

dependent upon personality, motivation and memory and it is necessary to examine the extent of the effect of these factors on the measurement of performance and to see how such influences might be controlled and minimised.

Eysenck (1963, 1972) and Claridge (1967, 1970) have shown that an inverted U relationship holds between some personality dimensions, e.g. neuroticism, and performance on sensori-motor tasks like the pursuit rotor. The inverted U relationship implies that high neuroticism subjects will have poorer performance than less neurotic ones, because of their personality. Inter-individual differences in performance, due to personality, are well illustrated in the different psychomotor test scores which have been observed in patient and 'normal' volunteer populations (Malpas, Legg & Scott, 1974; Tansella, Zimmermann-Tansella & Lader, 1974). Significant relationships between neuroticism, or anxiety levels, and performance changes with benzodiazepine derivatives have also been reported (Biehl, 1974; Leygonie, Rethone, Yuceyatak & Yuceyatak, 1975), and anxious patients have been shown to have significantly lower critical flicker fusion thresholds than age matched 'normals'. (Krugman, 1947; Goldstone, 1955; Bühler, 1955; Jones, 1958). The effects of personality on performance become more pronounced at the extremes of affectual dimensions. In studies of the effect of a psychoactive drug in normal volunteers, the interaction of personality and performance can be minimised by a pre-selection of subjects i.e. including only those scoring within a standard deviation of the normative score for their age and sex. The Middlesex Hospital Questionnaire (MHQ) (Crown & Crisp, 1970), Eysenck Personality Inventory (EPI) (Eysenck & Eysenck, 1964) and Spielberger State-Trait Anxiety Inventory (STAI) (Spielberger, Gorsuch & Lushene, 1968) are all suitable tests for screening subjects. The same principles apply to clinical studies especially where different groups of patients are to be compared. As patients will probably already have impaired psychomotor performance it is most necessary to establish adequate entry criteria to ensure the homogeneity of the experimental group.

Motivational factors can affect the results obtained in performance studies. The intentions of volunteers, the level of payment of subjects and the expectations of the experimenter and subject can all have a profound influence on experimental results (Ayd, 1972). These extraneous variables can only be controlled by the use of double-blind experimental designs, a careful screening of volunteers, the use of experienced experimenters and a thoroughly reasoned protocol to govern the pragmatics of the test situation.

The intrinsic motivation of the task situation is an important determinant of performance. Drug action on a performance measure can also be affected by the nature of the assessment task. Fargus & Hindmarch (1974) were unable to show any decrement of reaction time performance following temazepam 30 mg or placebo in a car driving simulator. However, Hindmarch (1975) was able to show a significant impairment of reaction time produced by temazepam 30 mg in contrast to placebo, on a laboratory based reaction time task. The protocols, dose, regimen and subject populations were similar for both studies and the contrary results are due to the different test situations. The car driving simulator presented the task in a high interest situation, a computer controlled driving compartment with appropriate noises and movements. On the other hand the laboratory based reaction task was a straightforward light and button assembly with little intrinsic interest.

It is most important to realise that the disruptive effect of a drug on performance could be masked by the 'stimulating' nature of the assessment measure, particularly if the trial is aimed at assessing the safety of a drug in clinical use, e.g. the effects on car driving performance and related risk prone activities encountered by ambulant patients. The sensitivity of the performance measure can be ensured by including a verum, or positive internal control, in the drug treatment regimen along with the unknown compound and placebo. For example, amylobarbitone sodium is known to have sedative effects. If such effects are not obvious on an assessment measure following the experimental use of the drug, then it must be assumed that the test is insensitive and no credence can be given to any findings obtained in such an instance.

Any test of psychomotor performance involving the co-ordination of sensory and motor systems, e.g. the pursuit rotor, will be prone to practice and learning effects as, on repeated administration, the subject acquires the skills that facilitate performance. Standard tests of mental performance e.g. the digit symbol substitution test of the Wechsler Adult Intelligence Scale, (Wechsler, 1955), cannot be used on repeated administration schedules without modification, as many subjects are able to remember the digit-symbol code and so speed their task performance. Practice, learning and the effects of memory on performance measures are relatively easy to control. Prior to entry in a study relying on a sensori-motor measure of performance all subjects must be trained on the task until their 'learning curve' has reached a plateau, i.e. until the response measure has reached a limiting value and maintained such a value for several trials. When subjects are trained to a criterion, where no further increase in performance can be detected, they can then be admitted to a study. Such pre-training can completely eliminate learning effects, as evidenced in the unchanging placebo condition responses found in a model study by Taeuber, Badian, Brettel, Royen, Rupp, Sittig & Uihlein (1979).

In experiments using repeated assessments involving codes, mental arithmetic procedures, memorized material, letter cancellation and similar sequential stimuli it is necessary to change the code or letter to be cancelled or material to be memorized on each test occasion to prevent subjects' remembering or familiarizing themselves with the solution or response code. However, the change in code or letter should not follow any clearly defined sequence but should be random, as some subjects are very adept in

'reasoning out' such patterned variation. This relatively simple procedure for making parallel forms of the same test effectively controls for any memorizing or learning which could otherwise interfere with the performance assessment.

We are now in a position to examine the ways in which the activity of psychoactive drugs on psychomotor performance can be measured. A consideration of Figure 1 shows that there are four essential components of psychomotor behaviour viz. the sensory processing aspects, the central integration and processing mechanisms, the overt motor responses and the overall sensori-motor co-ordination. The total psychological response to a psychotropic compound is, as we have seen, a more complex interaction involving personality, motivational factors and even sociocultural habits and expectancies. However, the psychomotor response to a drug is due to the several or conjoint effects of the substance on the components of performance.

The assessment of sensory function and sensory processing ability

Purely sensory measures of the effects of centrally acting drugs have not proved very reliable. Van Houten & Zenhausern (1967) showed that meprobamate significantly affected absolute auditory thresholds but the direction of the change was not consistent. Wittenborn (1979) found no test of auditory perception to discriminate between the actions of various benzodiazepines and placebo. On the other hand, Evans, Martz, Rodda, Kiplinger & Forney (1974) showed an increasing impairment of delayed auditory feedback to be commensurate with an increase in blood alcohol concentration but Bernstein et al. (1967) were unable to show any differences between placebo and medazepam 10 mg on a colour naming task under delayed auditory feedback.

Suzumura (1968) developed a kinetic visual acuity test which Roden, Harvey & Mitchard (1977) showed to be sensitive to the effects of alcohol alone and alcohol in combination with either nitrazepam or methaqualone and diphenhydramine (Mandrax). Veldkamp et al. (1974) showed ocular convergence to be impaired by triazolam 0.5 and 1.0 mg and Aschoff et al. (1975) found saccadic velocity reduced by diazepam 10 mg but not by sulpiride 100 mg. A study by Gendreau et al. (1972) using the classical conditioning of the human eyelid response differentiated methamphetamine 20 mg from both placebo and diazepam 20 mg because of the observed improvement in discrimination produced by the psychostimulant. Gupta (1974) showed stimulant (dexamphetamine, 10 mg) and depressant (phenobarbitone, 100 mg) drugs could be discriminated on the duration of the kinaesthetic figural after effect, while Malpas & Joyce (1969) found that nitrazepam 5 and 10 mg increased the latency and shortened the duration of visual after-images.

Although some of these tests of sensory function are discriminating of the action of psychoactive drugs, they have limited usefulness and replicability due to the interaction of personality variables (Eysenck & Easterbrook, 1960) and inter-subject processing differences (Gray, 1967) with the performance scores obtained.

Detection, perception and recognition of a stimulus are three levels of information processing which together account for the majority of the sensory activity of the organism (Mashour & Devine, 1977). Changes in the level of activity of the sensory input brought about by the administration of a drug can have a disruptive effect on total psychomotor performance and reduce the responsiveness of an individual to changes in his environment.

Changes in stimulus detection performance or vigilance have been produced by a variety of psychoactive drugs e.g., hyoscine and meclozine (Colquhoun, 1962), methylphenidate (Cohen, Douglas & Morgenstern, 1971), chlorpromazine and secobarbital (Kornetsky & Orzack, 1964), amphetamine (Mackworth, 1965); bromazepam (Saario, 1976), diazepam (Kleinknecht & Donaldson, 1975) and clobazam (Wittenborn et al., 1979).

Orzack, Taylor & Kornetsky (1968) devised a non-motivated continuous attention task given over a 3 h period. Subjects were required to press the key which matched a number display, the motor component was small and the task not paced. The number of errors made following magnesium pemoline 50 mg, caffeine 200 mg and methylphenidate 15 mg were all significantly less than those produced by placebo, showing the central stimulating activity of the three drugs. In the continuous attention task of Rosvold, Mirsky, Sarason, Bransome & Beck (1956) subjects have to detect a critical stimulus, usually a letter X, from random sequences of letters presented at a constant rate. Using this procedure Mirsky & Kornetsky (1964) were able to distinguish the activity of phenothiazines from the action of barbiturates. Wittenborn et al. (1979) describe both a simple and a complex vigilance task. The latency of the subjects' responses to the critical stimulus, as well as the errors made, are scored in both tests. The tests have proved sensitive enough to discriminate between the effects of different benzodiazepines (op. cit.). However, the use of letter stimuli and the task requirements of the conjoint recognition of two elements will involve higher mental coding processes. Observed drug effects can not then be directly attributed to disturbance of a sensory process alone. To avoid the interaction of coding and attentional systems with

letter recognition, Williams, Lubin & Goodnow (1959) produced an auditory version of the continuous performance test which was later refined and developed by Wilkinson (1968) into one of the most sensitive tests of vigilance. Subjects listen to 1kHz tones of 82dB against a background white noise of 76dB. The duration of the tone is usually 0.5 s but shorter tones of 0.4 s are randomly presented as critical stimuli to be recognized by pressing a button. Hart, Hill, Bye, Wilkinson & Peck (1976) showed the number of correct detections was significantly reduced by diazepam 2.5 mg, while Bye, Munro-Faure, Peck & Young (1973) found a significant improvement in the auditory vigilance task following dexamphetamine in a dose range 1 mg to 7.5 mg. The sensitivity of the task and the separation of the effects of sedative and stimulant drugs make it a most useful screen for potential psychotropic agents. Bye et al. (1973) were able to conclude that 1-benzyl-piperazine had psychostimulant actions because of its similar profile of action to dexamphetamine on the auditory vigilance task. Peck, Bye, Clubley, Henson & Riddington (1979) found that amitriptyline 25 mg impaired auditory vigilance but that bupropion 50 and 100 mg a potential antidepressant was indistinguishable from placebo in a study where dexamphetamine 5 and 10 mg, as a positive internal control, improved performance. In a study of the effects of nitrazepam 5 and 10 mg on sound and light sleepers Peck, Bye & Claridge (1977) found that the auditory vigilance of sound sleepers was unaffected by the drug treatment. However, light sleepers had an impaired performance the morning following nocturnal treatment with nitrazepam 10 mg but not following 5 mg.

Millar (1979) investigated the change of vigilance efficiency through the day following placebo, chlorpheniramine 10 mg and chlorpheniramine 10 mg plus ephedrine 15 mg. There was a significant contrast between the two drug conditions. Chlorpheniramine alone exhibited the sedative activity characteristic of an antihistamine and impaired vigilance. The addition of ephedrine to chlorpheniramine counteracted the effect and the combination was no different to placebo in its action on vigilance efficiency.

The perceptual processing of sensory information can be readily assessed by using a letter or number cancellation task, providing the motor component is not too great. Bond, James & Lader (1974a) provide a typical example of a number cancellation task where the number to be checked appears 40 times in 400 digits. Zimmermann-Tansella et al. (1976) have shown an adverse effect on cancellation 12 h after chlordesmethyldiazepam 1 and 2 mg. Cancellation tasks seem to be quite sensitive to low doses of sedative drugs as File & Bond (1979) found lorazepam 1 and 2.5 mg to reduce the total numbers cancelled in a 90 s period. Letter cancellation scores of subjects treated with diazepam 5 mg were significantly worse than those of subjects receiving placebo (Lawton & Cahn, 1963). Bond & Lader (1972) found the hypnotic nitrazepam 5 and 10 mg decreased the rate of cancellation when compared to placebo while both Stitt et al. (1977) and Jones et al. (1978) showed a significant impairment of letter search and cancellation tasks following diazepam 5 mg. Consroe, Carlini, Zwicker & Lacerda (1979) found the interactive effect of cannabidiol and alcohol to reduce performance on a cancellation test.

However, Bond & Lader (1975) were unable to show any significant effect of flunitrazepam 1 and 2 mg on a number cancellation task and Hindmarch & Clyde (1980a) found a letter cancellation task insensitive to the effects of a benzodiazepine hypnotic, HR158. In an attempt to increase the sensitivity of the letter cancellation task Hindmarch & Gudgeon (1980) had subjects cancel 1, 2, 3, or 4 letters from pages of random letters. The low information processing loads involved in cancelling 1 or 2 letters did not enable any discrimination to be made between lorazepam 1 mg, clobazam 10 mg or matching placebo 1 capsule, each given three times daily for 3 days. However, significant impairments of perceptual processing compared to placebo were found following repeated doses of lorazepam 1 mg when higher information loads, i.e. the cancellation of four letters, were used.

Recognizing sensory information involves the matching of the perceptual figuration with a pre-existing or stored stimulus pattern. The identification of current information and matching with previously stored patterns is obviously a function of the central sensory recoding and processing systems. Stroop (1935) drew attention to an anomalous feature of this recoding mechanism when he found that there was a large disruption and delay in colour naming when letters of one colour were formed into the name of an incongruous colour. This so called Stroop Phenomenon, i.e. a delay in colour naming under the unusual stimulus processing conditions described above, has been widely used in the study of personality (Uherik, 1973), perceptual (Shor, 1971), cognitive (Schiller, 1966), and response (Dyer, 1973) processes. The latency of the colour name response under Stroop conditions has been neglected as a measure of sensory performance within psycho-pharmacology. This is unfortunate as it would seem to be a reliable and sensitive index of the effect of psychoactive drugs on cognitive and perceptual systems. An interaction between Mandrax and alcohol was demonstrated (Roden et al., 1977) using a Stroop test, but no interaction between nitrazepam and alcohol could be shown. Nakano, Gillespie & Hollister (1978) used a mirror drawing and a Stroop test in an experimental model of anxiety to investigate

the effects of nabilone 2 mg and diazepam 5 mg; anxiety was reduced by both drugs.

Ambiguous figures with two distinct perspectives, as in the 'falling staircase' or Necker cube, also provide an assessment measure for sensory processing ability. Wittenborn et al. (1979), using the spontaneous reversals reported by subjects while gazing at a Necker cube for a 1 min period, were able to show an impairment of processing following diazepam 5 mg. More interestingly they were able to discriminate between the effects of clobazam 10 mg and diazepam 5 mg on the Necker cube reversal rate the former drug was no different to placebo while diazepam 5 mg significantly reduced the reversal rate.

It is convenient to discuss the effects of drugs upon time judgment under the central coding of sensory information without entering into any debate as to the neurological or psychological basis of temporal estimation. Frankenhaeuser (1959), Goldstone, Boardman & Lhamon (1958), Hormia (1956) and Goldstone & Kirkham (1968) have all shown consistent findings with central depressants and stimulants and the subjective estimation of time. Amphetamines and related stimulants produce a subjective over estimation of a standard time interval while barbiturates produce an under estimation. Wittenborn et al. (1976, 1979) have used the estimation of short temporal intervals, 8–15 s, in their studies of benzodiazepines and antidepressants. The natural tendency to over estimate the time required to produce a short time interval, without the benefit of a standard, was reduced by prazepam 30 mg and imipramine but not by clobazam 10 mg three times daily. The reduction of the 'normal' over estimate by prazepam and imipramine is evidence of their sedative activity on temporal processing.

Recoding and recognition of sensory information is well illustrated in the performance of the digit symbol substitution test. The DSST forms part of the performance scale of the Wechsler Adult Intelligence Test (Wechsler, 1955), and many researchers have used it to measure drug activity on perceptual coding skills. There is a motor component in the task but as the principal determinant of performance is the recoding of visual information we will consider the DSST here.

Table 1 shows that the DSST is a useful indicator of drug produced changes in sensory processing performance. The use of parallel forms for repeated administration is necessary to avoid interference from practice and learning effects.

The assessment of CNS function and central processing ability

A consideration of the psychomotor performance model shows that there are two major components of central nervous system activity, *viz.* integration and processing. We must also consider drug effects on memory and learning as these two systems have an extensive influence in determining the overall activity of a psychoactive substance on the brain and central nervous system.

Central integration

The relationship between the electrical activity of the brain as measured on the electroencephalogram and cognitive behaviour is, as yet, unclear. However, the development of techniques correlating drug induced changes in behaviour with electrophysiological changes in EEG variables (Goldstein & Stoltzfus, 1973), and the evoked potential (Näätänen, 1975), will no doubt provide, in the future, the most sensitive index of central nervous system activity. For example, Saletu & Taeuber (1980) used EEG for the assessment of antidepressant drug effects and found the pharmacokinetics of nomifensine did not correspond with the pharmacodynamics of the drug in producing changes in brain activity.

There have been many attempts at measuring the level of arousal or integration potential of the CNS. Guest, Duncan & Lawther (1970) used auditory flutter fusion threshold, Croucher & Hindmarch (1974) and Saletu & Grunberger (1979) used the duration of the spiral after effect. Marjerrison, Neufeldt, Holmes & Ho (1973) measured integrated EEG amplitude and two flash threshold and Smith & Misiak (1976) reviewed 33 studies which used the critical flicker fusion threshold to assess the changes in CNS arousal produced by a variety of psychotropic agents.

It is this last measure that must be regarded as the assessment of choice for investigating the change in overall integrative activity of the CNS produced by psychoactive drugs.

Smith & Misiak (1976) found the CFF threshold to be altered to a statistically significant degree ($P < 0.05$) in 65% of the studies they reviewed. They concluded that stimulants (amphetamines) increased the threshold and sedative-hypnotics (barbiturates, chloral hydrate, glutethimide) reduced the threshold. As with all review papers, the authors found difficulty in making absolute conclusions since the various studies employed different methodologies, controls, treatment regimens and subjects. Table 2 presents findings from studies published since, or not included in, the review.

These later studies confirm the general findings relating to stimulant and sedative drugs but also show the general sedative activity of the 1, 4 benzodiazepines which was somewhat equivocal in the earlier papers.

As yet there does not exist any standard for the rating of an individual's absolute CFF threshold so the technique should be used only for the monitoring of drug induced change. The CFF measure is dependent upon a number of experimental variables (Keesey, 1970), including ambient illumination, size of image, luminance of stimulus, viewing distance and pupil size. The easiest way to control the majority of these variables is to fix the conditions under which the measurement takes place and to hold them constant

Table 1 Performance on the DSST task following treatment with a variety of drugs, showing the sensitivity of the measure to the effects of sedative compounds

Studies where an impairment of DSST performance was found following psychoactive medication

Amylobarbitone	50 and 100mg	Hart *et al.* (1976)
Flunitrazepam	1 and 2mg	Bond & Lader (1975)
Flurazepam	15mg	Bond & Lader (1973)
	30mg	Bond & Lader (1973); Church & Johnson (1979)
Nitrazepam	5mg	Bond & Lader (1972); Malpas (1972)
	10mg	Malpas & Joyce (1969); Walters & Lader (1971); Bond & Lader (1972); Malpas (1972); Peck *et al.* (*1977*)
Diazepam	5mg	Hart *et al.* (1976)
	10mg	Jäättelä *et al.* (1971)
	17–28mg	Shira (1978)
Chlordiazepoxide	20mg	Shaffer *et al.* (1963); Besser & Steinberg (1967)
Lorazepam	1 and 2.5mg	File & Bond (1979)
Imipramine	50mg	Wittenborn (1977)

Studies where an improvement of DSST performance was found following treatment

Clobazam	10mg	Salkind *et al.* (1979)

Table 2   The sensitivity and range of the CFF measure as an index of drug activity on the central nervous system is shown in the changes, against placebo, found in the above studies

Drugs producing a reduction in CFF threshold

Chlorpromazine	25mg	Turner (1973)
	50mg	Parrott & Hindmarch (1975a,c)
Haloperidol	1mg	Parrott & Hindmarch (1975c)
Doxepin	25–75mg	Grundström *et al.* (1977)
Mianserin	15mg	Fink *et al.* (1977)
	10 and 20mg	Crome & Newman (1978)
Mianserin + alcohol	10mg + 0.5g/kg	Seppälä (1977)
Amitriptyline + alcohol	25mg + 0.5g/kg	
Amitriptyline + chlordiazepoxide	25mg + 10mg	Hindmarch *et al.* (1980)
Meperidine	75mg	Korttila & Linnoila (1975)
Phenobarbitone	100mg	Guest *et al.* (1970)
Quinalbarbitone	100mg	Turner (1973)
Amylobarbitone	100mg	Hindmarch (1975, 1976b, 1979a, c); Parrott & Hindmarch (1975a, b); Turner (1973)
Promethazine	25mg	Turner (1973)
Chlorpheniramine	4mg	Hindmarch & Parrott (1978b)
Ethanol	0.7g/kg	Tarter *et al.* (1971)
	0.48 – 0.67g/kg	Rosketh & Lorentzen (1954)
	0.8g/kg	Ideström & Cadenius (1968)
	0.32 – 1.29g/kg	Enzer *et al.* (1944)
	0.63 – 0.8g/kg	Goldberg (1943)
	0.44g/kg	Rizzo (1957)
Chlordiazepoxide	10mg	Hindmarch (1979a)
Diazepam	5mg	Hedges *et al.* (1971) Hindmarch (1979a)
	7.5 – 22.5mg	Grundström *et al.* (1978)
	8.8 – 22.8mg	Haffner *et al.* (1973)
	10mg	Mørland *et al.* (1974); Korttila & Linnoila (1975); Seppälä *et al.* (1976)
Medazepam	15mg	Seppälä *et al.* (1976)
Oxazepam	20 and 40mg	Molander & Duvhök (1976)
Lorazepam	0.5mg	Hedges *et al.* (1971)
	1mg	Hedges *et al.* (1971); Turner (1973)
	2.0mg	Ogle *et al.* (1976); Farhoumand *et al.* (1979)
	2.5mg	Seppälä *et al.* (1976)
Temazepam	30mg	Hindmarch (1975, 1976a, 1979c)
Nitrazepam	5mg	Hindmarch (1975)
	5 – 15mg	Grundström *et al.* (1978)
	10mg	Fell *et al.* (1973); Hindmarch & Clyde (1980b)

Drugs producing an elevation of CFF threshold

Amphetamine	10mg	Parrott & Hindmarch (1975b)
	15mg	Turner (1973); Taeuber *et al.* (1979)
Methylphenidate	20mg	Parrott & Hindmarch (1975a, b)
Phenmetrazine	25 and 30mg	Turner (1973)
Diethylproprion	25mg	Turner (1973)
Pemoline	20mg	Parrott & Hindmarch (1975b)
Dimethylxanthine	400mg	Parrott & Hindmarch (1975b)
Hydergine	12mg	Hindmarch *et al.* (1979)
Nomifensine	25mg	Hindmarch *et al.* (1980)
	75mg	Hindmarch & Parrott (1977)
Nomifensine + clobazam	25 + 7.5mg	Hindmarch *et al.* (1980)
Clobazam	10mg	Hindmarch (1979a, b)
	20mg	Hindmarch & Parrott (1980b)
	30mg	Hindmarch & Parrott (1979)

from test to test. Repeated measures of the threshold should be taken using one of the standard psychophysical methods; e.g. limits, paired comparison or frequency to collect the data (Woodworth & Schlosberg, 1958).

Changes in pupil diameter will result in alteration of the CFF threshold due to the change in retinal illumination. This pupillary change of CFF threshold could well mask any drug induced change in brain activity but the use of an artificial pupil, a 2 mm viewing aperture, will control such effects.

As individual CFF thresholds vary due to personality, motivational state and circadian cyclicity it is best to use each subject as his own control and to ensure that repeated testing is conducted at the same time of day—safeguards which apply to all psychometric assessments.

Central processing

The range of tasks to assess mental performance as processing ability is extensive. A concept identification task has been used in several studies (Hindmarch & Parrott, 1978; 1979; 1980a; 1980b) but performance ratings were found to be too dependant upon the experience of the test administrator to warrant the more general usage of such a measure. Symbol arrangement (Liljequist, Seppälä & Mattila, 1978) has proved to be a less sensitive test than either the DSST or symbol cancelling tasks described earlier.

Symbol copying as employed in studies by File & Bond (1979) and Bond & Lader (1973; 1975) is sensitive to drug induced changes but practice and learning effects make the results obtained variable. The most reliable and certainly the easiest way of measuring cognitive 'processing' ability is by an arithmetic or number handling task. Bond, James & Lader (1974a, b), Ashton *et al.* (1972) and Keuchel, Kohnen & Lienert (1979) used arithmetic addition tasks to show changes in performance due to amylobarbitone, oxypertine, and nicotine and caffeine respectively. Masuda & Bakker (1966) showed mathematical performance was reduced by diazepam 10 and 20 mg and similar impairments following repeated doses of diazepam 10-20mg were found by Frostad *et al.* (1966). Using the serial subtraction of numbers technique Hindmarch (1977b) was able to show the sedative effects of flunitrazepam 1 mg and flurezepam 15 mg. Disruptive effects and a lowering of task performance have also been shown using the sequential subtraction of numbers technique following clorazepate 15 mg, Hindmarch & Parrott (1979); lorazepam 1 mg, Hindmarch & Gudgeon (1980); triazolam 0.5 mg and nitrazepam 10 mg, Hindmarch & Clyde (1980b); HR158, a benzodiazepine hypnotic at doses of 1 and 2 mg, Hindmarch & Clyde (1980a); and amitriptyline

25 mg with chlordiazepoxide 10 mg, Hindmarch *et al.* (1980). Taeuber *et al.* (1979) found that nomifensine 100 mg increased the number of correct solutions obtained on a continuous arithmetic calculation test compared to placebo.

In numerical ability tests measurement of the time taken to complete the task and the number of errors made enables the separation of the effects of psychostimulants, which shorten task latency but increase the errors made, from the action of drugs which improve performance, i.e. shorter task latency without increasing errors. The two response measures also enable individual differences to be observed as some subjects sacrifice accuracy for speed. The confounding effects of individual styles on arithmetic tasks are controlled by careful instructions to the subjects and adequate pre-experimental training.

Memory and learning.

It is not proposed to enter a debate as to the theoretical basis for distinguishing between long and short term memory. A parsimonious definition of short term memory (STM) would indicate that it is a limited capacity store of processed information which functions for a variable time period, dependent on the demands of the task situation, to assist stimulus recognition and processing. Items in the STM store can be easily displaced by new stimuli or information. The likelihood of STM store being disrupted by new stimuli and the decay of the memory trace are the basis of most tasks designed to measure the effects of drugs on short term recognition or recall of learned information. A consideration of some relevant tasks and comments on methodology are given in a useful paper by Squitieri, Mazzola, Lazzari, Cervone & Agnoli (1977). Short term memory can be conveniently measured using the digit span technique of the Wechsler Adult Intelligence Test (Wechsler, 1955). It should be remembered that scores on digit span measures do relate to intelligence and mental performance ratings and subjects should, therefore, act as their own controls when such assessments are made.

Miller & Dolan (1974) were able to show the disruptive effect of alcohol, 1.2 mg kg^{-1} body weight, on a WAIS digit span test and Davis *et al.* (1976) showed a significant decrement in STM following physostigmine 3 mg. Digit span measures also showed an impairment of STM following both hyoscine 0.3 mg and nitrazepam 5 mg (Jones *et al.*, 1979). Haffner, Mørland, Setekleiv, Strømsaether, Danielsen, Frivik & Dybing (1973) found diazepam 10 and 20 mg to impair STM and Shira (1978) showed diazepam 17 to 28 mg to produce STM deficits. Anterograde amnesia has been found (Clarke, Eccersley, Frisby & Thornton, 1970) following intravenous diazepam 0.24 mg/kg and

Ghoneim, Mewaldt & Thatcher (1975) found immediate and delayed recall of words significantly impaired following diazepam 20 mg.

The lack of impairment of digit span performance following chlordiazepoxide 10 and 25 mg (Ogle & Ditman, 1966) and meprobamate 800 mg (Melikian, 1961) is due to differences in experimental protocols between these two studies and those more recent investigations given above.

The learning and subsequent recall or recognition of words, numbers and nonsense trigrams have been widely used to test the effects of drugs on immediate memory. Performance on four short term retention tasks was impaired following whisky 2 ml/kg body weight (Dornič, Myrsten & Frankenhäuser, 1971), and File & Bond (1979) showed lorazepam 1 and 2.5 mg interfered with the learning and retention of random digits. Using free recall and recognition of word lists Ghoneim & Mewaldt (1977) concluded that injected diazepam 0.3 mg/kg and scopolamine 8 mg/kg impaired the learning of new information. More esoteric measures of verbal rote learning (Andersson & Post, 1972; Andersson & Hockey, 1975) have been able to detect the effects of cigarette smoking on performance efficiency. Using verbal conditioning procedures, Gupta (1973) has separated the facilitatory effect of dexedrine from the inhibitory activity of chlorpromazine and phenobarbitone. Using both digit span and paired-associate learning techniques Liljequist et al. (1978) have shown that amitriptyline 25 mg, but not mianserin 10 mg or placebo impaired performance.

The inconsistencies between some of the results from different studies on digit span assessments are due to different methodologies and test conditions for Andersson (1975) has shown that STM performance can readily be affected by task induced arousal and situational novelty. However, with suitable controls for experimental variations it would seem that digit span and verbal material as employed by Brown, Lewis, Brown, Horn & Bowes (1978) are useful measures for estimating drug activity on short term memory and/or learning processes.

The assessment of motor function and behavioural co-ordination

Motor activity and co-ordination can be classified under four headings, viz. ballistic, gross body balance, fine motor control and motor manipulative activity. Centrally acting drugs have been shown to affect performance on measures of each type of motor activity.

Ballistic activity

The rate of finger tapping is one of the simplest of human motor activities and has been widely used to measure drug changes of motor performance. Even this simple task is subject to other than drug induced changes of which prospective users should be aware. Wilson, Tunstall & Eysenck (1971) have shown clear motivational and personality variables operating on finger tapping performance especially if the time on the task is prolonged. These extraneous variables should be isolated by limiting the test tapping period to a maximum of 60 s.

Most studies have used the technique described by Frith (1967) and tapping performance has been shown to be impaired following nitrazepam 10 mg (Peck et al., 1977), diazepam 10 mg (Černý et al., 1973; Ghoneim et al., 1975), butobarbitone 200 mg (Walters & Lader, 1971), flurazepam 30 mg (Salkind & Silverstone, 1975), oxazepam 10 mg (Di Mascio & Barrett, 1965) and nitrazepam 5 and 10 mg (Bond & Lader, 1972). Černý et al. (1973) have also shown that methylphenidate 20 mg significantly increases tapping performance compared to placebo, and Zimmermann-Tansella et al. (1976) have suggested that tapping rate is facilitated by chlordesmethyl-diazepam 1 mg. Although these findings suggest that finger tapping is useful in discriminating performance across the sedative—stimulant range of psychoactive drugs, Vogel (1979) found 19 of 22 instances of tests of finger tapping with a range of 7 anxiolytic drugs to show no placebo contrasted effects.

Gross body movement

The ability to walk along a straight line without undue deviation is a well known assessment of the effects of alcohol on body movement and balance systems. This simple assessment has not been widely used in experimental situations although Korttila, Saarnivaara, Tarkkanen, Himburg & Hytonen (1978) report its usefulness in monitoring the residual effects on sedation of diazepam and flunitrazepam used during bronchoscopy.

The stabilometer is the most widely used assessment of body movement. It is a motor learning task (Wade & Newell, 1972) in which a subject has to balance on a pivoted support. Taeuber et al. (1979) provide details of an automated body sway test and Wittenborn et al. (1979) details of a balance beam procedure which fulfil the same purpose as the stabilometer. Hindmarch (1979a) found both nitrazepam 5 mg and clobazam 20 mg significantly increased the balance time compared to placebo on a stabilometer test, but attributed these findings to the effectiveness of the drugs in reducing the perceived effects of physical fatigue inherent in that particular test. Wittenborn et al. (1979) found fewer instances of missteps using the balance beam technique following clobazam 10 mg than either placebo or diazepam 5 mg, and Taeuber et al. (1979) showed their body sway technique to be sensitive to the interaction of clobazam and alcohol. Orr, Dussault, Chappel, Goldberg & Reggiani (1976) found a clear impairment of standing steadiness following both 10 and 20 mg diazepam. Penttilä, Lehti & Lönnquist (1975) demonstrated the usefulness of stabilometer measures in screening patients for psychotropic effects and Evans *et al.* (1974) have shown the wobble board to be sensitive to alcohol induced impairment of body movement. Orr *et al.* (1976) found high dose related correlations between diazepam produced changes on stabilometer performance and drug plasma levels.

Fine motor control

Using a hand steadiness task and a Whipple Tracing Board, Doongaji *et al.* (1979) were able to show improved motor co-ordination following repeated dosing with clobazam 10 mg in a group of anxious patients. Trail making tests (Reitan, 1958) have shown both dexamphetamine 30 mg/kg body weight and psilocybin 0.2 mg/kg impair trail making performance (Duke & Keeler 1968). A variety of writing speed tasks have been shown to be sensitive to both stimulant and sedative drugs (Nash & Stone, 1974), and hand steadiness has been shown to be sensitive enough to discriminate the effects of pemoline and caffeine (Henert & Janke, 1957).

Motor manipulation

Pegboard and 'rivet with washer' techniques provide reasonable measures of motor manipulative skill. May, Childs & Urquhart (1976) found the performance of alcoholics on manipulative tests was significantly impaired and Knights & Hinton (1969) found a pegboard completion task sensitive to the effects of methylphenidate in children with learning problems. Roth *et al.* (1977) used a pegboard in an evaluation of the side effects of flurazepam, triazolam and secobarbital. Differences between the drugs on sleep variables were found to be consistent with the differences obtained on the pegboard and related measures. Lahtinen *et al.* (1978) using simple motor manipulations were able to show an impairment of performance following both 5 and 10 mg nitrazepam and Lawton & Cahn (1963) found pegboard performance reduced by diazepam 5 mg, but Hindmarch & Gudgeon (1980) were unable to detect changes in pegboard performance following repeated doses of lorazepam 1 mg, clobazam 10 mg and placebo although the two drugs were clearly differentiated by other tests administered at the same time.

In general measures of motor function are contaminated by the great inter-individual differences in performance which exist prior to the administration of a drug. Statistical control of between subject differences in pre-experimental performance can be effected through the use of analysis of covariance, but there is no better way of minimizing such differences than the adequate training of experimental subjects prior to the commencement of an investigation.

The assessment of sensori-motor performance

The co-ordination of sensory and motor systems is the basis of most skilled behaviours. It is easier to develop laboratory analogues of everyday behaviour than to control the real life situation to the level necessary for obtaining reliable information about drug interaction with performance skills. However, Harper & Kidera (1972) tested flurazepam and glutethimide in a twin-turbo jet flight simulator and found that both drugs impaired performance. Haward (1968) also showed improvement of concentration on an air traffic control simulation following phenytoin sodium 150 mg. In car handling tasks Betts *et al.* (1972) showed performance decrements following chlordiazepoxide 10 mg but using similar tasks Hindmarch, Hanks & Hewitt (1977) were unable to show any decrement in performance due to the administration of clobazam 20 mg nocte for six nights or clemastine 1 mg twice daily for three days (Hindmarch, 1976a).

Recent studies using similar low speed car handling tasks have shown significant performance impairments produced by lorazepam 1 mg three times daily for 3 days (Hindmarch & Gudgeon, 1980) and by chlordiazepoxide 10 mg with amitriptyline 25 mg three times daily for 2 days (Hindmarch, Parrott & Stonier, 1980). Biehl (1979) using dual control cars in traffic was able to show that diazepam 10 mg significantly impaired subjects' brake response readiness while clobazam 20 mg produced a significant increase in responsiveness compared to placebo values. Berry, Burtles, Grubb & Hoare (1974) found clobazam 10 mg did not increase brake reaction time although diazepam 10 mg produced a significant increase compared to placebo. Although there is great inter-study variability there is also consistency in the findings of impaired performance of real life tasks following sedative drugs. Such impairment emphasises the accident risks patients prescribed such drugs might encounter in the everyday work situation (Edwards, 1978).

Sensori-motor activity has also been assessed on a variety of tasks which have some relevance to performance of real life activities, particularly car driving. Linnoila & Hakkinen (1974) found that diazepam 10 mg caused professional drivers to 'collide' significantly more frequently than when treated with placebo, on a car driving simulator. On a set of skills related to car driving Seppälä, Korttila,

Häkkinen & Linnoila (1976) found that diazepam 10 mg, medazepam 15 mg and lorazepam 2.5 mg all produced significant impairments of one or more experimental measures when compared to placebo. Korttila (1977) showed lack of impairment of driving related skills following intramuscular injection of prilocaine or mepivacaine but found impairments following lidocaine, bupivacaine and etidocaine. Korttila, Tammisto, Ertama, Pfaffli, Blomgern & Hakkinen (1977) also showed an impairment of driving skills following halothane anaesthesia. Liljequist & Mattila (1979) were able to demonstrate the impairment of co-ordination and reaction time following nitrazepam 10 mg and temazepam 10 and 20 mg while Palva & Linnoila (1978) found that the main metabolites of chlordiazepoxide and diazepam significantly enhanced alcohol induced impairment of psychomotor tasks relating to car driving.

Landauer et al. (1974) failed to show any impairment of simulated car driving following 10 or 20 mg medazepam and Dureman & Norrman (1975) failed to find any impairment of simulated car driving after diazepam 15 mg or clorazepate 30 mg. However, the inter-subject pre-test differences in performance were not controlled in the first study and a patient population of neurasthenic, vegetative neurotics were subject to a 3 h testing sequence in the second investigation. It is most likely that such experimental artefacts have interfered with drug effects in these instances as, in general, tests of psychomotor skills related to car driving are sensitive to both psychostimulant and sedative drug activity.

The most basic measure of visuo-motor performance is the pursuit rotor or its pencil-and-paper counterpart, the spiral maze. Performance on these tasks is subject to practice effects which must be carefully controlled and personality has been shown to determine pursuit rotor scores (Eysenck, 1972). None of the 10 studies reviewed by Vogel (1979) showed any change in pursuit rotor performance following chlordiazepoxide 10–15 mg, diazepam 5–10 mg, meprobamate 200–800 mg, prazepam 10 mg and medazepam 10 mg. Salkind, Hanks & Silverstone (1979) found that pursuit rotor performance was significantly improved by placebo in a group of anxious patients showing the clear effects of practice but Salkind & Silverstone (1975) found impairment of tracking following 30 mg flurazepam. In a three way comparison of hexobarbital 250 mg, caffeine 200 mg and pemoline 40 mg against placebo, Busch et al. (1979) found no significant changes in pursuit rotor performance although there were drug effects observable on other tests of concentration and memory. Dexamphetamine 5 mg and etifoxine 300 mg have both improved pursuit rotor performance compared to placebo (Córsico et al., 1975). Ogle et al. (1976) found propranolol 240 mg, diazepam 5 mg and

lorazepam 2 mg to significantly impair pursuit rotor performance. Ashton et al. (1972) showed oxypertine 20 mg reduced the time on target in a pursuit rotor task and Macleod, Giles, Patzalek, Thiessen & Sellers (1977) showed impairment after alcohol and diazepam mixtures and Evans et al. (1974) for alcohol alone. However, the pursuit rotor cannot be regarded as a reliable index of drug effects on the visuo-motor system unless practice effects are controlled.

The Gibson spiral maze (Gibson, 1965) has been used with a certain degree of success to detect performance changes produced by diazepam in anxious patients (Zimmermann-Tansella et al., 1978). As with the pursuit rotor, practice effects on repeated administration over a short time period make the spiral maze too unreliable to discriminate other than profound sedatives and psychostimulants from placebo. Bond et al. (1974a) found it insensitive to the performance differences of anxious and volunteer populations.

The adaptive tracking task is a more refined pursuit and tracking test, which has been shown by Borland & Nicholson (1974) to be sensitive to the effects of heptabarbitone 200, 300 and 400 mg, and Nicholson (1979) has shown the residual sedative activity of flurazepam 30 mg, nitrazepam 10 mg, oxazepam 30 and 45 mg, temazepam 20 mg and diazepam 10 mg. Muller-Oerlinghausen, Bauer, Girke, Kanowski & Goncalves (1977) have also used adaptive tracking tests to detect the impairment of performance produced by lithium salts in both patient and volunteer populations. It is clear that adaptive tracking is a reliable index of the effects of sedative drugs.

Other visuo-motor tasks e.g. the automated rotated designs test (Sambrooks, Macculloch, Birtles & Smallman, 1972: Sambrooks, Macculloch & Rooney, 1975) and the continuous performance reading task (Stern, Bremer & McClure, 1974) have been used too infrequently for any estimate of their sensitivity to drug induced changes in performance to be made.

Card sorting is an excellent example of a performance task which embraces sensory, motor and central components. Berry, Gelder & Summerfield (1965) provide an excellent description of the experimental methodology of a card sorting task using conventional playing cards where task difficulty can be manipulated by altering the complexity of the sorting criteria. It is possible, using the card sorting technique, to isolate changes in performance due to motor activity alone. Card sorting assessments are widely used and sensitive to a range of psychoactive drugs. Zimmermann-Tansella et al. (1976) showed card sorting to be impaired following chlordesmethyldiazepam 10 and 20 mg and Tansella et al. (1974) found similar impairment with N-desmethyldiazepam 20 mg. Malpas & Joyce (1969)

Table 3 Simple reaction time as a measure of psychoactive drug activity

Studies which have shown an impairment of reaction time following psychoactive medication

Meprobamate	800mg	Huffman *et al.* (1963)
	1600mg	Kornetsky (1958); Uhr *et al.* (1963)
Butobarbitone	200mg	Walters & Lader (1971)
Amylobarbitone	100mg	Hart *et al.* (1976)
Nitrazepam	5 and 10mg	Peck *et al.* (1977)
Flurazepam	15 and 30mg	Bond & Lader (1973)
Flunitrazepam	1 and 2mg	Bond & Lader (1975)
Lorazepam	1.0mg	Hedges *et al.* (1971)
	2.0mg	Hedges *et al.* (1971), Harry & Richards (1972)
	2.5mg	File & Bond (1979)
	4.0mg	Harry & Richards (1972)
Diazepam	2.5mg	Hart *et al.* (1976)
	5mg	Hedges *et al.* (1971); Hart *et al.* (1976); Uhlenhuth *et al.* (1977)
	17 – 28mg	Shira (1978)
	20mg	Harry & Richards (1972)
Amitriptyline	25mg	Peck *et al.* (1979); Crome & Newman (1978)
Mianserin	20mg	Crome & Newman (1978)

Studies which have shown an improvement of reaction time following drug treatment

Nicotine	2.0mg	Frankenhaeuser *et al.* (1970)
	2.2mg	Myrsten *et al.* (1971)
Nomifensine	100mg	Hindmarch (1977a)
Amphetamine	15mg	Taeuber *et al.* (1979)

Table 4 The choice reaction time (CRT) task and the action of some psychotropic substances

Studies where a decrement in CRT performance has followed psychoactive medication

Amylobarbitone	100mg	Broadhurst & Arenillas (1975)
Dichloralphenazone	1300mg	Hindmarch *et al.* (1977b)
Meperidine	75mg	Korttila & Linnoila (1975)
Diphenhydramine	100mg	Moser *et al.* (1978)
Flurazepam	15mg	Broadhurst & Arenillas (1975)
	30mg	Church & Johnson (1979)
Nitrazepam	5mg	Hindmarch (1979a)
	10mg	Liljequist & Mattila (1979); Hindmarch & Clyde (1980b)
Temazepam	30mg	Hindmarch (1975, 1976b, 1979c)
Bromazepam	1.5mg	Richter & Hobi (1976)
	6.0mg	Saario (1976)
Lorazepam	2.0mg	Ogle *et al.* (1976)
Chlordiazepoxide	10mg	Hindmarch (1979a)
Diazepam	5mg	Ogle *et al.* (1976); Hindmarch (1979a)
	0.3mg/kg i.v.	Korttila *et al.* (1976)
	10mg	Korttila & Linnoila (1975); Mattila *et al.* (1978)
Amitriptyline + chlordiazepoxide	25mg + 10mg	Hindmarch *et al.* (1980)
Mianserin + alcohol	10mg + 0.5g/kg	Seppälä (1977)
Mianserin	10mg	Seppälä (1977)

Studies where an improvement in CRT performance has followed psychoactive medication

Clobazam	10mg	Hindmarch (1979a)
Nomifensine	25mg	Hindmarch *et al.* (1980)

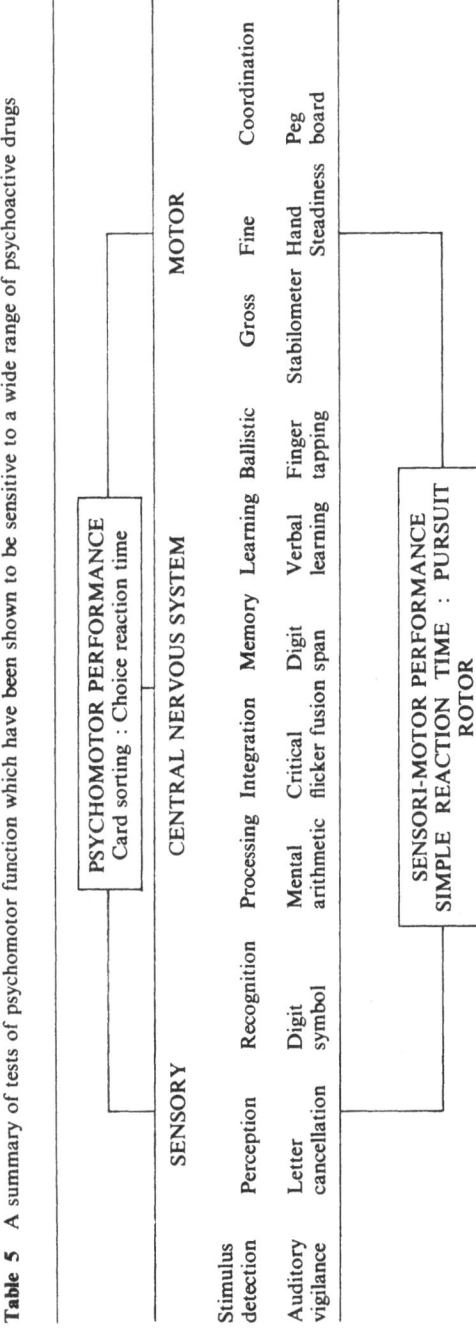

Table 5 A summary of tests of psychomotor function which have been shown to be sensitive to a wide range of psychoactive drugs

and Malpas (1972) found with nitrazepam 10 mg impaired card sorting time and Veldkamp et al. (1974) found triazolam 0.5 and 1.0 mg adversely affected card sorting performance. Berry et al. (1965) showed the sorting technique to be sensitive to changes in information processing brought about by three sub-anaesthetic doses of nitrous oxide and Haffner et al. (1973) have shown coloured card sorting to be impaired by ethanol 1.22 ml/kg and diazepam 10 and 20 mg. The card sorting technique as described by Berry et al. (1965), is a useful measure of sensori-motor performance which has been shown to be sensitive to a wide range of drugs. It has the added advantage, relative to other equipment based assessments, of being cheap and easy to score and administer.

Perhaps the most popular measure of sensori-motor performance is reaction time to a critical stimulus. Response or reaction time features in many assessments but it is useful to distinguish two varieties, viz. simple and complex, or choice, reaction time. The theoretical basis for both measures and valuable methodological comments are to be found in Teichner & Krebs (1972, 1974).

Simple reaction time involves a motor response, say button press, to an expected stimulus in the visual or auditory modality. The latency of the response is the reaction time. A choice reaction time is also a measure of the latency of a motor response but the critical stimulus is one of a number of alternatives and performance in the choice situation is, therefore, more dependant upon attentional monitoring abilities than it is in the simple response situation.

Table 3 presents details of simple reaction time findings and Table 4 presents studies where complex reaction time has been used.

It is clear from Tables 3 and 4 that reaction time is a sensitive measure of drug induced changes in sensori-motor performance. However, it is important to control for variability in motor response characteristics, i.e. the distance moved by the finger, arm or foot in making the response must be constant.

We have found it convenient to arrange the response buttons of a choice reaction time task about the arc of a circle and equidistant from a start button (Hindmarch & Parrott, 1978). Using this arrangement it is possible to measure three components of reaction time viz. the total reaction time from stimulus onset to completion of response, the movement time between start and response buttons and the processing time, obtained by subtracting the motor from the total reaction times.

The reaction time assessment whether it be simple or complex is only of use in psychopharmacological assessments of performance if the subject has received sufficient pre-test training to eliminate practice and learning effects. Under circumstances where subjects are at a performance plateau before they enter the study, the reaction time measure can be used to discriminate drugs along a psychostimulant-sedative continuum.

The assessment of psychomotor function following the administration of psychoactive drugs

Psychoactive drugs act upon the mood, feelings and states of awareness of subjects or patients receiving them. The clinician has little to assess the course of drug action other than the verbal reports of patients receiving the treatment. Subjective reports of drug action on performance are valuable and sensitive to drug induced changes providing they are collected and collated in a meaningful and controlled manner.

The literature is replete with scales for the measurement of mood, depression, anxiety and affect. However, the majority of published scales are to aid diagnosis in a clinical situation and many of the questionnaires have low test/re-test reliability. As subjective awareness of drug activity is an important determinant of behavioural response it is necessary to discuss reliable ways of evaluating the activity of psychotropics on an individual's feelings.

Aitken (1969) produced strong arguments in favour of a 10 cm line visual analogue scale based on the earlier work of Freyd (1923) and Hayes & Patterson (1921) and Bond & Lader (1974) demonstrated the usefulness of line analogue rating scales in drug evaluation studies. Luria (1975) has reported the validity and reliability of visual analogue mood scales in psychiatric populations and Oswald, Lewis, Dunleavy, Brezinova & Briggs (1971) and Hindmarch (1975, 1976b, 1977b) the usefulness in measuring the integrity of early morning performance following the nocturnal administration of hypnotics. Březinová (1974) demonstrated the sensitivity of visual analogue scales to the stimulant effects of caffeine 300 mg and Hindmarch & Gudgeon (1980) have shown a differentiation of lorazepam and clobazam on line analogue ratings of alertness. The line analogue scale remains a useful index of drug activity, which can be tailored to the experimental goals of a particular study by choosing the bipolar qualifiers carefully.

The labels at the ends of the line must be semantic opposites. Useful lists of dimensions upon which to rate mood are to be found in Bond & Lader (1974), Hindmarch & Gudgeon (1980) and Hindmarch & Clyde (1980a, b). Visual analogue rating scales should be included in all studies of psychoactive drug activity along with a selection of the tests presented above. It is best to adopt a multi-assessment approach using one or more tests for each component part of psychomotor performance to maximise the detection of the effects of a psychoactive drug.

A scheme for conducting an investigation of the effects of a psychoactive drug on human psychomotor function is given below (Table 5), after a consideration of the tests and assessments reviewed above.

Any study which utilises measures from each of the above divisions of human psychomotor performance will produce relevant, valid and reliable results only if the experimental conditions, methodology and selection of subjects are carefully controlled.

On the completion of a study the effects observed, statistically significant or not, must be treated with caution as they are limited by the sensitivity of the assessments employed and the experimental sets operating in the particular instance. More credibility can be given to results which fit the findings of other researchers and complement the corpus of knowledge relating to a particular drug but adverse effects do not necessarily mean a drug is of no clinical value. Nicholson (1976) summarises the difficulties in interpreting data from performance studies but also indicates the relevance of performance studies both to psychopharmacology and to clinical practice. Although there are no simple answers to the questions generated by performance studies it is clear that only by carefully controlled experimentation will the effects of psychoactive drugs on psychomotor function be elucidated.

References

ADAMS, R.G. (1974). Pre-sleep ingestion of two hypnotic drugs and subsequent performance. *Psychopharmacologia (Berl)*, **40**, 185–190.

ADAMSON, G.T. & FINLAY, S.E. (1966). A comparison of the effects of varying dose levels of oxypertine on mood and physical performance of trained athletes. *Br. J. Psychiat.*, **112**, 1177–1180.

AITKEN, R.C.B. (1969). Measurement of feelings using visual analogue rating scales. *Proc. Roy. Soc. Med.*, **62**, 989–997.

ANDERSSON, K. (1975) Cigarette smoking, arousal and performance in a complex memory task. *Reports from Psychology Dept.*, Univ. Stockholm. No 454 pp 1–7.

ANDERSSON, K. & HOCKEY, G.R. (1975) Effects of cigarette smoking on incidental memory. *Reports from Psychology Dept.*, Univ. Stockholm. No 455 pp 1–6.

ANDERSSON, K. & POST, B. (1972). Effects of cigarette smoking on verbal rote learning and physiological arousal. *Reports from Psychology Dept.*, Univ. Stockholm. No 364 pp 1–8.

ASCHOFF, J.C., BECKER, W. & WEINERT, D. (1975). Computer analysis of eye movements: evaluation of the state of alertness and vigilance after sulpiride medication. *J. Pharmac. Clin.,* **11,** 93–97.

ASHTON, H., HALL, E.H., SAVAGE, R.D., TELFORD, R. & THOMPSON, J.W. (1972). A small controlled study to determine the time of onset of action of oxypertine after oral administration in normal subjects. *Postgrad. med. J.,* (Sept. Suppl), 14–18.

AYD, F.J. (1972). Motivations and rewards for volunteering to be an experimental subject. *Clin. Pharmac. Ther.,* **13,** 771–781.

BERNSTEIN, M.E., HUGHES, F.W. & FORNEY, R.B. (1967). The influence of a new chlordiazepoxide analogue on human mental and motor performance. *J. clin. Pharmac.,* **7,** 330–335.

BERRY, P.A., BURTLES, R., GRUBB, D.J. & HOARE, M.V. (1974). An evaluation of the effects of clobazam on human motor co-ordination, mental activity and mood. *Br. J. clin. Pharmac.,* **1,** 346.

BERRY, C., GELDER, M.G. & SUMMERFIELD, A. (1965). Experimental analysis of drug effects on human performance using information theory concepts. *Br. J. Psychol.,* **56,** 255–265.

BESSER, G.M., STEINBERG, H. (1967). L'interaction du chlordiazepoxide et du dexamphetamine chez l'homme. *Therapie,* **22,** 977–990.

BETTS, T.A., CLAYTON, A.B. & MACKAY, G.M. (1972). Effects of four commonly-used tranquillizers on low-speed driving performance tests. *Br. med. J.,* **4,** 580–584.

BIEHL, B. (1974). The effects of two tranquillisers on driving performance as measured in the normal driving task. *Proceedings 8th Congress of International Association of Applied Psychology:* Montreal.

BIEHL, B. (1979). Studies of clobazam and car-driving. *Br. J. clin. Pharmac.,* **7,** 85s–90s.

BOND, A.J., JAMES, D.C. & LADER, M. (1974a). Physiological and psychological measures in anxious patients. *Psychological Med.,* **4,** 364–372.

BOND, A.J., JAMES, D.C. & LADER, M. (1974b). Sedative effects on physiological and psychological measures in anxious patients. *Psychological Med.,* **4,** 374–380.

BOND, A.J. & LADER, M.H. (1972). Residual effects of hypnotics. *Psychopharmacologia (Berl.),* **23,** 117–132.

BOND, A.J. & LADER, M.H. (1973). The residual effects of flurazepam. *Psychopharmacologia (Berl.),* **32,** 223–235.

BOND, A. & LADER, M. (1974). The use of analogue scales in rating subjective feelings. *Br. J. med. Psychol.,* **47,** 211–218.

BOND, A.J. & LADER, M.H. (1975). Residual effects of flunitrazepam. *Br. J. clin. Pharmac.,* **2,** 143–150.

BORLAND, R.G. & NICHOLSON, A.N. (1974). Human performance after a barbiturate (heptabarbitone). *Br. J. clin. Pharmac.,* **1,** 209–215.

BŘEZINOVA, V. (1974). Effect of caffeine on sleep: EEG study in late middle age people. *Br. J. clin. Pharmac.,* **1,** 203–208.

BROADHURST, A.D. & ARENILLAS, L. (1975). A clinical and psychometric evaluation of flurazepam as a hypnotic in psychiatric patients. *Curr. med. Res. Opin.,* **3,** 413–416.

BROWN, J., LEWIS, V., BROWN, M.W., HORN, G. & BOWES, J.B. (1978). Amnesic effects of intravenous diazepam and lorazepam. *Experientia,* **34,** 501–502.

BÜHLER, R.A. (1955). Flicker fusion threshold and anxiety level. *Psychol. Abstr.,* **39,** 701.

BUSCH, Von M., KLAPPROTH, H.E., LÜCKER. & SCHMITZ, H. (1979). Ein neues psychometrisches Testmodell auf der Basis des "tailored Testing" zur ökonomischen und effizienten Erfassung psychopharmakologischer Effekte. *Arzneim-Forsch/Drug Res.,* **29,** 859–863.

BYE, C., MUNRO-FAURE, A.D., PECK, A.W. & YOUNG, P.A. (1973). A comparison of the effects of 1-benzylpiperazine and dexamphetamine on human performance tests. *Eur. J. clin. Pharmac.,* **6,** 163–169.

ČERNÝ, M., JIRÁK, R., KRULÍK, A., LUKÁŠOVA, A., PAULÄT, J. & POKORNÁ, A. (1973). Comparison of the effect of methylphenidate, diazepam and their combination on some psychophysiological variables. *Activ. nerv. sup.* (Praha), **15,** 123–124.

CHURCH, M.W. & JOHNSON, L.C. (1979). Mood and performance of poor sleepers during repeated use of flurazepam. *Psychopharmacology.,* **61,** 309–316.

CLARIDGE, G.S. (1967). *Personality and arousal.* Oxford: Pergamon.

CLARIDGE, G.S. (1970). *Drugs and human behaviour.* London: Allen Lane.

CLARKE, P.R.F., ECCERSLEY, P.S., FRISBY, J.P. & THORNTON, J.A. (1970). The amnesic effect of diazepam. *Br. J. Anaesth.,* **42,** 690–697.

COHEN, N.J., DOUGLAS, V.I. & MORGENSTERN, G. (1971). The effect of methylphenidate on attentive behaviour and autonomic activity in hyperactive children. *Psychopharmacologia (Berl.),* **22,** 284–294.

COLQUHOUN, W.P. (1962). Effects of hyoscine and meclozine on vigilance and short-term memory. *Br. J. indust. Med.,* **19,** 287–296.

CONSROE, P., CARLINI, E.A., ZWICKER, A.P. & LACERDA, L.A. (1979). Interaction of cannabidiol and alcohol in humans. *Psychopharmacology,* **66,** 45–50.

CORSICO, R., MOIZESZOWICZ, J., BURSUCK, L. & ROVARO, E. (1976). Evaluation of the psychotropic effect of etifoxine through pursuit rotor performance and GSR. *Psychopharmacologia (Berl.),* **45,** 301–303.

CROME, P. & NEWMAN, B. (1978). A comparison of the effects of single doses of mianserin and amitriptyline on psychomotor tests in normal volunteers. *J. Int. med. Res.,* **6,** 430–434.

CROUCHER, T. & HINDMARCH, I. (1974). The spiral after effect as a measure of motion sickness susceptibility and the effect of the SAE on an antimotion sickness drug and a central nervous system depressant. *Psychopharmacologia (Berl.),* **32,** 15–22

CROWN, S. & CRISP, A.H. (1970). *Manual of the Middlesex Hospital Questionnaire.* Barnstaple: Psychological Test Publications.

DAVIS, K.L., HOLLISTER, L.E., OVERALL, J., JOHNSON, A. & TRAIN, K. (1976). Physostigmine: effects on cognition and affect in normal subjects. *Psychopharmacology,* **51,** 23–27.

DiMASCIO, A. & BARRETT, J. (1965). Comparative effects of oxazepam in 'high' and 'low' anxious student volunteers. *Psychosomatics,* **6,** 298–302.

DOONGAJI, D.R., SHETH, A., APTE, J.S., LAKDAWALA, P.D., KHARE, C.B. & THATTE, S.S. (1979). Clobazam versus diazepam: a double-blind study in anxiety neurosis. *Br. J. clin. Pharmac.,* **7,** 119S.

DORNIC, S., MYRSTEN, A-L. & FRANKENHAEUSER, M.

(1971). Effects of alcohol on short-term memory. *Reports from Psychology Dept.*, Univ Stockholm. No 336 pp 1–11.

DUKE, R.B. & KEELER, M.H. (1968). The effects of psilocybin, d-amphetamine and placebo on performance of the trail making task. *J. clin. psychol.*, **24**, 316–317.

DUREMAN, I. & NORRMAN, B. (1975). Clinical and experimental comparison of diazepam, clorazepate and placebo. *Psychopharmacologia (Berl.)*, **40**, 279–284.

DYER, F.N. (1973). The Stroop phenomenon and its use in the study of perceptual, cognitive and response processes. *Memory and Cognition*, **1**, 106–120.

EDWARDS, F. (1978). Risks at work from medication. *J. Roy. Coll. Phys.*, **12**, 219–229.

ENZER, N., SIMONSON, E. & BALLARD, G. (1944). The effects of small doses of alcohol on the central nervous system. *Am. J. clin. Path.*, **14**, 333–341.

EVANS, M.A., MARTZ, R., RODDA, B.E., KIPLINGER, G.F. & FORNEY, R.B. (1974). Quantitative relationship between blood alcohol concentration and performance. *Clin. Pharmac. Ther.*, **15**, 253–260.

EYSENCK, H.J. (1963). *Experiments with drugs*. Oxford: Pergamon.

EYSENCK, H.J. (1972). *Handbook of abnormal psychology*. London: Pitman Medical.

EYSENCK, H.J. & EASTERBROOK, J.A. (1960). Drugs and personality: the effect of stimulant and depressant drugs upon visual and kinaesthetic after-effects. *J. ment. Sci.*, **106**, 845–854.

EYSENCK, H.J. & EYSENCK, S.B.G. (1964). *Eysenck personality inventory*. London: University of London Press.

FARGUS, P.C.G. & HINDMARCH, I. (1974). A 1, 4 benzodiazepine, temazepam: effect on reaction time related to car driving. *IRCS Med. Sci.*, **2**, 1173.

FARHOUMAND, N., HARRISON, J., PARE, C.M.B., TURNER, P. & WYNN, S. (1979). The effect of high dose oxprenolol on stress induced physical and psychophysiological variables. *Psychopharmacology*, **64**, 365–369.

FELL, P.J., QUANTOCK, D.C. & VANDER BURGH W.J. (1973). The human pharmacology of GB94- a new psychotropic agent. *Eur. J. clin. Pharmac.*, **5**, 166–173.

FILE, S.E. & BOND, A.J. (1979). Impaired performance and sedation after a single dose of lorazepam. *Psychopharmacology*, **66**, 309–313.

FINK, M., IRWIN, P., GASTPAR, M. & DE RIDDER, J.J. (1977). EEG, blood level and behavioural effects of the antidepressant mianserin. *Psychopharmacology*, **54**, 249–254.

FLEISHMAN, E.A. & HEMPEL, W.E. (1956). Factorial analysis of complex psychomotor performance and related skills. *J. appl. Psychol.*, **40**, 96–104.

FRANKENHAEUSER, M. (1959). *Estimation of time*. Stockholm: Almquist and Wiksell.

FRANKENHAEUSER, M., MYRSTEN, A-L., POST, B. & JOHANSSON, G. (1970). Behavioural and physiological effects of cigarette smoking in a monotonous situation. *Reports from Psychological Dept.*, Univ Stockholm. No 301, pp 1–7.

FREYD, M. (1923). The graphic rating scale. *J. ed. Psychol.*, **14**, 83.

FRITH, C.D. (1967). The effects of nicotine on tapping. *Life Sci.*, **6**, 321–326.

FROSTAD, A.L., FOREST, G.L. & BAKKER, C.B. (1966). Influence of personality type on drug response. *Am. J. Psychiat.*, **14**, 1153–1158.

GAGNÉ, R.M. & FLEISHMAN, E.A. (1959). *Psychology and human performance*. New York: Holt.

GENDREAU, P., SHERLOCK, D., PARSONS, T., McLEAN, R., SCOTT, G.D. & SUBOSKE, M.D. (1972). Effects of methamphetamine on well-practiced discrimination conditioning of the eyelid response. *Psychopharmacologia (Berl.)*, **25**, 112–116.

GHONEIM, M.M., MEWALDT, S.P. & THATCHER, J.W. (1975). The effect of diazepam and fentanyl on mental, psychomotor and electroencephalographic functions and their rate of recovery. *Psychopharmacologia (Berl.)*, **44**, 61–66.

GHONEIM, M.M. & MEWALT, S.P. (1977). Studies on human memory: the interactions of diazepam, scopolamine and physostigmine. *Psychopharmacology*, **52**, 1–6.

GIBSON, H.B. (1965). *Manual of Gibson Spiral Maze*. London: University of London Press.

GOLDBERG, L. (1943). The influence of ethyl alcohol on sensory, motor and psychological functions referred to blood alcohol in normal and habituated individuals. *Acta Physiol. Scand.*, **5**, 1–128.

GOLDSTEIN, L. & STOLTZFUS, N.W. (1973). Psychoactive drug-induced changes of interhemispheric EEG amplitude relationships. *Agents and Actions*, **3**, 124–132.

GOLDSTONE, S. (1955). Critical flicker fusion measurements and anxiety level. *J. expt. Psychol.*, **49**, 200–202.

GOLDSTONE, S., BOARDMAN, W.K. & LHAMON, W.T. (1958). Effects of quinalbarbitone, d-amphetamine and placebo on apparent time. *Br. J. Psychol.*, **49**, 324–328.

GOLDSTONE, S. & KIRHAM, J.E. (1968). The effects of secobarbital and d-amphetamine upon time judgement: Intersensory factors. *Psychopharmacologia* (Berl.), **13**, 65–73.

GRAY, J.A. (1967). Strength of the nervous system, introversion — extraversion, conditionability and arousal. *Behav. Res. Ther.*, **5**, 151–170.

GRUNDSTRÖM, R., HOLMBERG, G., & HANSEN, T. (1977). Degree of sedation obtained with various doses of diazepam and nitrazepam. *Acta Pharmac. Tox.*, **43**, 13–18.

GUEST, A.D.L., DUNCAN, C. & LAWTHER, P.J. (1970). Carbon monoxide and phenobarbitone: a comparison of effects on auditory flutter fusion threshold and critical flicker fusion threshold. *Ergonomics*, **13**, 587–594.

GUPTA, B.S. (1973). The effects of stimulant and depressant drugs on verbal conditioning. *Br. J. Psychol.*, **64**, 553–557.

GUPTA, B.S. (1974). Stimulant and depressant drugs on kinaesthetic figural after-effects. *Psychopharmacologia (Berl.)*, **36**, 275–280.

HAFFNER, J.F.W., MØRLAND, J., SETEKLEIV, J., STRØM-SAETHER, C.E., DANIELSEN, A., FRIVIK, P.T. & DYBING, F. (1973). Mental and psychomotor effects of diazepam and ethanol. *Acta Pharmac. Tox.*, **32**, 161–178.

HARPER, C.R. & KIDERA, G.J. (1972). Aviator performance and the use of hypnotic drugs. *Aerospace Med.*, **43**, 197–199.

HARRY, T.V.A. & RICHARDS, D.J. (1972). Lorazepam — a study in psychomotor depression. *Br. J. clin. Prac.*, **26**, 371–373.

HART, J., HILL, H.M., BYE, C.E., WILKINSON, R.T. & PECK, A.W. (1976). The effects of low doses of amylobarbitone sodium and diazepam on human performance. *Br. J. clin. Pharmac.*, **3**, 289–298.

HAWARD, L.R.C. (1968). Effects of sodium diphenylhydantoinate upon concentration. Paper presented to British Psychology Society Conference: London (mimeograph).

HAYES, M.H. & PATTERSON, D.G. (1921). Experimental development of the graphic rating method. *Psychol. Bull.*, **18**, 98.

HEDGES, A., TURNER, P. & HARRY, T.V. (1971). Preliminary studies on the central nervous effects of lorazepam, a new benzodiazepine. *J. clin. Pharmac.*, **16**, 423–427.

HENERT, G.A. & JANKE, W. (1957). Pharmacological and psychological investigation into 5-phenyl-2-amino-4-oxo-oxazolidine. *Arzneim. Forsch. (Drug Res.)*, **7**, 352–355.

HINDMARCH, I. (1975). A 1, 4-benzodiazepine, temazepam (K3917): its effect on some psychological parameters of sleep and behaviour. *Arzneim. Forsch. (Drug Res.)*, **25**, 1836–1839.

HINDMARCH, I. (1976a). The effects of the sub-chronic administration of an anti-histamine, clemastine, on tests of car driving ability and psychomotor performance. *Curr. med. res. Opin.*, **4**, 197–206.

HINDMARCH, I. (1976b). A sub-chronic study of the subjective quality of sleep and psychological measures of performance on the morning following night time medication with temazepam. *Arzneim. Forsch. (Drug Res.)*, **26**, 2113–2116.

HINDMARCH, I. (1977a). Laboratory investigation of effect of acute doses of nomifensine on a simulated aspect of night-time car driving performance. *Br. J. clin. Pharmac.*, **4**, 167s–178s.

HINDMARCH, I. (1977b). A repeated dose comparison of three benzodiazepine derivatives (nitrazepam, flurazepam and flunitrazepam) on subjective appraisals of sleep and measures of psychomotor performance the morning following night-time medication. *Acta Psychiatrica Scand.*, **56**, 373–381.

HINDMARCH, I. (1979a). Some aspects of the effects of clobazam on human psychomotor performance. *Br. J. clin. Pharmac.*, **7**, 77s–82s.

HINDMARCH, I. (1979b). A preliminary study of the effects of repeated doses of clobazam on aspects of performance, arousal and behaviour in a group of anxiety rated volunteers. *Eur. J. clin. Pharmac.*, **16**, 17–21.

HINDMARCH, I. (1979c). Effects of hypnotic and sleep-inducing drugs on objective assessments of human psychomotor performance and subjective appraisals of sleep and early morning behaviour. *Br. J. clin. Pharmac.*, **8**, 43s–46s.

HINDMARCH, I. & CLYDE, C.A. (1980a). A preliminary investigation of the effects of a 1, 4 benzodiazepine derivative (HR158) on subjective aspects of sleep and objective measures of early morning performance. *Drugs Exptl. Clin. Res.*, **2**, 61–70.

HINDMARCH, I. & CLYDE, C.A. (1980b). The effects of triazolam and nitrazepam on sleep quality, morning vigilance and psychomotor performance. *Arzneim. Forsch (Drug Res.)*, **30**, 1163–1166.

HINDMARCH, I. & GUDGEON, A.C. (1980). The effects of clobazam and lorazepam on aspects of psychomotor performance and car handling ability. *Br. J. clin. Pharmac.*, **10**, 145–150.

HINDMARCH, I., HANKS, G.W. & HEWITT, A.J. (1977). Clobazam, a 1, 5 benzodiazepine derivative, and car driving ability. *Br. J. clin. Pharmac.*, **4**, 573–578.

HINDMARCH, I. & PARROTT, A.C. (1977). Repeated dose comparisons of nomifensine, imipramine and placebo on subjective assessments of sleep and objective measures of psychomotor performance. *Br. J. clin. Pharmac.*, **4**, 167s–173s.

HINDMARCH, I. & PARROTT, A.C. (1978). The effect of a sub-chronic administration of three dose levels of a 1, 5 benzodiazepine derivative, clobazam, on subjective aspects of sleep and assessments of psychomotor performance the morning following night time medication. *Arzneim. Forsch. (Drug Res.)*, **28**, 2169–2172.

HINDMARCH, I. & PARROTT, A.C. (1979a). The effects of repeated nocturnal doses of clobazam, dipotassium clorazepate and placebo on subjective ratings of sleep and early morning behaviour and objective measures of arousal, psychomotor performance and anxiety. *Br. J. clin. Pharmac.*, **8**, 325–329.

HINDMARCH, I. & PARROTT, A.C. (1979b). A repeated dose comparison of the side effects of five anti-histamines on objective assessments of psychomotor performance, central nervous system arousal and subjective appraisals of sleep and early morning behaviour. *Arzneim. Forsch., (Drug Res.)*, **28**, 483–486.

HINDMARCH, I. & PARROTT, A.C. (1980a). The effects of combined sedative and anxiolytic preparations on subjective aspects of sleep and objective measures of arousal and performance the morning following nocturnal medication. I: Acute Doses. *Arzneim. Forsch. (Drug Res.)*, **30**, 1025–1028.

HINDMARCH, I. & PARROTT, A.C. (1980b). The effects of combined sedative and anxiolytic preparations on subjective aspects of sleep and objective measures of arousal and performance the morning following nocturnal treatment. II: Repeated doses. *Arzneim. Forsch. (Drug Res.)*, **30**, 1167–1170.

HINDMARCH, I., PARROTT, A.C. & ARENILLAS, L. (1977b). A repeated dose comparison of dichloralphenazone, flunitrazepam and amylobarbitone sodium on some aspects of sleep and early morning behaviour in normal subjects. *Br. J. clin. Pharmac.*, **4**, 229–233.

HINDMARCH, I., PARROTT, A.C. & LANZA, M. (1979). The effects of an ergot alkaloid derivative (Hydergine) on aspects of psychomotor performance, arousal and cognitive processing ability. *J. clin. Pharmac.*, **19**, 726–731.

HINDMARCH, I., PARROTT, A.C. & STONIER, P.D. (1980). The effects of nomifensine and HOE8476 on car driving and related psychomotor performance. *Roy. Soc. Med. Int. Cong. Symp. Ser.*, No 25, 47–54.

HOLMBERG, G. & WILLIAM-OLLSON, U. (1963). The effect of benzquinamide, in comparison with chlordiazepoxide and placebo, on performance in some psychological tests. *Psychopharmacologia (Berl.)*, **4**, 402–417.

HORMIA, A. (1956). On the sensation of duration. *Ann. Acad. Sci. Fenn.*, **58**, 1–81.

HUFFMAN, W.J., FLORIO, A., PAYNE, J.L. & BOYS, F.E.

(1963). The influence of two selected tranquillisers on driving skills. *Am. J. Psychiat.*, **119**, 885–886.

HUGHES, F.W., FORNEY, R.B. & RICHARDS, A.B. (1965). Comparative effect in human subjects of chlordiazepoxide, diazepam and placebo on mental and physical performance. *Clin. Pharmac. Ther.*, **6**, 139–145.

IDESTRÖM, C-M. & CADENIUS, B. (1963). Chlordiazepoxide, dipiperon and amobarbital: Dose effect studies. *Psychopharmacologia (Berl.)*, **4**, 235–246.

IDESTRÖM, C.M. & CADENIUS, B. (1968). Time relations of the effects of alcohol compared to placebo. *Psychopharmacologia (Berl.)*, **13**, 189–200.

JÄÄTTELA, A., MÄNNISTÖ, P., PAATERO, H. & TUOMISTO, J. (1971). The effects of diazepam or diphenhydramine on healthy human subjects. *Psychopharmacologia (Berl.)*, **4**, 235–246.

JONES, O. (1958). Relationship between visual and auditory discrimination and anxiety level. *J. gen. Psychol.*, **59**, 111–118.

JONES, D.M., LEWIS, M.J. & SPRIGGS, T.L.B. (1978). The effects of low doses of diazepam on human performance in group administered tasks. *Br. J. clin. Pharmac.*, **6**, 333–337.

JONES, D.M., JONES, M.E.L., LEWIS, M.J. & SPRIGGS, T.L.B. (1979). Drugs and human memory: effects of low doses of nitrazepam and hyoscine on retention. *Br. J. clin. Pharmac.*, **7**, 479–483.

KEESEY, U.T. (1970). Variables determining flicker sensitivity in small fields. *J. Optical Soc. Amer.*, **60**, 390–398.

KEUCHEL, I., KOHNEN, R. & LIENERT, G.A. (1979). The effects of alcohol and caffeine on concentration test performance. *Arzneim. Forsch.* (Drug Res.), **29**, 973–975.

KLEINKNECHT, R.A. & DONALDSON, D. (1975). A review of the effects of diazepam on cognitive and psychomotor performance. *J. nerv. ment. Dis.*, **161**, 399–414.

KNIGHTS, R.M. & HINTON, G.C. (1969). The effects of methylphenidate on the motor skills and behaviour of children with learning problems. *J. nerv. ment. Dis.*, **148**, 643–654.

KORNETSKY, C. (1958). Effects of meprobamate, phenobarbital and dextroamphetamine on reaction time and learning in man. *J. Pharmac. exp. Ther.*, **123**, 216–219.

KORNETSKY, C. & ORZACK, M.H. (1964). A research note on some of the critical factors on the dissimilar effects of chlorpromazine and secobarbital on the digit symbol substitution and continuous performance test. *Psychopharmacologia (Berl.)*, **6**, 79–86.

KORTTILA, K. (1977). Lack of impairment in skills related to driving after intramuscular administration of prilocaine or mepivacaine. *Acta Anaesthesiol. Scand.*, **21**, 31–36.

KORTTILA, K. & LINNOILA, M.(1975). Psychomotor skills related to driving after intramuscular administration of diazepam and meperidine. *Anaesthesiology*, **42**, 685–691.

KORTTILA, K., MATTILA, M.J. & LINNOILA, M. (1976). Prolonged recovery after diazepam sedation: the inference of food, charcoal ingestion and injection rate on the effects of intravenous diazepam. *Br. J. Anaesth.*, **48**, 333–340.

KORTTILA, K., TAMMISTO, T., ERTAMA, P., PFAFFLI, P., BLOMGREN, E. & HAKKINEN, S. (1977). Recovery, psychomotor skills and simulated driving after brief inhalational anaesthesia with halothane or enflurane combined with nitrous oxide and oxygen. *Anaesthesiology*, **46**, 20–27.

KORTTILA, K., SAARNIVAARA, L., TARKKANEN, J., HIMBERG, J.J. & HYTONEN, M. (1978). Comparison of diazepam and flunitrazepam for sedation during anaesthesia for bronchoscopy. *Br. J. Anaesth.*, **50**, 281–287.

KRUGMAN, H. (1947). Flicker fusion frequency as a function of anxiety reaction: an exploratory study. *Psychosom. Med.*, **4**, 269–272.

LAHTINEN, U., LAHTINEN, A. & PEKKOLA, P. (1978). The effect of nitrazepam on manual skill, grip strength and reaction time with special reference to subjective evaluation of effects on sleep. *Acta Pharmac. Tox.*, **42**, 130–134.

LANDAUER, A.A., POCOCKE, D.A. & PLOTT, F.W. (1974). The effect of medazepam and alcohol on cognitive and motor skills used in car driving. *Psychopharmacologia (Berl.)*, **37**, 159–168.

LAWTON, M.P. & CAHN, B. (1963). The effects of diazepam and alcohol on psychomotor performance. *J. nerv. ment. Dis.*, **136**, 550–554.

LEYGONIE, F., RETHONE, A., YUCEYATAK, F. & YUCEYATAK, A. (1976). Anxiolytique nouveau, le clobazam, action sur le sommeil de nuit et le niveau de performance au réveil. *Gaz. Méd. France*, **82**, 1303.

LILJEQUIST, R. & MATTILA, M.J. (1979). Acute effects of temazepam and nitrazepam on psychomotor skills and memory. *Acta Pharmac. Tox.*, **44**, 364–369.

LILJEQUIST, R., SEPPÄLÄ, T. & MATTILA, M.J. (1978). Amitriptyline and mianserin induced changes in acquisition of paired-association learning task. *Br. J. clin. Pharmac.*, **5**, 149–153.

LINNOILA, M. & HAKKINEN, S. (1974). Effects of diazepam and codeine alone and in combination with alcohol on simulated driving. *Clin. Pharmac. Ther.*, **15**, 368–373.

LURIA, R.E. (1975). The validity of the visual analogue mood scale. *J. Psychiat. Res.*, **12**, 51–57.

MACKWORTH, J.F. (1965). The effects of amphetamine on detectability of signals in a vigilance task. *Canad. J. Psychol.*, **19**, 104–110.

MACLEOD, S.M., GILES, H.G., PATZALEK, G., THIESSEN, J.J. & SELLERS, E.M. (1977). Diazepam actions and plasma concentrations following ethanol ingestion. *Eur. J. clin. Pharmac.*, **11**, 345–349.

MALPAS, A. (1972). Subjective and objective effects of nitrazepam and amylobarbitone sodium in normal human beings. *Psychopharmacologia (Berl.)*, **27**, 373–378.

MALPAS, A. & JOYCE, C.R.B. (1969). Effects of nitrazepam, amylobarbitone and placebo on some perceptual, motor and cognitive tasks in normal subjects. *Psychopharmacologia (Berl.)*, **14**, 167–177.

MALPAS, A., ROWAN, A.J., JOYCE, C.R.B. & SCOTT, D.F. (1970). Persistent behavioural and electroencephalographic changes after single doses of nitrazepam and amylobartitone sodium. *Br. med. J.*, **2**, 762–764.

MALPAS, A., LEGG, N.J. & SCOTT, D.F. (1974). Effects of hypnotics on anxious patients. *Br. J. Psychiat.*, **124**, 482–484.

MARJERRISON, G., NEUFELDT, A.H., HOLMES, V. & HO, T. (1973). Comparative psychophysical and mood effects of diazepam and dipotassium clorazepate. *Biol. Psychiat.*, **7**, 31–41.

MASHOUR, M. & DEVINE, B. (1977). Detection performance and its relationship with human capacity for information processing. *Reports from Dept. of Psychology*, Univ. Stockholm. No 495, pp 1–14.

MASUDA, M. & BAKKER, C.B. (1966). Personality, catecholamine metabolites and psychophysical response to diazepam. *J. Psychiat. Res.*, **4**, 221–234.

MATTILA, M.J., PALVA, E., SEPPÄLÄ, T. & OSTROVSKAYA, R.U. (1978). Actions and interactions with alcohol of drugs on psychomotor skills: comparison of diazepam and gamma-hydroxybutyric acid. *Arch. int. Pharmac. Ther.*, **234**, 236–246.

MAY, A.E., CHILDS, D.J. & URQUHART, A. (1976). Intropunitiveness and finer dexterity in alcoholics. *J. Alcoh.*, **11**, 21–23.

MELIKIAN, L. (1961). The effect of meprobamate on the performance of normal subjects on selected psychological tasks. *J. Gen. Psychol.*, **65**, 33–38.

MICHON, J.A. (1976), Human information processing — with and without drugs. *Psychiat. Neurol. Neurochir.*, (Amst.), **76**, 163–174.

MILLAR, K. (1979). An objective assessment of vigilance following ingestion of a new controlled-release antihistamine preparation. *Med. Dig.*, *3*, 52–57.

MILLER, L.L. & DOLAN, M.P. (1974). Effects of alcohol on short term memory as measured by a guessing technique. *Psychopharmacologia (Berl.)*, **35**, 353–364.

MIRSKY, A.F. & KORNETSKY, C. (1964). On the dissimilar effects of drugs on the digit symbol substitution and continuous performance tests. *Psychopharmacologia (Berl.)*, **5**, 161–177.

MOLANDER, L. & DUVHÖK, C. (1976). Acute effects of oxazepam, diazepam and methylperone alone and in combination with alcohol on sedation co-ordination and mood. *Acta Pharmac. Tox.*, **38**, 145–160.

MØRLAND, J., SETEKLEIV, J., HAFFNER, J.F.W., STRØMSAETHER, C.E., DANIELSEN, A. & WETHE, G.H. (1974). Combined effects of diazepam and ethanol on mental and psychomotor functions. *Acta Pharmac. Tox.*, **34**, 5–15.

MOSER, L., HÜTHER, K.J., KOCH-WESER, J. & LUNDT, P.V. (1978). Effects of terfenadine and diphenhydramine alone or in combination with diazepam or alcohol on psychomotor performance and subjective feelings. *Eur. J. clin. Pharmac.*, **14**, 417–423.

MULLER-OERLINGHAUSEN, B., BAUER, H., GIRKE, W., KANOWSKI, S. & GONCALVES, N. (1977). Impairment of vigilance and performance under lithium-treatment: studies in patients and volunteers. *Pharmakopsychiatr. Neuropsychopharmakol.*, **10**, 67–68.

MYRSTEN, A-L., POST, B., FRANKENHAEUSER, M. & JOHANSSON, G. (1971). Enhanced behavioural efficiency induced by cigarette smoking. *Reports from Psychological Labs.*, Univ. Stockholm. No 337, pp 1–10.

NÄÄTÄNEN, R. (1975). Selective attention and evoked potentials in humans — a critical review. *Biol. Psychiat.*, **2**, 237–307.

NAKANO, S., GILLESPIE, H.K. & HOLLISTER, L.E. (1978). A model for the evaluation of anti-anxiety drugs with the use of experimentally induced stress: comparison of nabilone and diazepam. *Clin. Pharmac. Ther.*, **23**, 54–62.

NASH, H. & STONE, G.C. (1974). Psychological effects of drugs. *J. nerv. ment. Dis.*, **159**, 444–447.

NICHOLSON, A.N. (1976). Performance and impaired performance. *Br. J. clin. Pharmac.*, **3**, 521–522.

NICHOLSON, A.N. (1979). Performance studies with diazepam and its hydroxylated metabolites. *Br. J. clin. Pharmac.*, **8**, 39S–42S.

ORR, J. DUSSAULT, C., CHAPPEL, C., GOLDBERG, L. & REGGIANI, G. (1976). Relation between drug-induced central nervous system effects and plasma levels of diazepam in man. *Mod. Probl. Pharmacopsych.*, **11**, 57–67.

ORZACK, M.H., TAYLOR, C.L. & KORNETSKY, C. (1968). A research report on the anti-fatigue effects of magnesium pemoline. *Psychopharmacologia (Berl.)*, **13**, 413–417.

OSWALD, I., LEWIS, S.A. DUNLEAVY, D.L.F., BREZINOVA, V. & BRIGGS, M. (1971). Drugs of dependence though not of abuse: Fenfluramine. *Br. med. J.*, **3**, 70–73.

PALVA, E.S. & LINNOILA, M.J. (1978). Effects of active metabolites of diazepam and chlordiazepoxide alone and in combination with alcohol on psychomotor skills related to driving. *Eur. J. clin. Pharmac.*, **13**, 345–350.

PARROTT, A.C. & HINDMARCH, I. (1975a). Arousal and performance — the ubiquitous inverted U relationship. Comparison of changes in response latency and arousal levels in normal subjects induced by CNS stimulants, sedatives and tranquillisers. *IRCS Med. Sci.*, **3**, 176.

PARROTT, A.C. & HINDMARCH, I. (1975b). Clobazam, a 1, 5-benzodiazepine derivative: effects on anxiety, arousal and performance compared with those of CNS stimulants, sedatives and tranquillizers. *IRCS Med. Sci.*, **3**, 177.

PARROTT, A.C. & HINDMARCH, I. (1975c). Haloperidol and chlorpromazine — comparative effects upon arousal and performance. *IRCS Med. Sci.*, **3**, 562.

PARROTT, A.C. & HINDMARCH, I. (1978). Clobazam; a 1, 5 benzodiazepine derivative: effects upon human psychomotor performance under different levels of task reinforcement. *Arch. int. Pharmacodyn. Ther.*, **232**, 261–268.

PECK, A.W., ADAMS, R., BYE, C. & WILKINSON, R.T. (1976). Residual effects of hypnotic drugs: evidence for individual differences on vigilance. *Psychopharmacologia (Berl.)*, **47**, 213–216.

PECK, A.W., BYE, C.E. & CLARIDGE, R. (1977). Differences between light and sound sleepers in the residual effects of nitrazepam. *Br. J. clin. Pharmac.*, **4**, 101–108.

PECK, A.W., BYE, C.E., CLUBLEY, M., HENSON, T. & RIDDINGTON, C. (1979). A comparison of bupropion hydrochloride with dexamphetamine and amytriptyline in healthy subjects. *Br. J. clin. Pharmac.*, **7**, 469–478.

PENTTILÄ, A., LEHTI, H. & LÖNNQUIST, J. (1975). Psychotropic drugs and impairment of psychomotor function. *Psychopharmacologia (Berl.)*, **43**, 75–80.

REITAN, M. (1958). The comparative effects of placebo, ultran and meprobamate on psychologic test performances. *Antibiol. Med. Clin. Ther.*, **4**, 158–165.

RICHTER, R. & HOBI, V. (1976). Personality specific actions of a tranquillizer. *Arzneim. Forsch.*, **26**, 1136–1138.

RIZZO, P. (1957). Study of the modifications induced by the ingestion of ethyl alcohol in the critical flicker frequency of light stimuli. *Riv. Med. Aeronaut. Spaz.*, **20**, 249–261.

RODEN, S., HARVEY, P. & MITCHARD, M. (1977). The

influence of alcohol on the persistent effects on human performance of the hypnotics Mandrax and nitrazepam. *Int. J. clin. Pharmac.*, **15**, 350–355.

ROSKETH, R. & LORENTZEN, F.V. (1954). Combined effect of alcohol and hypoxia on flicker fusion frequency. *J. appl. Physiol.*, **69**, 559–565.

ROSVOLD, H.E., MIRSKY, A., SARASON, I., BRANSOME, E.D. & BECK, L.H. (1956). A continuous performance test of brain damage. *J. Cons. Psychol.*, **20**, 343–350.

ROTH, T., KRAMER, M. & LUTZ, T. (1977). The effects of hypnotics on sleep, performance and subjective state. *Drugs Exp. Clin. Res.*, **1**, 279–286.

SAARIO, I. (1976). Psychomotor skills during subacute treatment with thioridazine and bromazepam and their effects combined with alcohol. *Ann. Clin. Res.*, **8**, 117–23.

SALETU, B. & GRUBERGER, J. (1979). Evaluation of pharmacodynamic properties of psychotropic drugs: quantitative EEG, psychometric and blood levels investigations in normals and patients. *Pharmakopsychiatr. Neuropsychopharmakol.*, **12**, 45–58.

SALETU, B. & TAEUBER, K. (1980). Serum levels of nomifensine and pharmacodynamics. *Roy. Soc. Med. Int. Cong. Symp. Ser.*, **25**, 31–38.

SALKIND, M. & SILVERSTONE, J.T. (1975). A clinical and psychometric evaluation of flunitrazepam. *Br. J. clin. Pharmac.*, **2**, 223–226.

SALKIND, M.R., HANKS, G.W. & SILVERSTONE, J.T. (1979). Evaluation of the effects of clobazam, a 1, 5 benzodiazepine, on mood and psychomotor performance in clinically anxious patients in general practice. *Br. J. clin. Pharmac.*, **7**, 113s–118s.

SAMBROOKS, J.E., MACCULLOCH, M.J., BIRTLES, C.J. & SMALLMAN, C. (1972). Assessment of the effect of flurazepam and nitrazepam on visuo-motor performance using an automated assessment technique. *Acta Psychiat. Scand.*, **48**, 443–454.

SAMBROOKS, J.E., MACCULLOCH, M.J. & ROONEY, J.F.F. (1975). The automated assessment of the effect of flurazepam and nitrazepam on mood state. *Acta Psychiat. Scand.*, **51**, 201–209.

SCHILLER, P.H. (1966). Developmental study of colour-word interference. *J. exp. Psychol.*, **72**, 105–108.

SEPPÄLÄ, T. (1977). Psychomotor skills during acute and two week treatment with mianserin and amitriptyline and their combined effects with alcohol. *Ann. Clin. Res.*, **9**, 66–72.

SEPPÄLÄ, T., KORTTILA, K., HÄKKINEN, S. & LINNOILA, M. (1976). Residual effects and skills related to driving after a single oral administration of diazepam, medazepam or lorazepam. *Br. J. Pharmac.*, **3**, 831–841.

SHAFFER, J.W., FREINEK, W.R., WOLF, S., FOXWELL, N.H. & KURLAND, A.A. (1963). A controlled evaluation of chlordiazepoxide in the treatment of convalescing alcoholics. *J. nerv. ment. Dis.*, **137**, 494–507.

SHIRA, R.B. (1978). A technique for investigating the intensity and duration of human psychomotor impairment after intravenous diazepam. *Oral Surg.*, **45**, 493–502.

SHOR, R.E. (1971). Symbol processing speed differences and symbol interference effects in a variety of concept domains. *J. gen Psychol.*, **85**, 187–205.

SMITH, J.M. & MISIAK, H. (1976). Critical Flicker Frequency (CFF) and psychotropic drugs in normal

human subjects — a review. *Psychopharmacology*, **47**, 175–182.

SPIELBERGER, C.D., GORSUCH, R.L. & LUSHENE, R.E. (1968). *Manual for the State-Trait Anxiety Inventory*. Tallahassee: Florida State University.

SQUITIERI, G., MAZZOLA, M.D., LAZZARI, R., CERVONE, A. & AGNOLI, A. (1977). Methodology for assessing the effect of drugs acting upon the human memory. *Drugs Exp. Clin. Res.*, **1**, 325–332.

STERN, J.A., BREMER, D.A. & McCLURE, J. (1974). Analysis of eye movements and blinks during reading: effects of valium. *Psychopharmacologia (Berl.)*, **40**, 171–175.

STITT, F.W., LATOUR, R. & FRANE, J.W. (1977). A clinical study of naproxen-diazepam drug interaction on tests of mood and attention. *Curr. Ther. Res.*, **21**, 149–156.

STROOP, J.R. (1935). Studies of interference in serial verbal reactions. *J. exp. Psychol.*, **18**, 643–662.

SUZUMURA, A. (1968). Annual report of the Research Institute of Environmental Medicine. Nagoya University, **16**, 77–89.

TAEUBER, K. (1977). Dynamic interaction of nomifensine with alcohol. *Br. J. clin. Pharmac.*, **4**, 147S–151S.

TAEUBER, K., BADIAN, M., BRETTEL, H.F., ROYEN, Th., RUPP, W., SITTIG, W. & UIHLEIN, M. (1979). Kinetic and dynamic interaction of clobazam and alcohol. *Br. J. clin. Pharmac.*, **7**, 91S–97S.

TAEUBER, K., ZAPF, R., RUPP, W. & BADIAN, M. (1976). Pharmacodynamic comparison of the acute effects of nomifensine, amphetamine and placebo in healthy volunteers. *Int. J. clin. Pharmac. Biopharm.*, **17**, 32–37.

TANSELLA, M., ZIMMERMANN-TANSELLA, C. & LADER, M. (1974). The residual effects of N-desmethyldiazepam in patients. *Psychopharmacologia*, **138**, 81–90.

TARTER, R.E., JONES, B.M., SIMPSON, C.D. & VEGA, A. (1971). Effects of task complexity and practice on performance during acute alcohol intoxication. *Percept. Mot. Skills*, **33**, 307.

TEICHNER, W.H. & KREBS, M.J. (1972). Laws of simple reaction time. *Psychological Review*, **79**, 344–358.

TEICHNER, W.H. & KREBS, M.J. (1974). Laws of visual choice reaction time. *Psychological Review*, **81**, 75–98.

TURNER, P. (1973). Clinical pharmacological studies on lorazepam. *Curr. med. Res. Opin.*, **1**, 262–264.

UHERIK, A. (1973). Methodological problems of psychophysiological research on human subjects. *Studia Psychologica*, **15**, 213–228.

UHR, L., MILLER, J.G. & PLATZ, A. (1963). Time and dosage effects of meprobamate on simple behavioural tasks. *J. gen. Psychol.*, **68**, 317–323.

UHLENHUTH, E.H., TURNER, D.A., PURCHATZKE, G., GIFT, T. & CHASSAN, J. (1977). Intensive design in evaluating anxiolytic agents. *Psychopharmacology*, **52**, 79–85.

VAN HOUTEN, P.L. & ZENHAUSERN, R. (1967). Meprobamate and absolute auditory thresholds. *J. Aud. Res.*, **7**, 253–257.

VELDKAMP, W., STRAW, R.N., METZLER, C.M. & DEMISSIANOS, H.V. (1974). Efficiency and residual effect evaluation of a new hypnotic, triazolam. *J. clin. Pharmac.*, **14**, 102–111.

VOGEL, J.R. (1979). Objective measurement of human performance changes produced by anxiolytic drugs.

Anxiolytics, eds Fielding, J. & Lal, S. pp 343–374. New York: Futura.

WADE, M.G. & NEWELL, K.M. (1972). Performance criteria for stabilometer learning. *J. Mot. Behav.,* **4,** 231–239.

WALTERS, A.J. & LADER, M.H. (1971). Hangover effects of hypnotics in man. *Nature,* **229,** 637–638.

WECHSLER, D. (1955). *A manual for the Wechsler Adult Intelligence Scale.* New York: Psychological Corporation.

WILKINSON, R.T. (1968). Sleep deprivation: performance tests for partial and selective sleep deprivation. *Prog. Clin. Psychol.,* **8,** 28–43.

WILLIAMS, H.L., LUBIN, A. & GOODNOW, J.J. (1959). Impaired performance with acute sleep loss. *Psychol. Mon.,* **73,** 1–26.

WILSON, G., TUNSTALL, O.A. & EYSENCK, H.J. (1971). Individual differences in tapping performance as a function of time on the task. *Percep. Mot. Skills.,* **33,** 375–378.

WITTENBORN, J.R. (1977). Contrasts in anti-depressant medications. *Br. J. clin. Pharmac.,* **4,** 153s–156s.

WITTENBORN, J.R. (1979). Benzodiazepines and psychomotor performance. *Br. J. clin. Pharmac.,* **7,** 61s–67s.

WITTENBORN, J.R., FLAHERTY, C.F., HAMILTON, L.W., SCHIFFMAN, H.R. & McGOUGH, W.E. (1976). The effect of minor tranquillizers on psychomotor performance. *Psychopharmacology,* **47,** 281–286.

WITTENBORN, J.R. FLAHERTY, C.F., McGOUGH, W.L.E. & NASH, R.J. (1979). Psychomotor changes during the initial day of benzodiazepine medication. *Br. J. clin. Pharmac.,* 69s–76s.

WOODWORTH, R.S. & SCHLOSBERG, H. (1958). *'Experimental Psychology'.* London: Methuen.

ZIMMERMANN-TANSELLA, C., TANSELLA, M. & LADER, M. (1976). The effects of chlordesmethyldiazepam on behavioural performance and subjective judgement in normal subjects. *J. clin. Pharmac.,* **16,** 481–488.

ZIMMERMANN-TANSELLA, C., TANSELLA, M. & LADER, M. (1978). Psychological performance in patients treated with diazepam. Paper read at *11th CINP Congress,* Vienna (mimeograph).

SLEEP STUDIES IN CLINICAL PHARMACOLOGY

IAN OSWALD

University Department of Psychiatry, Royal Edinburgh Hospital,
Morningside Park, Edinburgh EH10 5HF, Scotland

Introduction

Prescriptions for drugs that alter sleep are, with those for antibiotics, the commonest prescriptions of clinical practice. Some drugs that alter sleep are intended so to do and others, prescribed in the hope of altering mood, will generally alter sleep too, while yet others, prescribed for somatic ailments, may have unsuspected effects on the brain observable during sleep. I shall below take as a primary example the study in man of a drug expected to have hypnotic actions, following studies in animals and preliminary human testing.

There are methods for subjective evaluation and others for objective evaluation. It is the former that are of first interest for clinical practice and, although imprecise where any one individual is concerned, these methods are relatively cheap. In the case of hypnotic drugs, more than any other class of compound, one must take an interest not only in the effects of their administration, but in the effects of their withdrawal, and if one is to conduct relevant studies then one will be influenced by the fact that in clinical practice these drugs will be taken not only as occasional single doses, but often too for consecutive nights during many weeks or even years. During these weeks of intake there will be time for cumulative actions and time for the development of tolerance, with then the certainty of withdrawal effects after the drug ceases.

Subjective evaluation of sleep

A worth-while study must embody the principles of the double-blind trial. The pills containing the active drug or drugs should not only look like the blanks, they should also taste like them. They should preferably be capsules that are properly sealed, made available in individual blister packs for each individual subject, and to cover a period of days. A pharmaceutical company that gives an impression of professionalism in these matters gives confidence to the investigator that they can also be relied upon to have put active and inert pills in those parts of the design that the written schedule says they should have appeared in.

The subjective judgements can be very simple, such as saying that night 2 was or was not better than night 1 and this is perhaps all that can be asked of ill patients in hospital. Most people who take sleeping pills are, however, not in hospital but living active lives, and greater sophistication can be sought by the use of ratings, for example, into five categories, from sleeping 'excellently' to 'very badly', having 'no dreams at all' to dreaming 'very much and vividly', and so on (e.g. Spiegel, 1973). In this case there should be subsequent use of non-parametric statistics for these rankings by each individual.

Visual analogue scales

Visual analogue scales provide another valuable method. In these the patient or volunteer is presented with a line of 100 mm length across a page, one end bearing a statement such as 'Best sleep ever' and the other end a statement such as 'Worst night ever'. The instructions request him to make a mark in the middle of the scale for what he considers to have been for him a normal night and to make his mark some way towards one or other end of the line if he feels the night was a particularly good one or a particularly poor one. He thus creates his own scale and range of values. Like all methods that rely on introspection and the use of abstract concepts for displaying introspection, the method prospers when there is an average or better level of intelligence and education. It is wise to use any potential subjects in a small pilot study before a main study, as there are occasional individuals, albeit intelligent and educated, who will jump from one extreme of the scale to the other in a seemingly insightless manner. Most people, however, find the method simple and acceptable and will fill in these ratings day after day for many months.

In the use of visual analogue scales for research it is helpful to have a top copy of flimsy but opaque paper and a lower card copy that will be marked simultaneously, bearing a feint scale of numbered mm, so that the point of the mark along the scale can easily be read off and then written into a box on the lower copy, for eventual computer handling. If a reasonably large number of subjects is used then the raw data in mm are suitable for later calculations. If only small numbers of persons have been used, then it means that those who make only small excursions from the

52

mid-point contribute less to the eventual scores than those who are more ready to make flamboyant excursions. One approach to overcoming this problem is to determine each individual's standard deviation during one sequence of nights, such as placebo nights, and then to express every single night of the study as a percentage of that standard deviation, and to use these percentages for the eventual analysis. Figure 1 shows an example of a study in which 12 people made ratings each morning of the quality of sleep they had experienced the previous night and did so for six weeks, during which they received placebos each night for the first two weeks, lormetazepam 1 mg nightly for the next three weeks, and placebo again for each night of the final week. Statistical analysis, using Friedman's analysis of variance and the Wilcoxon test showed a significant change in subjective evaluation in the direction of better sleep during the drug period, compared with the baseline, and a significant impairment or rebound of sleep quality, to a degree worse than that of baseline during the withdrawal period (Oswald, Adam, Borrow & Idzikowski, 1979).

As a further illustration of the use of such methods, my colleagues and I recently extended them to one hundred middle-aged volunteers, selected because of their subjectively poor sleep, who each took a capsule at bedtime each night for 32 weeks. In the first 4 weeks the capsules were blanks for all subjects, as they were in the final 4 weeks. In the other 24 weeks, 50 of the subjects received lormetazepam 2 mg, 25 received nitrazepam 5 mg, and 25 received blanks throughout. Subjective sleep quality, assessed by a visual analogue scale, was improved by both drugs throughout the whole of the 24 weeks of administration, with a rebound on withdrawal that, on graphical display, appeared to have a duration of about 3 weeks before it ended.

In order to assess the time taken to fall asleep, the scale shown in Figure 2 was used, being a modified log scale. In the case of lormetazepam there was once again a significant improvement throughout the period of drug intake, and both lormetazepam and nitrazepam were associated with a significant lengthening of sleep latency after withdrawal, again persisting for an

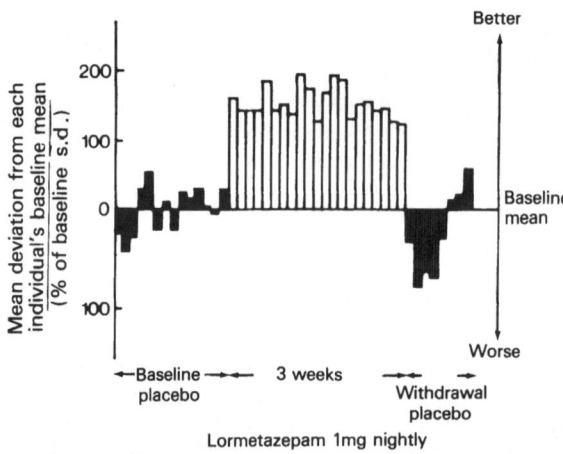

Figure 1 Display of data originally derived from visual analogue scale self-ratings of the quality of sleep by 12 subjects, mean age 53 years. Data are expressed as percentages of the baseline standard deviation (see text). Lormetazepam 1 mg nightly significantly improved the subjective quality of sleep but there was a significant impairment compared with baseline following withdrawal of the drug.

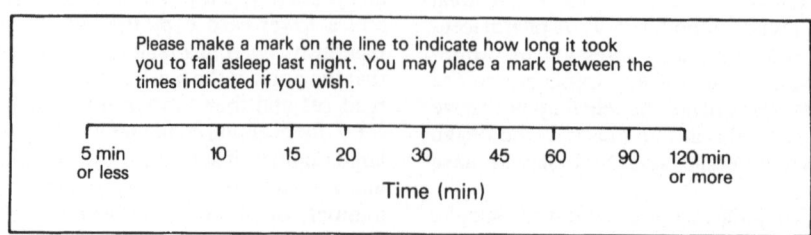

Figure 2 A scale that has proved of practical value for the self-rating of how long it takes to fall asleep.

apparent period of 3 weeks. In handling data such as these, graphical display, by 5-point moving means to smooth the curves was helpful in conveying the outcome. In order to obtain a more precise and economical method of handling the data for statistical comparison it had been decided in advance to compare the first 4 days of the fourth baseline (placebo) week with the first 4 days during the fifth week (lormetazepam, nitrazepam, or continued placebo), the first 4 days of the 28th week (lormetazepam, nitrazepam or continued placebo) and the first 4 days of the 29th week, this last being the first week of withdrawal. The mean of each 4-night period for each individual was found and his or her mean value for the baseline period was subtracted from each of the later mean values. The resultant data, being then normally distributed, were used for analysis of variance and Scheffé tests, to examine the null hypothesis that there would be no difference between behaviour in the case of those receiving placebo throughout and those receiving active drug. Visual analogue scales, used as here, can be confidently recommended as a method, there being many reports in the literature of their successful use (e.g. Zealley & Aitken, 1969; Oswald, Lewis, Dunleavy, Brezinová & Briggs, 1971; Bond & Lader, 1974; Hindmarch, Parrott & Arenillas, 1977).

Other subjective judgements

There are of course, other subjective features of sleep that can be sought. In the above-mentioned study of 100 subjects, Yes/No answers were given to whether they felt they had experienced vivid dreams during each night. Again, at the end of the study, the interviewing physician, who had remained blind to the nature of the pill taken during the weeks 5–28, was asked to make a subjective judgement of whether the subject's sleep would benefit by continuing or not continuing on the same medication. In this particular study these subjective judgements by the observer discriminated significantly in favour of lormetazepam. Discriminations such as these could only be hoped for when a large number of subjects had been used. In the same study the subjects completed a 25-item check list each evening concerning the simple alternative of the absence or the presence of such possible side-effects as lethargy, dizziness, irritability, dry mouth, diarrhoea and so on, all side-effects that might be associated with hypnotics, and there was no increase in the rate of any of these subjective experiences in association with either of the drugs. This conclusion that there was no increase was possible, however, only because of the large number of subjects employed and the fact that a placebo was included in the design for continuous intake throughout the whole period.

Daytime skills and feelings

Apart from seeking subjective estimates of unwanted side-effects of hypnotic drugs, it is important to undertake day-time objective testing of as comprehensive as possible a range of performance skills (Hindmarch, 1980). Many of the published studies in this field are unsatisfactory. Too many have reported on studies involving only about six subjects, often much younger in age than those who usually take hypnotic drugs, often after only a single-dose instead of sustained intake over a week or more, and often with perhaps a dozen or more comparisons being the subject of statistical examination, with one or two of these described as having reached the $P<0.05$ criterion, or all results being reported as negative. In this field, as indeed in all research, it is important first to demonstrate that the instruments of measurement are sensitive. Unless it is shown that tests of the kind used, on the sort of population used, are sensitive to some standard drug, then negative findings carry no weight and sporadic comparisons reaching the $P<0.05$ criterion are difficult to interpret as other than attributable to chance.

Hypnotic drugs make people sleepy, and the Wilkinson vigilance test, originally developed for people who were sleepy owing to brevity of sleep, is one that requires the subject to sustain alertness for at least 30 min and one that I regard as important in the evaluation of hypnotic drugs and their effect on daytime performance. Tasks of this duration have rarely been used in drug studies, though my colleagues and I found the vigilance test to be a task sensitive in discriminating between the intake of flurazepam 30 mg nightly during 3 weeks, compared with placebo or lormetazepam in doses of 2.5 mg or 1 mg nightly. Visual analogue scale ratings each morning of how vigilant or alert the same subjects felt themselves showed that they recognized that during their period of flurazepam intake they were aware of impairment for the first 10 days, but they thought they had returned to normal thereafter. The objective measures, however, showed a greater degree of impairment in the third week on intake of flurazepam than in the first week, confirming the value of concurrent subjective and objective evaluation and that subjective evaluation alone is not to be relied upon (Oswald et al., 1979).

Hypnotic drugs are also anti-anxiety drugs, and drugs that are sold for the treatment of anxiety are drugs that can also be used as hypnotics. It is therefore of value to combine any study that involves the subjective evaluation of hypnotic efficacy with subjective ratings of anxiety, that can be made each evening using visual analogue scales. By this means drugs such as diazepam have been shown to reduce anxiety in anxious patients (Tansella, Tansella &

Lader, 1979). The withdrawal of a modern benzodiazepine, fosazepam, after 3 weeks of nightly intake has been shown to cause significant increase of daytime anxiety above withdrawal levels as a rebound sustained during a three-week period (Allen & Oswald, 1975).

Electrophysiological measures of sleep

The electroencephalogram or EEG is currently the best available indicator of the presence of sleep. As sleep succeeds wakefulness there are progressive changes in the appearance of the EEG and these appearances are divided into stages 1 (drowsiness), 2, 3 and 4 on the basis of their appearance (Rechtschaffen & Kales, 1968). This staging has a validity beyond the EEG technique. Sleep is a state of unresponsiveness and there are diminishing degrees of responsiveness associated with the EEG defined stages, for example, motor responses to auditory signals during sleep (Williams, Morlock & Morlock, 1966), amounts of spontaneous scratching by itchy patients (Savin, Paterson, Adam & Oswald, 1979), whole-body oxygen consumption (Brebbia & Altschuler, 1968) and a variety of other measures, all fall with, and consistently follow, the sequential EEG stages 1, 2, 3 and 4. They rise again, to about the same level as stage 2, during paradoxical sleep, also known as rapid eye movement or REM sleep. The latter is a different state of the organism, characterised by rapid, jerky eye movements, by profound loss of skeletal muscle tone, high cerebral blood flow, penile erections and irregularities of respiration and heart rate. Recordings of eye-movements and muscle tone customarily accompany the EEG recording throughout the night, while measurements of respiration, or spontaneous electrical potentials in the skin (Haider & Oswald, 1971), or other measures may be made according to special interest.

Methods

The use of the EEG is a method suited to the detailed study of small numbers of subjects. It is precise but expensive. The techniques make heavy demands on the energies of the investigators and the co-operation of the subjects. Subjects may have to forgo home comforts, renounce alcohol and come repeatedly at night for months to an expensive, hotel-like laboratory in the study of the effect of a drug on sleep compared with that of a placebo. The patients or volunteers would be expected to attend the laboratory at perhaps 21.30 h, to have the necessary electrodes fixed to the head and to go to bed with lights out for some fixed period of time, perhaps from 22.30 h till 07.00 h. A fixed duration available for sleep is important in order to keep down the variance in a measure like total

sleep duration, one of the important measures to be made. It seems to be the practice in some laboratories to give subjects only 7 h or less in bed, but it will be found that if a longer period is given, more sleep is taken, and it is desirable not to curtail the available duration compared with what would be taken at home merely for the convenience of technicians who may be eager to get away to their families in the mornings. It may be remarked that chronic all-night sleep studies need a high degree of dedication on the part of the research workers and at Edinburgh we rely upon graduate research workers with a direct personal involvement in the successful completion of the project and its eventual publication. Where sleep studies are such that individual subjects attend during many months, it is the special relationship between subject and research workers that sustains the subject's confidence and her willingness to continue, and it is this that makes drop-outs rare.

The eventual all-night recordings, still most reliably made on paper, are again still generally scored by visual inspection. Those unfamiliar with the field often assume that this takes an undue amount of time, but the time involved is small compared with the investment of time in marshalling subjects, being there in the evening and at night with them, and generally shepherding them through a study. It may be that in the coming years the recording of the data on tape and their visual display on a screen may come to have the proven reliability that is necessary in this kind of research, but that time has not yet come. Likewise the data can be analysed by computers more expensive that those housed within the human cranium, but the computer cannot be expected to recognize unusual features that may appear as a result of the action of a drug, such as when the human eye enabled the observation to be made that fenfluramine caused nocturnal bruxism (Lewis, Oswald & Dunleavy, 1971). Monoamine-oxidase inhibitors (Akindele, Evans & Oswald, 1970) and clomipramine (Dunleavy, Brezinová, Oswald, Maclean & Tinker, 1972) are examples of drugs that cause anomalous pictures during sleep, combining some of the appearances of REM sleep with a sustained high level of muscle tone, a combination that would have defeated a naive computer. Nevertheless, there are useful functions for computer analysis that cannot be matched by the unaided human. Thus, Johnson, Hanson & Bickford (1976) used an automatic technique for the measurement of total sleep spindle activity (waves between 12.25 and 15.5 Hz) of amplitude at least 5 μV, and they used an automatic detector for counting K-complexes. They were then able to quantify the large increase in spindle activity and the diminution in the rate of appearance of K-complexes caused by flurazepam. Subsequently Johnson, Seales, Naitoh, Church & Sinclair (1979) used off-line computer analysis to determine the amount and distribution of delta waves (slow waves of between 0.5 and 2 Hz) with a peak-to-trough amplitude of at least 10 μV. They were thereby able to confirm that the slow wave components of sleep are considerably reduced by the intake of flurazepam and not merely redistributed through the night as had been suggested by others. It will be realized that these examples are refinements of sleep scoring only of interest to the research worker, for the clinician will want to know the answers to the simple questions of how a drug affects the duration and brokenness of sleep. There are advanced methods being developed for automatic scoring that cover nearly all the requirements, such as that of Gaillard and Aubert (1975) and there are other computer-assisted techniques primarily for the automatic analysis of brain electrical rhythms after drug intake, (e.g. Saletu, Allen & Itil, 1974) that do not bear a close relation to the more conventional scoring of sleep states. The more a technique analyses data in a form difficult for clinicians to understand, the more it is simply a research tool, and even such standard measurements as the percentage or duration of REM sleep in the night, or the periodicity of the ultradian rhythm (the NREM-REM cycle) during the night, and the effects of drugs on these measures, cannot at the present time be interpreted in terms of immediate clinical relevance. It can be supposed only that sleep having natural characteristics is better than sleep that is in some ways distorted. The clinician would probably recognize the value of the EEG in indicating that a drug he may prescribe for other than its actions on the CNS may yet have an action on the brain, shown, by, for example, reduction of REM sleep (e.g. debrisoquine, Dunleavy, Maclean & Oswald, 1971).

Subjects

The subjects of greatest relevance will be patients, but many of these will already have been receiving CNS-acting drugs and such drugs or their withdrawal will be bound to complicate any possible effects being looked for from a new drug and, because clinical progress cannot be predicted with confidence, it is not usually possible to predict that most patients will be able to change from one drug regime to another or to placebo at fixed times in the future.

If one is testing a sleeping pill then certainly patients who complain of insomnia are ideal, but it has to be remembered that most such complaining patients sleep much longer than they think and take much less time to fall asleep than they believe (Carskadon, Dement, Mitler, Guilleminault, Zarcone & Spiegel, 1978). There is always uncertainty about how reliably such patients will give up any sleeping pills they may have been having in recent times. In the study by Frankel, Coursey, Buchbinder & Snyder (1976) a group of patients with 'primary insomnia' was compared with a group of controls and the authors simply reported that all the insomniacs had 'agreed to discontinue' hypnotic drugs during the 4 weeks preceding the start of the study. Experienced clinicians would expect a high proportion of patients of this kind to be unreliable and likely to go on taking their drugs secretly. They will even do so when they come to the laboratory—a fact that can be betrayed by the increased fast activity at about 20 Hz in the drowsy and REM sleep EEG records, as well as some enhancement of the spindle activity. These disadvantages and uncertainties must be balanced by the thought that volunteers who say they are poor sleepers but do not use drugs will be a less-relevant population. The greatest advantage of volunteers is the flexibility, to change them to placebo or another drug precisely in accord with a planned design.

Owing to the disruption of their lives, volunteers will expect payment, breakfasts when they have attended the laboratory, taxis to and from their homes and conditions of comfort equivalent to those at home. Young men of student age generally sleep so well that it is not easy to disturb their sleep and their sleep is so prolonged and continuous there is little scope for determining whether an hypnotic drug might improve it. The older brain seems more sensitive to drugs, for example nitrazepam (Castleden, George, Marcer & Hallett, 1977) or flurazepam (Greenblatt, Allen & Shader, 1977). Middle-aged and older volunteers have the advantage of greater reliability and regularity in their habits of drinking, times of going to bed, amounts of exercise, and their relative immunity from unpredictable absences on account of transient romantic diversions. At Edinburgh we have found volunteers aged 40–70 years to be much more satisfactory than younger adults. We ask them to sign forms of consent after written and oral explanation of the study to them. We utilize their help with the agreement of their own family doctors and our hospital ethics committee.

Study design and analysis

As Kay, Blackburn, Buckingham & Karacan (1976) in their review of the human pharmacology of sleep emphasized, a great many of the published reports of the action of drugs on sleep have weaknesses in their design, often because of too few subjects, absence of cross-over procedures, absence of dose-response data or invalid statistics. It should not be assumed that this is simply because those who have undertaken the work have lacked competence or awareness of the limitations of their design, but rather because of the great labour and expense of the research.

An initial study will be exploratory and the design simple. Regard will be had to what little may be known about the likely time for absorption of the drug, the likelihood that it may be rapidly eliminated or cumulative in its effects. There may be little data to go on in the case of, for example, newer benzodiazepines that are active in very small dosage of the primary compound, and with no available information about the metabolites owing to the difficulty of measurement. A compromise is necessary between the conflicting desires for simplicity, for dose-response data, and for the desirability of some degree of chronic intake. The traditional approach would involve the use of a Latin square with multiple doses of the drug and placebo as one of the conditions, on single nights of each condition. Such designs were popular in the days before there was recognition of the rebound effects that follow the withdrawal of an hypnotic drug, with the consequence that so-called placebo nights were often really withdrawal nights. There is no perfect answer, but if one wanted to do some preliminary testing in man with a new hypnotic then one might decide on a sample of ten individuals and ask them to attend the sleep laboratory on three nights each on two successive weeks. On the first of each trio of nights they would always get placebo and the night would be treated as an adaptation night, though with all laboratory procedures. On both of the next two nights each subject would receive either active drug or placebo, and in the subsequent week would receive the other treatment, the order being balanced among the ten subjects, perhaps with subjects attending the laboratory in pairs, each member of the pair having the opposing conditions. The all-night recordings would eventually be coded and scored 'blind'. The code would be broken and the data treated by taking the mean of each condition, and a *t*-test then used for statistical comparison. Fewer than ten people would compromise the weight that could be attached to any statistical evaluation. The data could be further analysed by comparing the first and second nights of recording in relation to one another for the drug condition, or again the differences between the drug and placebo condition on the first night could be compared with the differences between the drug and placebo condition on the second night. Such a design would be reasonably likely to give an indication of whether the dosage that had been chosen for this first exploratory trial had some measurable effects and whether they looked about the same on the two nights.

A more ambitious exploratory study would utilize two or more doses, each dose again to be taken on two successive nights and if, for example, three different dose-levels were chosen, again for comparison with placebo, then one would use a 4×4 Latin square, with attendance at the laboratory on three consecutive nights during each of 4 weeks by each volunteer and using sixteen volunteers. The general rule is that if one asks a single, simple question one may get an answer. If one seeks to answer several questions from the one experiment, one may end up with equivocal answers to all the questions and the likelihood of getting definitive answers will depend on the use of an adequate number of subjects. The simple designs just mentioned ignore the potentially confusing effect of a drug that may persist for several days, or persisting withdrawal effects.

It will be noted that one night was allowed in the above design for purposes of adaptation to the laboratory. The first night in the laboratory is accompanied by more broken sleep, less REM sleep and less total sleep. A single night is not strictly sufficient for full adaptation and, of course, after a bad first night the second night would include heavier sleep to make up for the previous night's deficiency. Individuals may be expected to vary among themselves in how rapidly they adapt and anxious patients may be expected to adapt less quickly. The inclusion in the design of at least one adaptation night prior to actual recordings should help to reduce the variance.

Larger-scale designs

A more thorough study will allow more time for adaptation, time for the establishment of what might be considered to be a baseline for an individual, the opportunity for tolerance or cumulative effects to be seen during more or less prolonged intake of the drug, and a period after withdrawal of the active preparation. The withdrawal effects are likely to be detectable for a month whatever the drug, as a consequence of the slow turnover time of brain proteins, but the abruptness and the magnitude of the peak of the rebound will vary according to how slowly the drug is eliminated.

Rebound insomnia after withdrawal of paraldehyde, chloral or barbiturates has long been recognized (Oswald, 1970), and it certainly occurs after benzodiazepine hypnotics such as nitrazepam (Adam, Adamson, Brezinová, Hunter & Oswald, 1976a), though it is hardly a new syndrome as Kales, Scharf & Kales (1978) have lately proposed. The converse of less broken sleep is found after withdrawal of a sleep-disturbing drug (Lewis *et al.*, 1971).

A rapidly-metabolized drug means an almost immediate rebound of high intensity, while slowly-eliminated active compounds, as after phenobarbitone or flurazepam, mean persistence of the effects of drug for days after withdrawal and the slow emergence of a less extreme withdrawal effect, reaching a peak as late as 2 weeks after withdrawal. If only the first few withdrawal nights are studied, a sharp withdrawal effect may be seen after a short half-life hypnotic, whereas the delayed and more gently appearing rebound after flurazepam may not be discerned. Rebound effects appear after overdoses of drugs and if one is interested in the phenomenon, patients who have taken overdoses provide illustrations of the varying durations of time to the peak of the rebound (Haider & Oswald, 1970) and as may be seen in Figure 3, which illustrates the REM sleep rebound after an overdose of flurazepam hydrochloride, the peak of the withdrawal effect being seen as late as 16 days after the single dose.

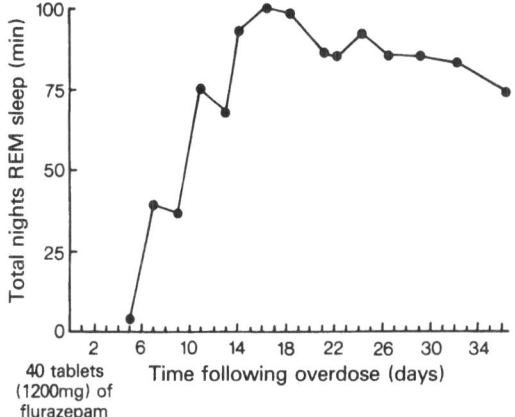

Figure 3 An illustration of the delay to the peak of a rebound where the drug is only slowly eliminated. A woman aged 58 years took an overdose of 1200 mg flurazepam and the peak of the REM sleep rebound is here delayed until 16 days later.

There is no evidence that placebo pills that are believed by the subject to contain an active drug will have any effect on the objective indices of sleep (Adam, Adamson, Brezinová & Oswald, 1976b), though one may suppose that the absence of placebo during a withdrawal period would mean that patients might be afraid of difficulty in getting to sleep and that this itself might keep them from sleeping. Consequently it is customary to use blank or placebo pills in a design that involves adaptation, baseline, active drug and withdrawal. The number of days of drug intake will vary according to the taste and resources of the experimenter. There is no merit in rigidity of design schedules. One may take as an example the following design:

Week 1   Nightly placebos, 2 adaptation nights
Week 2   Nightly placebos, 2 recorded baseline nights
Week 3   Active drug, nights 1 and 3 recorded
Week 4   Active drug, continued at home
Week 5   Adaptation on night 16 of active drug. Nights 19 and 21 of continued active drug recorded
Week 6   Withdrawal. Placebos nights 1, 2, 3, 5 and 7 recorded.

The above may be treated as a basic unit within a larger design so that, for example, in one of our own projects with nine volunteers of mean age 61 years, for each volunteer the drug was at one time flurazepam 30 mg nightly, at another time of year the drug was lormetazepam 1 mg nightly and at another time of year the drug was lormetazepam 2.5 mg. The design was a 3×3 Latin square, repeated three times, so that each volunteer attended the sleep laboratory on a total of 42 nights, each 6 week sequence being separated by a month of non-attendance. Naturally, each volunteer had been free of CNS drugs during the months prior to the study and continued to have no other drugs except those prescribed and no alcohol, except that modest amounts of alcohol were agreed to for the first three weeks of each rest period. It will be seen that each volunteer had to plan his life for 26 weeks and so it is necessary to take account of such times as Christmas, New Year and other holidays in planning.

The withdrawal period

A design such as this is reasonably satisfactory for statistical analysis, but there is no method that is fully informative for the evaluation of the withdrawal period. The course to recovery after withdrawal may involve an initial persistence of the drug and of, for example, continuing increased duration of sleep, then a night about equal to baseline, then several nights of reduced sleep as the full effects of withdrawal appear, and then a gradual return to baseline. If these withdrawal nights are all simply averaged, very little departure from baseline may be found. If nights in only the first week of withdrawal are recorded, then only if the hypnotic is a rapidly eliminated one can early rebound effects be expected to show up on statistical examination, by simply averaging. A graphical display of the data can convey a lot more than statistics, but statistics must be used, so that in the kind of example given above analysis of variance can be used, such as the non-parametric Friedman's analysis of variance and, where appropriate, a Wilcoxon matched pairs signed rank test to examine the difference between, for example, the two baseline nights and the two early drug nights, of any given drug regimen. Likewise there will be comparison of the baseline nights with the two late drug nights, and examination of the difference between the two early drug nights and the two late drug nights, and again the difference between the average of the baseline nights and the average of the withdrawal nights. It is then necessary to examine the data for any differences among the three drugs in their effects upon sleep. One way to do this is to average the two baseline values in each 6-week period of study for each variable and for each subject. For each subject this average may be deemed to equal 100%, and then the values for each night in that 6 week period can be converted to percentages by comparison with the baseline 100% for that variable and for that subject. The mean percentages for each period of the 6 weeks can then be compared among drugs by ranking them 1, 2 or 3 and the Friedman 2-way ANOVA then used to compare drugs, followed by the Wilcoxon test.

Special features of sleep

In evaluating the individual features of sleep it must be borne in mind that the sleep latency, or time taken to fall asleep, is a measure that has a skewed distribution. Parametric tests, though commonly-used, are invalid, but $\log_e$ transformation will give a normal distribution of the data and allow parametric tests (Johns, 1977). The large element of variability among these latencies means that if only a small sample of subjects is used there is little likelihood of getting a significant positive effect, and even less likelihood if the drug is a slowly absorbed one. Bixler *et al.* (1978) reported on temazepam and found no significant effect on sleep latency. This would not justify any conclusion that the drug is without effect on the time taken to fall asleep, it simply reflects the fact that only six subjects were employed.

The criterion of sleep latency that is usually taken is the duration of time from lights-out to the first stage 2 sleep, namely a sleep spindle at about 14Hz, usually most prominent over the front of the head, and of at least half a second in duration. The latency to the first stage 1 sleep is not satisfactory, since stage 1 is less clearly defined and comes and goes. Sometimes authors have used the latency to the beginning of that period of stage 1 that leads into sustained stage 2 sleep. In a recent study we used all three measures independently and failed to find any evidence to support the idea that 1 g of L-tryptophan would shorten sleep latency (Adam & Oswald, 1979).

The amount of accumulated sleep between first falling asleep and the onset of the first REM period of the night, or REM latency, is likewise not a measure that is normally distributed. It is not only skewed, it has a bimodal distribution, and once again parametric tests are not appropriate.

Distribution in the night

It is desirable to look not only at the total amount of any sleep stage in the night, but also at its distribution. It is common in hypnotic drug studies to find no change in the total amount of REM sleep in the night, but if then one one looks carefully it can be seen that REM sleep is suppressed in the early part of the night and enhanced above normal in the later part of the night.

Hour-by-hour cumulative curves offer a useful means of displaying data, as Figure 4 exemplifies. The figure shows the number of minutes of wakefulness and of stage 1 that were present in the course of accumulating a total of 60 min of actual sleep, likewise the number of minutes that intruded in the course of accumulating a total of a further 60 min of sleep for the second hour, and so on.

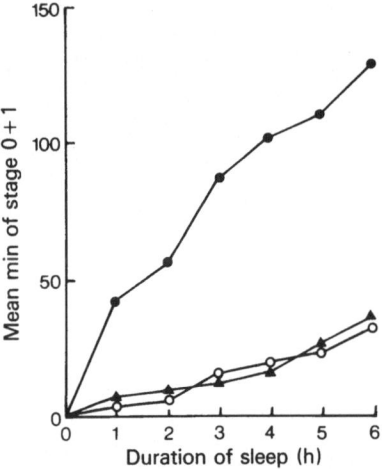

Figure 4 A method for displaying cumulative data, in this case the cumulative amounts of intervening wakefulness plus drowsiness. Figure by courtesy of Dr Vlasta Březinová, and data from Březinová (1974). Caffeine at bedtime makes sleep more broken. ● caffeine 300 mg; ▲ decaffeinated coffee; ○ no drink.

Other measures

The electrophysiological measures outlined above can be conducted concurrently with studies of body motility through the night, so that an hypnotic drug like flurazepam will be found to reduce motility, and to do so not only by night but by day also (Crowley & Hydinger-Macdonald, 1979). A novel approach has recently been adopted by Bonnet & Webb (1979), who deliberately awakened their subject at intervals through the night and measured how long it took to fall asleep again and found that prior flurazepam or pentobarbitone were associated with more rapid return to sleep.

Restorative function and hormones

In the U.S.A. many workers have adopted the term 'sleep efficiency' as an indication of the proportion of time in bed and available for sleep that has actually been spent asleep, but the term raises the further question of the efficacy or restorative function of sleep and whether drugs affect that restorative function (Adam, 1979). So far it has been hormonal indices that have especially been studied, to give some indication of the probable balance between anabolic and degradative processes in association with sleep and wakefulness. The hormone pattern of sleep is generally anabolic, while the hormone pattern of wakefulness favours catabolism. The catabolic corticosteroids are low during the early night and only rise towards the end of sleep, while growth hormone is high in the early part of the night, in association with EEG slow-wave sleep. In contrast, during wakefulness growth hormone is low, but the catecholamines and corticosteroids are relatively high.

A catheter can be inserted in a forearm vein at bedtime and an extension led out through a hole in the bedroom wall, so enabling blood to be sucked at intervals through the night without seriously disturbing sleep. The system can be kept filled with heparinized saline during the intervals between bloodsucking. It is advisable to sample every twenty minutes or so, spinning down samples of blood and putting the plasma as quickly as possible into a deep freeze. It is taxing work and it requires at least the nearby presence of medical personnel. Spasm in the vein is an occasional problem and sometimes the nights have to be repeated. Consequently, this kind of research is expensive and has not often been undertaken using substantial numbers of subjects. However, it has been shown that a modern minor tranquil-

lizer, benzoctamine, will bring about a significant fall in the concentration of corticosteriods in the plasma during sleep, with a rebound above normal following withdrawal (Ogunremi, Adamson, Brezinová, Hunter, Maclean, Oswald & Percy-Robb, 1973). Although the benzodiazepines in chronic use greatly reduce the proportion of slow-wave sleep, the secretion of growth hormone does not appear to be affected by nitrazepam (Adam et al., 1976a) or by benzoctamine or barbiturates (Ogunremi et al., 1973).

A less onerous avenue to knowledge of the hormone pattern during sleep and its modification, if any, by drugs, is possible with newer techniques for the measurement of urinary adrenaline and cortisol, but these will give only the catabolic side of the picture and research into the effects of drugs on the anabolic hormones will continue to require all-night blood sampling.

Conclusions

Studies of the effects of drugs on sleep are very much dictated in their design by matters of cost, for they require a lot of organization and dedication over long periods of time, both by subjects and staff. It is thus axiomatic that studies should be well-designed from the start and analysed using appropriate statistics. The exceptionally heavy use of hypnotic drugs throughout the world justifies a full assessment of a new hypnotic drug before it is introduced to general consumption.

References

ADAM, K. (1979). Do drugs alter the restorative value of sleep? In *Pharmacology of the States of Alertness*, ed. Passouant, P. & Oswald, I., pp. 105–111. Oxford: Pergamon Press.

ADAM, K., ADAMSON, L., BREZINOVÁ, V., HUNTER, W.M. & OSWALD, I. (1976a). Nitrazepam: lastingly effective but trouble on withdrawal. *Br. med. J.*, 1, 1558–1560.

ADAM, K., ADAMSON, L., BREZINOVÁ, V. & OSWALD, I. (1976b). Do placebos alter sleep? *Br. med. J.*, 1, 195–196.

ADAM, K. & OSWALD, I. (1979). One gram of L-tryptophan fails to alter the time taken to fall asleep. *Neuropharmac.*, 18, 1025–1027.

AKINDELE, M.O., EVANS, J.I. & OSWALD, I. (1970). Monoamine oxidase inhibitors, sleep and mood. *Electroenceph. clin. Neurophysiol.*, 29, 47–56.

ALLEN, S. & OSWALD, I. (1976). Anxiety and sleep after fosazepam. *Br. J. clin. Pharmac.*, 3, 165–168.

BIXLER, E.O., KALES, A., SOLDATOS, C.R., SCHARF, M.B. & KALES, J.D. (1978). Effectiveness of temazepam with short-, intermediate-, and long-term use: sleep laboratory evaluation. *J. clin. Pharmac.*, 18, 110–118.

BOND, A. & LADER, M. (1974). The use of analogue scales in rating subjective feelings. *Br. J. med. Psychol.*, 47, 211–218.

BONNET, M.H. & WEBB, W.B. (1979). The return to sleep. *Biol. Psychol.*, 8, 225–233.

BREBBIA, D.R. & ALTSHULER, K.Z. (1968). Stage related patterns and nightly trends of energy exchange during sleep. In *Computers and Electronic Devices in Psychiatry*, ed. Kline, N.S. & Laska, E., pp. 319–335. New York: Grune & Stratton.

BREZINOVÁ, V. (1974). Effect of caffeine on sleep: EEG study in late middle aged people. *Br. J. clin. Pharmac.*, 1, 203–208.

CARSKADON, M.A., DEMENT, W.C., MITLER, M.M., GUILLEMINAULT, C., ZARCONE, V.P. & SPIEGEL, R. (1976). Self-reports versus sleep laboratory findings in 122 drug-free subjects with complaints of chronic insomnia. *Am. J. Psychiat.*, 133, 1382–1388.

CASTLEDEN, C.M., GEORGE, C.F., MARCER, D. & HALLETT, C. (1977). Increased sensitivity to nitrazepam in old age. *Br. med. J.*, 1, 10–12.

CROWLEY, T.J. & HYDINGER-MACDONALD, M. (1979). Bedtime flurazepam and the human circadian rhythm of spontaneous motility. *Psychopharmacology*, **62**, 157–161.

DUNLEAVY, D.L.F., BREZINOVÁ, V., OSWALD, I., MACLEAN, A.W. & TINKER, M. (1972). Changes during weeks in effects of tricyclic drugs on the human sleeping brain. *Br. J. Psychiat.*, **120**, 663–672.

DUNLEAVY, D.L.F., MACLEAN, A.W. & OSWALD, I. (1971). Debrisoquine, guanethidine, propranolol and human sleep. *Psychopharmacologia (Berl.)* **21**, 101–110.

FRANKEL, B.L., COURSEY, R.D., BUCHBINDER, R. & SNYDER, F. (1976). Recorded and reported sleep in chronic primary insomnia. *Arch. gen. Psychiat.*, **33**, 615–623.

GAILLARD, J.M. & AUBERT, C. (1975). Specificity of benzodiazepines action on human sleep confirmed. Another contribution of automtic analysis of polygraphic recordings. *Biol. Psychiat.*, **10**, 185–197.

GREENBLATT, D.J., ALLEN, M.D. & SHADER, R.I. (1977). Toxicity of high-dose flurazepam in the elderly. *Clin. Pharmac. Ther.*, **21**, 355–361.

HAIDER, I. & OSWALD, I. (1970). Late brain recovery processes after drug overdose. *Br. med. J.*, **2**, 318–322.

HAIDER, I. & OSWALD, I. (1971). Effects of amylobarbitone and nitrazepam on the electrodermogram and other features of sleep. *Br. J. Psychiat.*, **118**, 519–522.

HINDMARCH, I. (1980). Psychomotor function and psychoactive drugs. *Br. J. clin. Pharmac.*, **10**, 189–210.

HINDMARCH, I., PARROTT, A.C. & ARENILLAS, L. (1977). A repeated dose comparison of dichloralphenazone, flunitrazepam and amylobarbitone sodium on some aspects of sleep and early morning behaviour in normal subjects. *Br. J. clin. Pharmac.*, **4**, 229–233.

JOHNS, M.W. (1977). Validity of subjective reports of sleep latency in normal subjects. *Ergonomics*, **20**, 683–690.

JOHNSON, L.C., HANSON, K. & BICKFORD, R.G. (1976). Effect of flurazepam on sleep spindles and K-complexes. *Electroenceph. clin. Neurophysiol.*, **40**, 67–77.

JOHNSON, L.C., SEALES, D.M., NAITOH, P., CHURCH, M.W. & SINCLAIR, M. (1979). The effects of flurazepam hydrochloride on brain electrical activity during sleep. *Electroenceph. clin. Neurophysiol.*, **47**, 309–321.

KALES, A., SCHARF, M.B. & KALES, J.D. (1978). Rebound insomnia: a new clinical syndrome. *Science*, **201**, 1039–1041.

KAY, D.C., BLACKBURN, A.B., BUCKINGHAM, J.A. & KARACAN, I. (1976). Human pharmacology of sleep. In *Pharmacology of Sleep*, ed. Williams, R.L. & Karacan, I., pp. 83–210. New York: John Wiley.

LEWIS, S.A., OSWALD, I. & DUNLEAVY, D.L.F. (1971). Chronic fenfluramine administration: some cerebral effects. *Br. med. J.*, **3**, 67–70.

OGUNREMI, O.O., ADAMSON, L., BREZINOVÁ, V., HUNTER, W.M., MACLEAN, A.W., OSWALD, I. & PERCY-ROBB, I.W. (1973). Two anti-anxiety drugs: a psychoneuroendocrine study. *Br. med. J.*, **2**, 202–205.

OSWALD, I. (1970). Dependence upon hypnotic and sedative drugs. *Br. J. hosp. Med.*, **4**, 168–172.

OSWALD, I., ADAM, K., BORROW, S. & IDZIKOWSKI, C. (1979). The effects of two hypnotics on sleep, subjective feelings and skilled performance. In *Pharmacology of the States of Alertness*, ed. Passouant, P. & Oswald, I., pp. 51–63. Oxford, Pergamon Press.

OSWALD, I., LEWIS, S.A., DUNLEAVY, D.L.F., BREZINOVÁ, V. & BRIGGS, M. (1971). Drugs of dependence though not of abuse: fenfluramine and imipramine. *Br. med. J.*, **3**, 70–73.

RECHTSCHAFFEN, A. & KALES, A. (1968). *A Manual of Standardized Terminology, Techniques and Scoring System for Sleep Stages of Human Subjects*. Washington, D.C.: U.S. Government Printing Office, NIH Publication, No. 204.

SALETU, B., ALLEN, M. & ITIL, T.M. (1974). The effect of coca-cola, caffeine, antidepressants, and chlorpromazine on objective and subjective sleep parameters. *Pharmakopsychiat.*, **254**, 307–321.

SAVIN, J.A., PATERSON, W.D., ADAM, K. & OSWALD, I. (1979). Effects of trimeprazine and trimipramine on noctural scratching in patients with atopic eczema. *Arch. Dermatol.*, **115**, 313–315.

SPIEGEL, R. (1973). Controlled clinical investigations with a phenothiazine derivative used as sleep-inducer in nonpsychotic insomniacs. In *Sleep: Physiology, Biochemistry, Psychology, Pharmacology, Clinical Implications*, ed. Koella, W.P. & Levin, P., pp. 91–101. Basel: Karger.

TANSELLA, C.Z., TANSELLA, M. & LADER, M. (1979). A comparison of the clinical and psychological effects of diazepam and amylobarbitone in anxious patients. *Br. J. clin. Pharmac.*, **7**, 605–611.

WILLIAMS, H.L., MORLOCK, H.C., & MORLOCK, J.V. (1966). Discriminative responses to auditory signals during sleep. *Psychophysiol.*, **2**, 208–215.

ZEALLEY, A.K. & AITKEN, R.C.B. (1969). Measurement of mood. *Proc. roy. Soc. Med.*, **62**, 993–996.

MEASUREMENT OF SERUM DRUG LEVELS IN THE ASSESSMENT OF ANTIDEPRESSANTS

STUART A. MONTGOMERY

Academic Department of Psychiatry,
St Mary's Hospital,
Harrow Road,
London W9 3RL

In the absence of a simple adequate or even promising biochemical or physiological marker for the presence of depressive illness it is necessary for researchers in this field to keep close to validated clinical criteria. Depression is a term which unfortunately means different things to different people and even has a different meaning to different researchers. It may indicate anything from some minor transient irritability or the lowering of spirits in the face of understandable setbacks to a profound and persistent melancholia preoccupied with delusions of guilt, ruin and utter despair.

In the presence of such a heterogenous variety of states described by the same term depression, it would be wiser to place less reliance on any research where an adequate description of the definition of depression is not given.

Early attempts to define depression more closely were based entirely on presenting psychopathological features and took no account of the history or other conditions. The Medical Research Council (1965) criterion requiring a persistent alteration of mood and only one other psychopathological feature is altogether too thin and unreliable. The Present State Examination (PSE) (Wing, Cooper & Sartorius, 1974), although based on a standardised interview to assess the signs and symptoms present, fails to distinguish between primary depression and depression secondary to alcohol, drugs etc.

The research criteria of Feighner, Robins, Guze, Woodruff, Winokur & Munoz (1972) of the St Louis group for primary affective disorder have been widely adopted. The Research Diagnostic Criteria of Spitzer, Endicott & Robins (1977) develop these somewhat but for their major definite depressive disorder they use a definition which leans very heavily on endogenous depression which is better defined and validated by the Newcastle scales (Carney, Roth & Garside, 1965; Gurney, Roth, Garside, Kerr & Schapira 1972).

The American Psychiatric Association developed this work in a series of cumbersome committees to produce the DSM III (1979) which appears to be an advance in schizophrenia and personality disorders but less so in depressive illness.

Angst (1980) compared the psychiatrist's diagnosis in his clinic with the diagnosis made using research criteria and reported good reliability with the criteria of Feighner et al. (1972) but not with the DSM III (1979). This same failure by committee is noticeable in the WHO 9th International Classification of Diseases (1978) where 20 different categories of depression are listed with considerable overlap and consequent confusion.

In a series of elegant studies Sir Martin Roth and the Newcastle group created weighted diagnostic scales to differentiate endogenous depression from reactive depression (Carney et al., 1965) and depression from the anxiety states (Gurney et al., 1972). These diagnostic scales, used in conjunction with a set of criteria e.g. Feighner et al. (1972) which separate primary from secondary depression, provide a sufficiently thorough categorisation of the depressed group studied to allow comparisons with other populations as well defined.

Table 1 Research criteria for studies in depression

Adequate	Feighner et al. (1972)
	Spitzer et al. (1977)
	Carney et al. (1965)
	Gurney et al. (1972)
Less than adequate	DSM III (1979)
Better than nothing	PSE
	WHO 9th Classification (1978)
	MRC (1965)

Failure to use careful diagnostic criteria may have the effect of increasing variance which may obscure interesting findings. In clinical psychopharmacological research where critical small differences may be the only indication of an interesting relationship the lack of careful methodology may obscure all but the most obvious result.

Varying levels of carefulness of clinical methodology probably account for some of the conflicting results which have been reported in the investigations into the relationship of antidepressant plasma concentrations and clinical response. To help understand some of these apparently conflicting results it may be helpful to review the plasma level antidepressant literature in relation to the clinical methodology involved.

A review of the plasma level antidepressant response literature provides an excellent example of the importance of the obvious influence that good or bad clinical methodology has on the results. For example in the studies on nortriptyline that failed to demonstrate a plasma concentration response relationship, Lyle, Brooks, Early, Leggett, Silverman, Braithwaite, Cuthill, Goulding, Pearson, Smith & Strang (1974) gave no definition of depression and reported no diagnostic criteria, Burrows, Davies & Scoggins (1972) and Burrows, Scoggins, Turecek & Davies (1974) specifically excluded severe depression and did not give diagnostic criteria. In the studies that demonstrated a relationship, Kragh-Sorensen, Asberg & Eggert-Hansen (1973) and Kragh-Sorensen, Eggert-Hansen, Baastrup & Hvidberg (1976) and Montgomery, Braithwaite, Dawling & McAuley (1978) used the Newcastle Scale (Gurney et al., 1972) to define endogenous depression. Indeed with mianserin Montgomery, Montgomery, McAuley & Rani (1978) reported that a plasma level response relationship could only be detected in endogenous depression defined in their study by the Newcastle Scale and not in the reactive depression group.

Nortriptyline which is the most easily measured tricyclic has been the subject of a number of plasma concentration response studies. Asberg, Cronholm, Sjoqvist & Tuck (1971); Kragh-Sorensen et al. (1973, 1976); Ziegler, Clayton, Taylor, Co & Biggs (1976); Ziegler, Clayton (1977); Montgomery, Braithwaite & Crammer (1977) and Montgomery, Braithwaite et al. (1978) have all reported a significant relationship between plasma nortriptyline concentrations and clinical response. Studies by Lyle et al. (1974); Burrows et al. (1972, 1974) and Fensbo (1976) did not demonstrate a significant relationship. There appears to be a concensus that in treating endogenous depression with nortriptyline the best clinical response is associated with steady state plasma concentrations approximately between 50–175 or 200 μg/l and that a poorer response is seen in patients with concentrations outside this range. In a double-blind study Kragh-Sorensen et al. (1976) demonstrated the significant clinical advantage of adjusting the dosage of patients to bring their plasma nortriptyline concentrations from above to within the optimum range between the fourth and sixth week of treatment.

Amitriptyline the most widely used antidepressant has also been the subject of many plasma response studies. A relationship has been reported by Braithwaite, Goulding, Theano, Bailey & Coppen (1972); Montgomery & Braithwaite (1975), Ziegler et al. (1977); Kupfer, Hanin, Spiker, Grau & Coble (1977); Vandel, Vandel, Sandoz, Allers, Bechtel & Volmat (1978); Montgomery, McAuley, Montgomery, Braithwaite & Dawling (1979 a,b); Moyes, Ray & Moyes (1980) and Corona, Fenoglio, Pinelli & Zerbi (1977). All of these with the exception of Kupfer et al. (1977) either reported a curvilinear relationship (Montgomery & Braithwaite, 1975; Vandel et al., 1978; Montgomery et al., 1979 a,b; Moyes et al., 1980) or had findings which were consistent with the curvilinear hypothesis that optimum antidepressant effect is associated with intermediate plasma concentrations of amitriptyline plus its active metabolite nortriptyline of between approximately 80–200 μg/l. Coppen, Ghose, Montgomery, Ramo Rao, Bailey, Christiansen, Mikklesen, van Praag, van de Poel, Minsker, Kozulja, Matussek, Kungkunz & Jorgensen (1978); Liisberg, Mose, Amdisen, Jorgensen & Hopfner-Petersen (1978) and Robinson, Cooper, Ravaris, Ives, Nies, Bartlett & Lamborn (1979) did not report the existence of a plasma level response relationship. In the study of Liisberg et al. (1978) two of the three patients with high levels were non-responders which is consistent with the curvilinear hypothesis. In the same way the study by Coppen et al. (1978) reported that high concentrations of amitriptyline were associated with a significantly poorer response measured as percentage change of Hamilton Rating Scale (HRS) (Hamilton, 1967). This observation that it is the high levels of the metabolite nortriptyline that are associated with the poorer response is seen also in other studies (Vandel et al., 1978; Montgomery et al., 1979 a,b: Moyes & Moyes, 1980) and suggests at least for endogenous depression that they should be avoided.

A curvilinear relationship has been demonstrated for mianserin by Montgomery, McAuley & Montgomery (1978) and a linear relationship consistent with this by Russell, Niaz, Wakeling & Slade (1978) and Perry, Fitzsimmons, Shapiro & Irwin (1978), but not by Coppen, Gupta, Montgomery, Ghose, Bailey, Burns & de Ridder (1976).

Likewise high levels of norzimelidine, the active metabolite of zimelidine, have been reported associated with a poor response by Montgomery, McAuley, Rani, Roy & Montgomery (1980); Coppen et al., (1979) in their study of zimelidine did not report a relationship.

From the results of Glassman, Kantor & Shostak (1975), Glassman, Perel, Shostak, Kantor & Fleiss (1977) and Gram (1977) who reported that best response was associated with higher plasma levels of imipramine it appears that an upper limit for best response with imipramine either does not exist or has not been determined. However the exclusion of psychotic depressives (Glassman et al., 1975) would have the effect of biassing the sample in the same way that it did for Burrows et al. (1972, 1974). In our sample of 30 patients we can detect no relationship between plasma levels and clinical response, (unpublished observations). Relationships have not been reported in small studies on maprotiline (Angst & Rothweiler, 1974; Mathur, Jones & Luscombe 1976;

Fensbo, 1976; Montgomery, McAuley, Montgomery, Dawling & Braithwaite, 1980a) or nomifensine (Montgomery, Roy, Rani, McAuley & Montgomery, 1980).

In our study of endogenous depression treated with clomipramine we found no relationship between plasma levels and response but there was a trend for patients with high levels of desmethylclomipramine (DMCL) to have a poorer response (Montgomery et al., 1980a). Steady state levels of DMCL were not observed in our study, they continued to rise throughout the six week period. Stern, Marks, Wright & Luscombe (1980) reported a curvilinear relationship between level and response in patients with obsessional neurosis treated with clomipramine. Half the patients in the study had secondary depression which complicates the analysis.

Most investigators now concur that there is a relationship between plasma concentration of nortriptyline and response. For amitriptyline there is now very strong evidence for a relationship but for the other antidepressants it remains a research interest.

It is useful therefore to comment on methodology used in these studies. Criticism must be levelled at those studies (Kupfer et al., 1977; Corona et al., 1977) which permitted alterations in the dosage of the drug during an investigation of 'steady state' concentrations and response. Response to antidepressants may take 4 weeks or longer in responders and alterations in dosage and steady state plasma concentrations during that time introduce a number of extra imponderable sources of variance which seriously interfere with analysis and interpretation.

A further serious criticism is of any investigation which is too short and forces a premature judgement of response. Any investigation which lasts less than 4 weeks should be viewed with caution. The first plasma concentration response study on nortriptyline (Asberg et al., 1971) lasted only 2 weeks and reported a curvilinear relationship. This finding at 2 weeks has not been confirmed in any other study and must be regarded as intriguing. The investigation was complicated by the concomitant use of barbiturates in some patients which have since been shown to induce microsomal enzymes and lower tricyclic plasma levels. It is for this reason that subsequent investigations have attempted to exclude patients known to have received or are receiving microsomal inducing or inhibiting drugs.

The longer trial period of up to 6 weeks allows the advantage or possible disadvantage of particular plasma concentrations to become apparent. For example in the studies of Montgomery et al (1979a) and Montgomery, McAuley, Montgomery, Dawling & Braithwaite (1980b) on amitriptyline a worsening of depression was observed in patients developing drug concentrations above the recommended range between 4 and 6 weeks.

A criticism of many investigations is that insufficient numbers of patients were studied. There are large inter-dividual differences in the drug clearance and therefore the steady state plasma concentrations achieved. In any group studied there may by chance be insufficient numbers of patients developing a particular range of drug concentrations to adequately test a particular plasma concentration response hypothesis. Large numbers of patients are needed to overcome this problem. It is of course possible that a comparatively small study may by chance have sufficient patients above and below a critical level to produce a significant result. It is also obviously true that to test for the presence of a more complex non-linear relationship even larger numbers of patients are required and a report that no relationship is seen in a relatively small study may simply mean that insufficient numbers of patients were studied to test the hypothesis. This would be a classical Type 2 error. It is for this reason that most weight is given to a well conducted study with a significant finding.

Since relationships between plasma concentration and response are sometimes complex and difficult to detect, patients should be selected who are thought likely to respond to the pharmacological actions of the drug. The inclusion of non-responders should be avoided as far as possible. Two recent large studies (Coppen et al., 1978; Robinson et al., 1979) on amitriptyline which reported no relationship are open to criticism because of the very low overall response rate achieved. Potter & Goodwin (1978) criticised the study by the WHO group (Coppen et al., 1978) which reported a response rate of 35% as being rather inept in the selection of patients thought likely to respond. When the same criterion of response in the WHO study (a final HRS of 6 or less) is applied to the study of Robinson et al. (1979) a response rate of only 16% is apparent.

Both studies are open to other criticisms. The multicentre WHO study did not report any inter-centre rater reliabilities. Since the centres were in different parts of Europe some differences in presenting psychopathology and rating attitudes would be expected (Montgomery, Asberg, Traskman & Montgomery, 1978) and these would increase variance. The study by Robinson et al. (1979) was conducted on out-patients who included as far as one can tell a relatively difficult group of patients with reactive depression who were not as likely to respond to pharmacotherapy.

The inclusion of out-patients who are known to have a poorer compliance with treatment introduces another source of variance. Ideally there should be adequate checks on compliance. In the study of Montgomery, Braithwaite, et al. (1978a) on nortriptyline all the patients had a single oral dose kinetic test which calculated half-life and clearance and from which steady-state plasma concentrations could be predicted. In the study on amitriptyline half the patients had a single oral dose kinetic dose. This enabled us to be relatively sure that the inter-individual differences in plasma concentrations reported were the product of differences in metabolism in patients and not due to failure to take the tablets. A less direct method of checking on compliance was used by Kragh-Sorensen and his colleagues (1973, 1976) in their study on nortriptyline. This involves the exclusion of patients with excess variance in steady state plasma concentrations achieved. Because of increased variance from these sources out-patient studies or those studies which do not check on compliance would be expected to produce rather less reliable data.

A few studies have reported inter-laboratory reliability of the measurement of the drug concentrations (Montgomery *et al.* 1978; Coppen *et al.*, 1978; Jones & Turner, 1980). Differences in measurements between laboratories have previously been advanced as a possible reason why the results of the Australian group were not in accord with the European groups. Our group and the Australian group have both now reported international reliability studies. In our view if the measurements are undertaken by good laboratories who participate in reliability studies this is unlikely to be the source of conflicting results.

If the improvement in the depression is to be attributed to particular drug plasma concentrations it is necessary to use the most sensitive and valid measures of the severity of depression. In the study by Montgomery, McAuley *et al* (1978b) (Figure 1) the relationship between mianserin plasma concentration and response was demonstrated on the Montgomery and Asberg Depression Rating Scale (MADRS) (Montgomery & Asberg, 1978) and the HRS (Hamilton, 1967) which are regarded as more sensitive than the Beck Self Rating Inventory (BSRI) (Beck, Ward, Mendelson, Mock & Erbaugh 1961) which does not show the relationship. Likewise in the study on amitriptyline (Montgomery *et al.*, 1980b) a significant difference in response above and below 200 μg/l was detected on the HRS but not on the BSRI. In the studies on nortriptyline which did not demonstrate a plasma level response relationship, Lyle *et al.* (1974) and Fensbo (1976) used global judgements which have been shown to be less sensitive to treatment change than either the HRS or MADRS (Montgomery & Asberg, 1979).

The difference in clinical methodology which we have reviewed in the plasma level studies in this paper

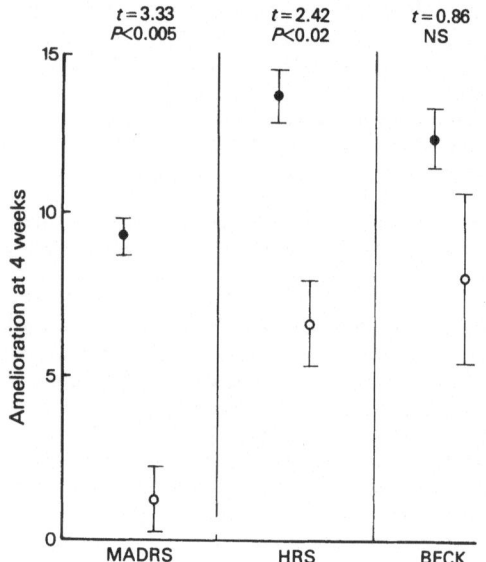

Figure 1 Relationship between plasma mianserin level and antidepressant response measured on the Montgomery & Asberg (1979) depression rating scale (MADRS), the Hamilton (1967) rating scale (HRS) and the Beck *et al.* (1961) self-rating inventory (BECK). Forty-seven patients were treated with mianserin 60 mg daily. The results are expressed as mean ± s.e. mean. ○ plasmal levels > 70 μg/l, ● plasma levels < 70 μg/l.

are likely to be a source of conflicting results.

In the assessment of the efficacy of antidepressants most weight must be attached to the results from those studies which have used a stringent clinical methodology. When combined with drug plasma levels these investigations may achieve an added sensitivity capable of demonstrating differing antidepressants effects at different drug plasma concentrations, of detecting the presence of possible plasma level related drug toxicity, and of assessing patient compliance by detecting the presence or absence of the drug in the plasma or by registering variations in steady state plasma levels achieved.

In studies which show no difference between a compound and a reference antidepressant the absence of plasma level determinations is a serious methodological flaw which detracts from the results. For the reasons outlined drug plasma levels should be measured in all comparative studies where an antidepressant effect may be attributed to a new compound.

References

ANGST, J. (1980). New perspectives in depressive illness. *Acta Psychiat. Scand.* (In press).

ANGST, J. & ROTHWEILER, R. (1974). Blood levels and clinical effects of maprotiline (Ludiomil). A preliminary study. Classification and prediction of outcome of depression. *Symposium Medicum Hoechst*, **8**, 237–244.

ASBERG, M., CRONHOLM, B., SJOQVIST, F. & TUCK, D. (1971). Relationship between plasma level and therapeutic effect of nortriptyline. *Br. med. J.*, **3**, 331–334.

BECK, A.T., WARD, C.H., MENDELSON, M., MOCK, J. & ERBAUGH, I. (1961). An inventory for measuring depression. *Arch. gen. Psychiat.* **4**, 561–571.

BRAITHWAITE, R.A., GOULDING, R., THEANO, G., BAILEY, J. & COPPEN, A. (1972). Plasma concentration of amitriptyline and clinical response. *Lancet*, **i**, 1297–1300.

BURROWS, G.D., DAVIES, B. & SCOGGINS, B.A. (1972). Plasma concentrations of nortriptyline and clinical response in depressive illness. *Lancet*, **ii**, 619–623.

BURROWS, G.D., SCOGGINS, B.A., TURECEK, L.T. & DAVIES, B. (1974). Plasma nortriptyline and clinical response. *Clin. Pharmac. Ther.* **16**, 639–644.

CARNEY, M.W.P., ROTH, M. & GARSIDE, R.F. (1965). The diagnosis of depressive syndromes and the prediction of ECT response. *Br. J. Psychiat.*, **111**, 659–674.

COPPEN, A., GUPTA, R., MONTGOMERY, S., GHOSE, K., BAILEY, J., BURNS, B. & DE RIDDER, J.J. (1976). Mianserin hydrochloride: a novel antidepressant. *Br. J. Psychiat.*, **129**, 342–345.

COPPEN, A., GHOSE, K., MONTGOMERY, S., RAMO RAO, V.A., BAILEY, J., CHRISTIANSEN, J., MIKKLESON, P.L., VAN PRAAG, H.M., VAN DE POEL, F., MINSKER, E.J., KOZULJA, V.G., MATUSSEK, N. KUNGKUNZ, G. & JORGENSEN, A. (1978). Amitriptyline plasma concentration and clinical effect. *Lancet*, **i**, 63–66.

COPPEN, A., RAMA RAO, V.A., SWADE, C. & WOOD, K. (1979). Zimelidine: A therapeutic and pharmacokinetic study in depression. *Psychopharmacology*, **63**, 199–202.

CORONA, G., FENOGLIO, L., PINELLI, P. & ZERBI, F. (1977). Amitriptyline, nortriptyline plasma levels and therapeutic response in depressed women. *Pharmakopsychiatrie*, **10**, 299–308.

DSM III (1979). *Diagnostic criteria*. American Psychiatric Association.

FEIGHNER, J.P., ROBINS, E., GUZE, S.B., WOODRUFF, R.A., WINOKUR, G. & MUNOZ, R. (1972). Diagnostic criteria for use in psychiatric research. *Arch. gen. Psychiat.*, **26**, 57.

FENSBO, C. (1976). A clinical trial of nortriptyline and maprotiline with cardiovascular monitoring and serum level estimates, Ludiomil Symposium. Horsham: Ciba.

GLASSMAN, A.H., KANTOR, S.J. & SHOSTAK, M. (1975). Depression delusions and drug response. *Am. J. Psychiat.*, **132**, 716–719.

GLASSMAN, S.H., PEREL, J.M. SHOSTAK, M., KANTOR, S.J. & FLEISS, J.L. (1977). Clinical implication of imipramine plasma levels for depressive illness. *Arch. gen. Psychiat.*, **34**, 197–204.

GRAM, L.F. (1977). Plasma level monitoring of tricyclic antidepressant therapy. *Clin. Pharmacokin.*, **2**, 237–251.

GURNEY, C., ROTH, M., GARSIDE, R.F., KERR, T.A. & SCHAPIRA, K. (1972). Studies in the classification of affective disorders. *Br. J. Psychiat.*, **121**, 162–166.

HAMILTON, M., (1967). Development of a rating scale for primary depressive illness. *Br. J. social clin. Psychol.* **6**, 278–296.

JONES, S. & TURNER, P. (1980). Interlaboratory variability in determination of serum antidepressant drug concentrations—results of a quality control programme. *Br. J. clin. Pharmac.*, **9**, 311P.

KRAGH-SORENSEN, P., ASBERG, M. & EGGERT-HANSEN, C. (1973). Plasma nortriptyline levels in endogenous depression. *Lancet*, **i**, 113–115.

KRAGH-SORENSEN, P., EGGER-HANSEN, C., BAASTRUP, P.C. & HVIDBERG, E.F. (1976). Self inhibiting action of nortriptyline's antidepressant effect at high plasma levels. *Psychopharmacologia*, **45**, 305–316.

KUPFER, D.J., HANIN, I., SPIKER, D.G., GRAU, T. & COBLE, P. (1977). Amitriptyline plasma levels and clinical response in primary depression. *Clin. Pharmac. Ther.*, **22**, 904–911.

LIISBERG, P., MOSE, H., AMDISEN, A., JORGENSEN, A. & HOPFNER-PETERSEN, H.E. (1978). A clinical trial comparing sustained release amitriptyline (Saroten Retard) and conventional amitriptyline tablets (Saroten) in endogenously depressed patients with simultaneous determination of serum levels of amitriptyline and nortriptyline. *Acta Psychiat. Scand.*, **57**, 426–435.

LYLE, W.H., BROOKS, P.W., EARLY, D.F., LEGGETT, W.P., SILVERMAN, G., BRAITHWAITE, R.A., CUTHILL, J.M., GOULDING, R., PEARSON, I.B., SMITH, R.P. & STRANG, G.E. (1974). Plasma concentration of nortriptyline as a guide to therapy. *Postgrad. med. J.*, **50**, 282–287.

MATHUR, N., JONES, R.B. & LUSCOMBE, D.K. (1976). Plasma maprotiline concentrations in depressive patients following an incremental dosage regime. Ludiomil Symposium. Horsham: Ciba.

MEDICAL RESEARCH CRITERIA. (1965). Clinical trial of the treatment of depressive illness. *Br. med. J.*, **1**, 881–886.

MONTGOMERY, S.A. (1978). *Measures of depression*. MD Thesis, Karolinska Institute, Stockholm.

MONTGOMERY, S.A. & ASBERG, M. (1979). A new depression scale designed to be sensitive to change. *Br. J. Psychiat.*, **134**, 382–389.

MONTGOMERY, S., ASBERG, M., TRASKMAN, L. & MONTGOMERY, D. (1978). Cross cultural studies on the use of CPRS in English and Swedish depressed patients. *Acta Psychiat. Scand.*, Supplement 271, 33–47.

MONTGOMERY, S.A. & BRAITHWAITE, R.A. (1975). Amitriptyline plasma levels and clinical response. Presented to joint British and Scandinavian Associations of Psychopharmacology, London.

MONTGOMERY, S.A., BRAITHWAITE, R.A. & CRAMMER, J. (1977). Routine plasma nortriptyline levels in the treatment of depression. *Br. med. J.*, **3**, 166–167.

MONTGOMERY, S.A., BRAITHWAITE, R., DAWLING, S. & McAULEY, R. (1978). High plasma nortriptyline levels in the treatment of depression. *Clin. Pharmac. Ther.*, **32**, 309–314.

MONTGOMERY, S.A., McAULEY, R. & MONTGOMERY, D.B. (1978). Relationship between mianserin plasma levels and antidepressant effect in a double-blind trial comparing a single night-time and divided daily dose regimens. *Br. J. clin. Pharmac.*, **5**, 71S–76S.

MONTGOMERY, S.A., McAULEY, R., MONTGOMERY, D.B., DAWLING, S. & BRAITHWAITE, R.A. (1980a). Plasma concentration of clomipramine and desmethyl-clomipramine and clinical response in depressed patients. *Postgrad. med. J.*, **56**, (Suppl. 1) 130–133.

MONTGOMERY, S.A., McAULEY, R., MONTGOMERY, D.B., DAWLING, S. & BRAITHWAITE, R.A. (1980b). Clinical efficacy, side effects, and plasma concentrations of maprotiline and amitriptyline. *Br. J. clin. Pract.*,

Suppl. 7, 60–66.

MONTGOMERY, S.A., McAULEY, R., RANI, S.J. MONTGOMERY, D.B., BRAITHWAITE, R.A. & DAWLING, S. (1979b). Amitriptyline plasma concentration and clinical response. *Br. med. J.*, **1**, 230–231.

MONTGOMERY, S.A., McAULEY, R., RANI, S.J., ROY, D., MONTGOMERY, D.B., DAWLING, S. & BRAITHWAITE, R.A. (1979a). High levels of amitriptyline and clinical response. In *Biological psychiatry today*, p. 980. Amsterdam: Elsevier.

MONTGOMERY, S.A., McAULEY, R., RANI, S.J., ROY, D. & MONTGOMERY, D.B. (1980). A double-blind comparison of zimelidine and amitriptyline in endogenous depression. *Acta Psychiat. Scand.* (in press).

MONTGOMERY, S.A., MONTGOMERY, D.B., McAULEY, R. & RANI, S.J. (1978). Mianserin plasma levels and differential clinical reponse in endogenous and reactive depression. *Acta Psychiat. Belg.*, **78**, 798–812.

MONTGOMERY, S:A., ROY, D., RANI, S.J., McAULEY, R., MONTGOMERY, D.B. (1980). A comparative clinical study of nomifensine, mianserin and imipramine. *Royal Soc. Med. Symposium*, **25**, 81–85.

MOYES, K.A., RAY, R.L., & MOYES, R.B. (1980). Plasma levels and clinical improvement—a comparative study of clomipramine and amitriptyline in depression. *Postgrad. med. J.*, **56**, (Suppl. 1) 127–129.

PERRY, G.F., FITZSIMMONS, B., SHAPIRO, L. & IRWIN, P. (1978). Clinical study of mianserin, imipramine and placebo in depression: blood level and HMG correlations. *Br. J. clin. Pharmac.*, **5**, 35S–41S.

POTTER, W. & GOODWIN, R. (1978). Antidepressant drug levels and clinical response. *Lancet*, **i**, 1049–1050.

ROBINSON, D.S., COOPER, T.B., RAVARIS, C., IVES, J.O., NIES, A. BARTLETT, D. & LAMBORN, K.R. (1979). Plasma tricyclic drug levels in amitriptyline treated depressed patients. *Psychopharmacology*, **63**, 223–231.

RUSSELL, G.F.M., NIAZ, U., WAKELING, A. & SLADE, P.D. (1978). Comparative double blind trial of mianserin hydrochloride (Organon GB94) and diazepam in patients with depressive illness. *Br. J. clin. Pharmac.* **5**, 57s–65s.

SPITZER, R.L., ENDICOTT, J., ROBINS, E. (1977). *Research diagnostic criteria for a selected group of functional disorders*. National Institute of Mental Health.

STERN, R.B., MARKS, I.M., WRIGHT, J. & LUSCOMBE, D.K. (1980). Clomipramine: plasma levels, side effects and outcome in obsessive-compulsive neurosis. *Postgrad. med. J.*, **56** (Suppl. 1), 134–139.

VANDEL, S., VANDE., B., SANDOZ, M., ALLERS, G., BECHTEL, P. & VOLMAT, R. (1978). Clinical response and plasma concentration of amitriptyline and its metabolite nortriptyline. *Eur. J. clin. Pharmac.*, **14**, 185–190.

WING, J.K., COOPER, J.E. & SARTORIUS, N. (1974). The measurement and classification of psychiatric symptoms: an instruction manual for the PSE and Catego program. Cambridge University Press.

ZIEGLER, V.E., CLAYTON, P.J., TAYLOR, J.R., CO, B.T. & BIGGS, J.T. (1976). Nortriptyline plasma levels and therapeutic response. *Clin. Pharmac. Ther.*, **20**, 458–463.

ZIEGLER, V.E., CLAYTON, P.J & BRIGGS, J.T. (1977). A comparison of amitriptyline and nortriptyline with plasma levels. *Arch. gen. Psychiat.*, **34**, 607.

BIOCHEMICAL ASSESSMENT OF ANTIDEPRESSIVE DRUGS

KARABI GHOSE

Lingfield Hospital School,
Lingfield,
Surrey RH7 6PN

Introduction

Biochemical assessment of antidepressive drugs in man is usually focused on the evaluation of these drugs' interactions with biogenic amines and their receptors. There are two main reasons for this. Firstly, almost all antidepressive drugs possess one or more effects on these amines. Monoamine oxidase (MAO) inhibitors reduce the rate of their metabolism (Glowinski, Hamon, Javoy & Morot Gaudry, 1972), tricyclic antidepressive (TCA) drugs inhibit their re-uptake at the nerve terminals (Iversen, 1965), and lithium salts increase the reuptake of noradrenaline (NA) by synaptosomes (Colburn, Goodwin, Bunney & Davis, 1967). It is generally believed that these drugs act by increasing the amount of functional monoamines present in the synaptic cleft, and indeed this had been the basis for 'biogenic amine hypothesis of depression' (Schildkraut, 1965; Coppen, 1970). Although during recent years many investigators have become doubtful about the validity of this simple hypothesis (Ghose & Coppen, 1977; Leonard, 1980), it is now being argued that depressive disorders are biochemically heterogenous conditions where deficiency of either 5-hydroxytryptamine (5-HT) or NA is the primary aetiological factor (Asberg, Thoren, Traskman & Bertilsson, 1975; Maas, 1975). Similar deficiency of dopamine (DA) has also been suggested (Randrup & Braestrup, 1977). Understandably, there is a growing trend in the pharmaceutical industry to introduce compounds which in animal pharmacological studies have been shown to possess significant effects on the central biogenic amines, for the evaluation of their putative antidepressive activity in man. Secondly, these drugs (particularly TCA) produce many autonomic side-effects (Osborne & Sigg, 1960) and may interact with other drugs simultaneously administered (Briant, Reid & Dollery, 1973). A clinician should have some guide regarding a drugls potential hazards.

In this article attention has mainly been given to the biochemical assessment of TCA and pharmacologically related non-MAO inhibitor drugs, as these drugs are not only in wide use but they are also considered to be the drugs of first choice to treat acute episodes of depression (Hollister, 1978). During the last two decades several such drugs have been marketed and there is still interest in the pharmaceutical industry to develop similar drugs. Apart from their central sedative, anticholinergic and weak antihistaminic properties, these drugs are known to inhibit the uptake of biogenic amines and to influence the release and metabolism of these amines in the central nervous system (CNS). At present, there is no direct method to study these CNS changes in man. Many investigators have studied the metabolism of biogenic amines by indirect methods namely by measuring the cerebrospinal fluid (CSF) amine concentrations (Asberg, Ringberger, Sjöqvist, Toren, Traskman & Tuck, 1977) or the urinary excretion of their metabolites (Beckmann & Goodwin, 1975; Perry, Fitzsimmons, Shapiro & Irwin, 1978). However, the drug-effects are not always demonstrable in these tests and the amine concentrations may be variable at different areas of brain. Hence, the peripheral effects of antidepressive drugs are mostly assessed in man. During recent years, interactions of these drugs are usually studied by determining,

1. Peripheral adrenergic interactions,
2. Uptake of monamines by platelets,
3. Biogenic amines and their metabolites in CSF/urine,
4. Other biochemical changes.

Peripheral adrenergic interactions

Sympathomimetic amines as pharmacological tools

The peripheral NA reuptake blocking and post-synaptic α-adrenergic receptor blocking activities of TCA and related non-MAO inhibitor drugs can be studied in man by using various sympathomimetic amines as pharmacological tools. Although these amines are routinely used in animal studies, their role in human investigation remained somewhat limited until Siwers and co-workers (Siwers, Tuck, Freyschuss, Azarnoff & Sjöqvist, 1969) introduced the tyramine (TY) pressor test to assess the adrenergic interactions of TCA drugs in man. TY is an indirectly acting sympathomimetic amine and evokes its pharmacological action by releasing intraneuronal NA (Burn & Rand, 1958). It is taken up actively by the same membrane pump which reaccumulates biogenic amines at the neuronal storage sites. Therefore, the pharmacological effect of TY is dependent on its uptake by the nerve terminals, release of NA from the storage sites and the post synaptic alpha adrenergic receptor sensitivity at the target site. Any change in these functions, like reuptake and/or receptor blocking effects of a drug, will be reflected as a diminished pharmacological response to TY, and it can be used as a pharmacological tool to study these effects of TCA and related drugs. Similarly, by assessing the pharmacological response to NA, it is possible to obtain information regarding receptor functions (Coppen & Ghose, 1978). However, in the presence of NA reuptake blocking effect of a drug, since the subject will be more sensitive to this amine, it will be difficult to comment on the activities of the post synaptic α-adrenergic receptors by using NA sensitivity test. In this situation, the use of another agonist which has no significant effect on the uptake mechanism may provide information regarding receptor sensitivity and phenylephrine can be used for this purpose (Ghose, 1980a). It should be emphasised that these amines are the substrate for MAO and any change in this enzyme's function will also be reflected in their pharmacological responses.

Sympathomimetic amines produce various pharmacological effects of which increase in blood pressure (BP), pupillary mydriasis and superficial venoconstrictor effect can be measured in man by simple methods and their modification by drugs can be assessed with reasonable reliability (Ghose, 1976; Ghose, Gifford, Turner & Leighton, 1976; Ghose, 1980a) and are discussed below.

a. *Pressor response tests*

Subjects Both male and female subjects (healthy volunteers or depressed patients) with no clinical evidence of cardiovascular or cerebrovascular disorders are selected for these investigations. Subjects suffering from certain neurological conditions like Parkinson's disease or disorders of autonomic nervous system should preferably be excluded. All subjects should remain drug-free for at least 7 days prior to the baseline assessment and no other medication apart from the test drug should be given during the drug assessment period. However, if a patient requires an hypnotic and/or tranquilliser, these should be administered during both baseline and drug assessment periods. Informed consent from patients should always be obtained prior to these studies.

Measurement of BP Following an intravenous injection of TY/NA/PE both systolic and diastolic BP are increased, but in view of the rapid change in BP,

attention is given only to the systolic BP. This is monitored in every 30 s by an indirect auscultatory method using a standard Hg sphygmomanometer and Korotkoff's first and fourth sounds are taken as systolic and diastolic BP respectively. In an earlier study, various automatic BP instruments were tried, but all of them failed to produce any consistent readings in six healthy drug-free resting individuals whose BP was measured every 30 s for 30 min (Ghose, 1977). Although the School of Tropical Hygiene sphygmomanometer (Mark IV) is ideal for this type of investigation (Raftery, 1979), the minimum time required to measure BP on a single occasion is approximately 2 min and hence is considered unsuitable for these pressor response studies.

TY pressor response test During this experiment, the subjects should rest comfortably in a supine position on an examination couch. A forearm vein is cannulated and is kept patent by flushing with 2 ml of normal saline injection, and BP is recorded on the other arm. The test should be commenced only when the BP has remained steady for more than 5 min and usually after 15–30 min rest. Heart rate should be monitored by an electrocardiogram or a cardiac monitor. TY is diluted just before the injection in normal saline to obtain a total volume of 2 ml. It is given as a short and rapid intravenous injection starting usually from a very small dose of 0.25 mg, as the possibility of silent phaeochromocytoma or impaired MAO activity should always be considered. The needle and the cannula are then flushed with another 2 ml of normal saline. Systolic BP should be measured every 30 s for at least 5 min or until the BP returns to the base level. The dose of TY is increased according to the BP response to the previous increment and

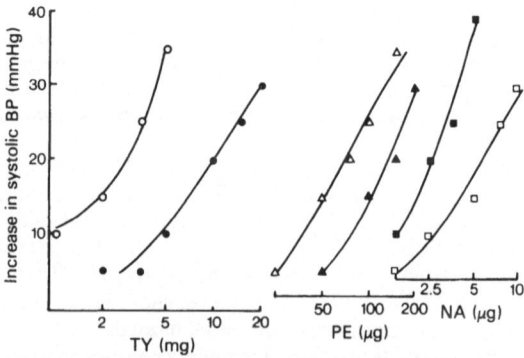

Figure 1 TY (O ●), PE (△ ▲) and NA (□ ■) dose-response curves in a male patient (55 years) before (open symbols) and during (closed symbols) amitriptyline therapy (150 mg daily for 2 weeks). The dose-response curves shifted to right indicating decreased sensitivity (NA). (From Ghose (1980a), reproduced by kind permission of the editor of the *Eur. J. clin. Pharmac.*).

should be injected only if the BP has remained steady for 5 min or more after the last injection. In order to avoid tachyphylaxis (Day & Rand, 1963), the dose of TY should be increased as quickly as prudent. No further amine is injected if the systolic BP has increased to 30 mm Hg or more. From the dose response curves, the amount of amine required to increase the systolic BP by 30 mm Hg is determined (Figure 1). *Basal response* is assessed by performing this test during drug-free or placebo treatment period and *drug response* is determined by repeating it following a drug treatment either during steady-state plasma concentrations of a drug (Ghose & Coppen, 1977) or after a single oral dose (Ghose *et al.*, 1976).

NA and PE pressor response tests The procedures are the same as above, but these amines are injected as a slow intravenous injection (2 ml/min), starting from a dose of 25 μg of PE and 1 μg of NA. These are diluted in normal saline to obtain a total volume of 2 ml just before use and ascorbic acid (0.1 mg/ml) should be added to the NA solution to prevent oxidation. Systolic BP is monitored as above, and no further injection should be given when the systolic BP has increased to 30 mm Hg or more.

Reproducibility It will be seen in Table 1 that these pressor response tests produce satisfactory reproducible results.

Table 1 Reproducibility of tyramine, noradrenaline and phenylephrine pressor response tests, as assessed in drug-free healthy volunteers for 2–4 consecutive weeks (Ghose, 1980a).

Pressor response tests	n	Weekly observations	F*
Tyramine	6	Wk I v Wk II	1.46
		Wk I v Wk III	1.18
		Wk I v Wk IV	1.13
		Wk II v Wk III	1.24
		Wk II v Wk IV	1.65
		Wk III v Wk IV	1.34
Noradrenaline	7	Wk I v Wk II	1.34
Phenylephrine	7	Wk I v Wk II	1.28

* *P* NS, i.e. no significant difference between observations.

Dose response curves Figure 1 illustrates the TY, NA and PE dose response curves in a male patient before (basal response) and during treatment with amitriptyline (drug response). The dose response curves were shifted to right (TY and PE) and left (NA) indicating decreased and increased sensitivities to the respective amines during this drug treatment. These changes in sensitivity are taken as an index of drug effect and are defined as follows:

Decreased TY-sensitivity (DTS) $= \dfrac{\text{Drug response}}{\text{Basal response}}$,

Decreased PE-sensitivity (DPS) $= \dfrac{\text{Drug response}}{\text{Basal response}}$,

Increased NA-sensitivity (INS) $= \dfrac{\text{Basal response}}{\text{Drug response}}$.

Implications Decreased TY sensitivity (DTS) following amitriptyline therapy (Figures 1 and 2) indicates uptake blocking and/or post-synaptic α-adrenergic receptor blocking activities. Associated increased NA sensitivity (INS) confirms this drug's NA reuptake blocking activity and decreased PE sensitivity (DPS) suggests post-synaptic α-adrenergic receptor blockade. Figure 2 summarises the interactions of these sympathomimetic amines in patients treated with various drugs and electroconvulsive therapies (ECT). TCA and related antidepressive drugs, in the recommended therapeutic dosage, produce variable degrees of reuptake and receptor blocking activity. It will be seen in Figure 2 that ciclazindol possesses reuptake blocking activity similar to amitriptyline but has much less receptor blocking effect, and some of the newer antidepressive drugs, like ECT (Freyschuss, Sjöqvist & Tuck, 1970), are devoid of these peripheral interactions (Ghose, 1980c). Although there is no significant change in TY sensitivity during lithium therapy, this drug appears to possess post synaptic alpha adrenergic receptor blocking activity (DPS) which has also been reported previously by other investigators (Fann, Davis, Janowsky, Kaufmann, Cavanaugh and Oates, 1974). In addition, lithium is known to stimulate monoamine uptake by human platelets (Murphy, Colburn, Davis & Bunney, 1969) and this increased uptake probably explains normal TY sensitivity with DPS in patients treated with lithium. However, it is difficult to comment from only DTS, as in the case of haloperidol and indoramin, whether this change is due to uptake blocking and/or receptor blocking effects. Hence, it is necessary to carry out all these three pressor response tests, otherwise incomplete or erroneous conclusions may be drawn.

Relationships with the plasma concentrations Figure 3 illustrates the correlation between the DTS and the plasma concentrations of desipramine in healthy volunteers following a single oral dose (Ghose *et al.*, 1976). Similar correlation with the plasma concentrations of nortriptyline during steady-state has previously been reported by others (Freyschuss *et al.*, 1970). Table 2 shows the relationships between the plasma concentrations of some antidepressive drugs and these pharmacodynamic measurements. Furthermore, in six depressed patients amitriptyline therapy was discontinued following 6 weeks treatment and

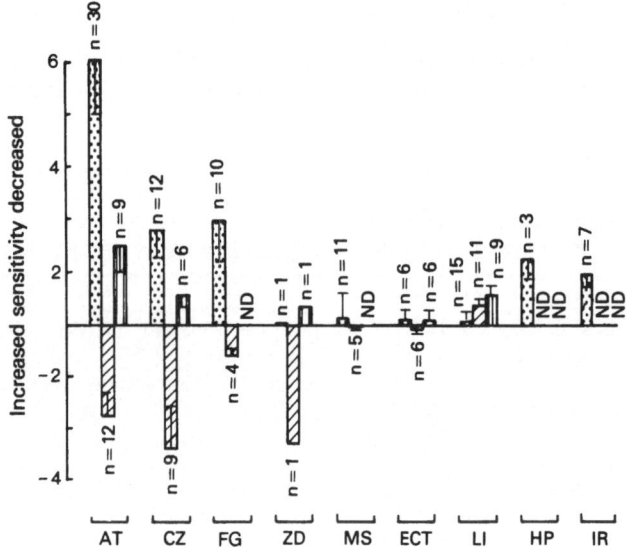

Figure 2 Summary of the pressor response tests|(TY⊡, NA⊠, PE▥) in patients during treatment with amitriptyline (AT), ciclazindol (CZ), FG4963 (FG), zimeldine (ZD), mianserin (MS), electroconvulsive therapy (ECT), lithium (Li), haloperidol (HP) and indoramin (IR). (From Ghose (1980a), reproduced by kind permission of the editor of the *Eur. J. clin. Pharmac.*).

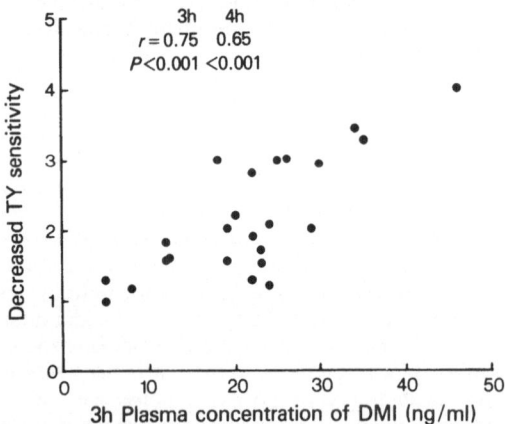

Figure 3 Correlation between the decreased TY sensitivity and plasma concentrations of desmethylimipramine (DMI) in healthy volunteers 3–4 h after a single 50 mg oral dose. (Plasma concentrations were estimated by Dr Gifford & Mr Witts).

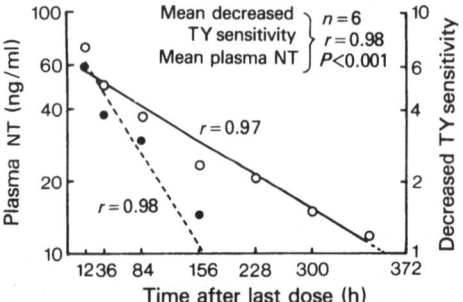

Figure 4 Relationship between the decline of pharmacodynamic effect (DTS, ○) with plasma concentrations of nortriptyline (NT, ●) following discontinuation of amitriptyline therapy in six depressed patients. (For details, Ghose (1980b). (Plasma concentrations were estimated by Dr Jorgensen.)

serial determinations of DTS were made after the last dose as illustrated in Figure 4. It is possible to assess DTS up to 372 h, although there is no measurable nortriptyline in plasma after 84 h, and the pharmacodynamic half-life (mean 139 h) correlates ($r = 0.91$) significantly with the plasma half-life of nortriptyline (mean 38 h) (Ghose, 1980b). However, DTS during

amitriptyline therapy has no correlation with the clinical outcome (Ghose & Coppen, 1977).

Unwanted effects These tests are relatively safe to carry out even in elderly patients, provided the subjects are selected carefully and the investigations are closely monitored. However, in 2–5% of subjects, the ECG may reveal ventricular/atrial ectopics which are more frequent during TCA drug therapy (Ghose, 1977), but the condition usually improves within

Table 2 Some correlations between plasma levels of antidepressive drugs and pharma-codynamic measurements

Variables	n	r	P	Reference
DTS v desipramine	24	0.75	<0.001	Ghose et al. (1976)
DTS v nortriptyline	16	0.80	<0.01	Ghose & Coppen (1977)
DTS v ciclazindol	12	0.59	<0.05	Ghose et al. (1978)
DPS v nortriptyline	6	0.56	NS	Ghose et al. (1978)
DPS v ciclazindol	8	0.66	<0.05	Ghose et al. (1978)
* $Pd_{1/2}$ (DTS) v nortriptyline	6	0.91	<0.01	Ghose (1980b)
* $Pd_{1/2}$ (DTS) v plasma clearance rate of nortriptyline	6	−0.60	NS	Ghose (1980b)
DTS v Inhibition of TY mydriasis	6	0.81	=0.05	Ghose (1976)
DTS v Decreased TY venoconstriction	6	0.87	<0.05	Ghose et al. (1976)

* $Pd_{1/2}$ Pharmacodynamic half-life
DTS Decreased tyramine sensitivity

15–30 min of the last injection. It is advisable to terminate the investigation even if occasional extra-systoles or other arrythmia appears in the electro-cardiogram. Sometimes there may be a paradoxical fall in BP as discussed elsewhere (Ghose, 1980c). These tests should never be performed without any facilities for cardiac resuscitation and drugs like phentolamine should always be ready at hand. Most subjects experience increased force of cardiac con-traction usually associated with increase in BP and bradycardia, lasting for approximately 1–2 min. This condition, unless continued for more than 5 min, does not require any intervention. Some subjects, usually with previous history of migraine may develop head-ache which may last for 1–24 h. Occasionally patients may suffer from transient pain and tightness across the chest with or without bronchospasm, and some may complain of vague symptoms of dizziness, shakiness and flushing attacks which occasionally may last for 24 h.

b. Assessment of pupillary mydriasis

The inhibitory effect of TCA and related antidepres-sive drugs on the mydriatic effect of TY (2%) can be studied in man by using a photographic method to measure pupil diameters (Turner, 1975). One drop of amine is instilled in one eye and the other eye acts as a control. This test is performed during the drug-free period and repeated following a drug treatment. The inhibitory effect can be taken as an index of drug action (Ghose, 1976), but the pupillary reaction is sluggish in elderly subjects, depends on the colour of the iris, and is sometimes difficult to assess in dark-eyed persons. However, this method correlates with DTS (Table 2) and can be used as an alternative technique in subjects where systemic pressor re-sponse tests are contraindicated, or in restless anxious patients.

c. Assessment of venoconstrictor effect

The venoconstrictor effect of TY can be studied on the dorsal hand vein. This is performed by continuous slow TY infusion and the venous diameter is measured by a method similar to that described by Nachev, Collier & Robinson (1971) and by using an electronic displacement transducer (Ghose et al., 1976). The inhibitory effect of a TCA drug on the venoconstric-tor effect of TY, although it correlates with the DTS (Table 2), has failed to show any correlation with the plasma concentrations. This effect is influenced by various non-pharmacological factors like ambient temperature and the subject's emotional state. Be-sides, slow TY infusion is likely to be associated with more tachyphylaxis than with rapid intravenous in-jection as performed in the pressor response test. This method, obviously, has limited use in the assess-ment of this type of drug interaction.

Comments

Of these three methods, pressor response tests appear to be the best technique to study the peripheral adrenergic interactions of antidepressive drugs. They are relatively safe, reproducible and provide reliable information regarding peripheral adrenergic inter-actions, even after a single oral dose of a drug. They can also be used to assess the pharmacodynamic half-life of a drug and to measure drug compliance especially in a centre where facilities to measure drug plasma levels are limited. However, these interaction studies have no predictive value as screening test for potential antidepressive activity of a drug, as many antidepressive drugs are devoid of these peripheral effects (Ghose, 1980c) and DTS has no correlation with the clinical response of an antidepressive drug (Ghose & Coppen, 1977).

Uptake of monoamines by platelets

Human platelets as models for monoaminergic neurones

TCA drugs which block the reuptake of 5-HT by nerve terminals centrally, usually also inhibit its uptake of blood platelets peripherally (Toddrick & Tait, 1969). Platelets have certain physicochemical characteristics which are in many ways comparable to those of central neurones. Like them, platelets take up 5-HT actively, store it in intracellular granules and release it with other platelet factors on stimulation (Weiss, 1975). Platelets, however, do not synthesise 5-HT or other biogenic amines. The platelet uptake system for 5-HT has kinetic constants similar to those reported for brain synaptosome preparations in animals (Shaskin & Snyder, 1970). Platelets also store other biogenic amines, but the significance of their (DA and NA) uptake is uncertain, as the concentration gradients are much less than for 5-HT. However, it has recently been suggested that the uptake of DA into platelets is mediated through a 5-HT uptake system, rather than through an independent transport mechanism for DA (Omenn & Smith, 1978), and can be inhibited by many drugs (Trenchard, Turner, Pare & Hills, 1975). Hence, human platelets may serve as a model for monoaminergic neurones and the uptake, binding and release of 5-HT/DA can be studied in man peripherally (Sneddon, 1973; Stahl & Meltzer, 1978). This model is not suitable for NA, as it is only taken up passively into platelets.

TCA and related antidepressive drugs block 5-HT uptake in the platelet by a competitive mechanism (Trenchard et al., 1975). In addition some of these drugs also inhibit 5-HT uptake in a non-competitive manner usually at lower concentrations and this uptake system is probably much more complicated than previously considered (Lingjaerde, 1979). However, this mechanism in man can be studied in platelet rich plasma by using labelled (^{3}H or ^{14}C) amines, and reliable information regarding interactions of antidepressive drugs in man may be obtained.

a. 5-HT/DA uptake by blood platelets

Subjects Both healthy volunteers and depressed patients can be selected for this study. There is no age restriction, but patients with certain neurological conditions like Parkinson's disease and Huntington's chorea should preferably be excluded. All subjects should remain drug-free for at least 7 days for in vitro, and in vivo basal response studies. They should be treated only with the test drug for in vivo drug response study, for a desired period. It is also advisable to collect blood under standard conditions, and it is usually taken in the morning from fasting subjects,

prior to their morning medication (in case of drug response study).

Preparation of platelet rich plasma (PRP) This is prepared by the method described by Coppen, Ghose, Swade & Wood (1978). Venous blood (10–20 ml) is collected and added immediately to one tenth its volume of a solution containing 27 mM disodium EDTA, 120 mM sodium chloride and 6 mM glucose (Shaw, McSweeney, Woodcock & Bevan-Jones, 1971). EDTA is selected as an anticoagulant because platelet counts and uptake are stable longer than with heparin or sodium citrate. The blood is then centrifuged at 350 g for 15 min to obtain PRP. The platelet concentration is measured by using an improved Neubauer Haemocytometer.

Measurement of platelet uptake of 5-HT Aliquots (usually 0.5 ml) of PRP are preincubated for 10 min at 37°C in a shaking water bath or at 4°C in an ice-water bath (Coppen et al., 1978). [^{14}C]-labelled 5-HT creatinine sulphate (specific activity 60.7 μci/mol) solutions are prepared at various concentrations (0.25, 0.5, 1.0, 2.0 and 4.0 mM) and 0.9% NaCl is added to make up the total volume to 50 μl. To these [^{14}C]-labelled 5-HT solutions, aliquots (0.5 ml) of PRP are added and the solutions are incubated for a further 2 min. The reaction is stopped by addition to each tube of 1 ml ice-cold 3% formaldehyde in 0.9% NaCl (Costa & Murphy, 1965). The platelet suspensions are then centrifuged at 2300 g at 0°C for 20 min, and the supernatant fractions are discarded. Each tube is then sealed after adding 1 ml of 1M KOH and is left overnight at 37°C. Aliquots (0.2 ml) of these preparations are added to 10 ml scintillation fluid and the radioactivity is counted for 30 min in an LKB ultra-beta spectrometer. The results are expressed as 5-HT accumulated/10^8 platelets/min. The active uptake of 5-HT is determined by subtracting the values obtained for passive diffusion of 5-HT into cells at 4°C from the total uptake values at 37°C. The overall uptake ($\bar{Y}$) is described as the mean uptake over the 5 concentrations. K_m (Michaelis' constant) indicates the concentration of the 5-HT giving half-maximum uptake and V_{max} is defined as the maximum entry rate. These parameters are determined by the double reciprocal plot of Lineweaver & Burk (1934) and serve to distinguish between competitive and non-competitive inhibition. Other kinetic parameters are calculated by standard methods. Figures 5a and 5b illustrate the time course of [^{14}C]-5-HT uptake (Figure 5a) and [^{14}C]-5-HT uptake at various substrate concentrations (Figure 5b) in human and rat platelets (Wielosz, Salmona, de Gaetano & Garattini, 1976). In Figure 5c, reciprocals of [^{14}C]-5-HT concentrations are plotted v reciprocals of amine accumulations into human and rat platelets.

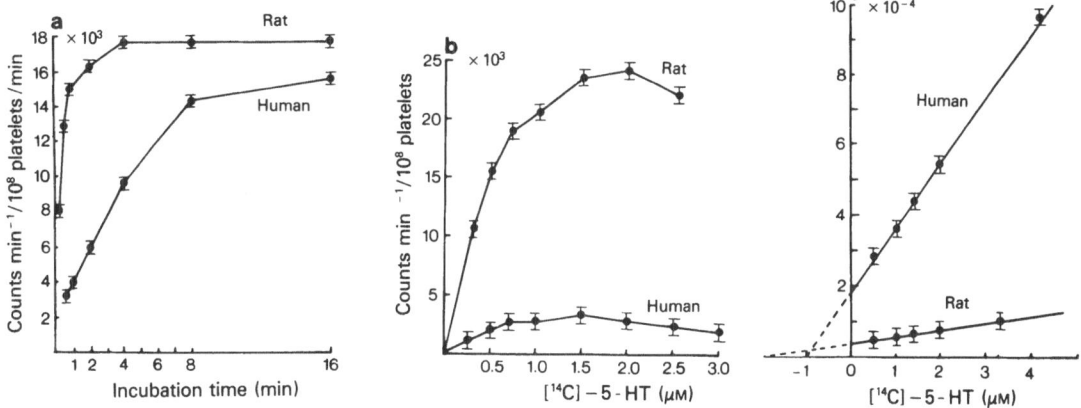

Figure 5 Differences in platelet uptake of [^{14}C]-5-HT and kinetic behaviour between human and rat platelets (From Wielosz *et al.* (1976), reproduced by kind permission of the authors and editor of *Naunyn-Schmiedeberg's Arch. Pharmac.*).

a) Time course of [^{14}C]-5-HT uptake by platelets, using a substrate concentration of 1μM.

b) [^{14}0]-5-HT uptake by platelets at various substrate concentrations. Rat platelets were incubated for 30 s whereas human platelets were incubated for 4 min.

c) Kinetic analysis of [^{14}C]-5-HT uptake. Reciprocals of [^{14}C]-5-HT concentrations were plotted *v* reciprocals of amine accumulation into platelets.

Kinetics of [^{14}C]-*5-uptake* Figure 5a (Wielosz *et al.*, 1976) illustrates the difference of kinetics in human and rat platelets. In the case of human platelets the uptake is linear up to 8 min (1 min for rat) and reaches the steady state after 15 min incubation and is much later than with rat platelets (4 min). The uptake of [^{14}C]-5-HT increases proportionally up to 1.5 μM then reaches a plateau in both human and rat platelets, but the uptake is much more in rat platelets, as shown in Figure 5b. These results are expressed as double reciprocal plots in Figure 5c. As shown in these illustrations, the apparent K_m value is approximately 1.6 times higher and V_{max} is about five times lower in human than in rat platelets. These differences in 5-HT uptake kinetics highlight the species variation and indicate the importance of conducting drug interaction studies in man.

Measurement of 5-HT uptake inhibition: The effect of drugs on platelet uptake kinetics can be studied in both *in vitro* experiments or in platelets obtained from subjects who are receiving an antidepressive drug (*in vivo*). During *in vitro* studies, aliquots of PRP prior to the incubation with ^{14}C-labelled 5-HT creatinine sulphate, are preincubated with an antidepressive drug for 10 min at 37°C in a shaking water bath. The concentrations of drug added to this solution should preferably be similar to the range of plasma levels achieved following oral administration of that drug in recommended therapeutic dose. The effect of a drug on uptake kinetics is compared with control values as shown in Figure 6.

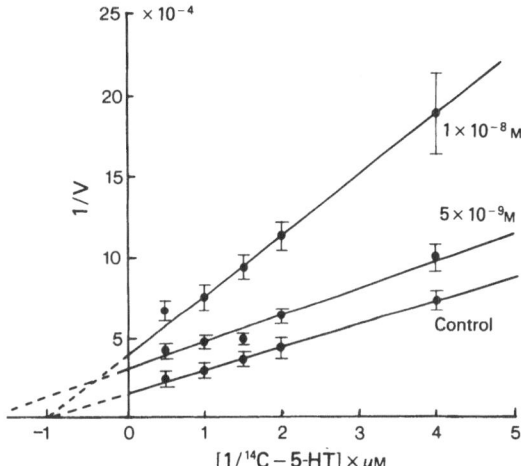

Figure 6 Kinetic analysis of [^{14}C]-5-HT uptake inhibition by chlorimipramine in human platelets. (From Wielosz *et al.* (1976), reproduced by kind permission of the authors and editor of *Naunyn-Schmiedeberg's Arch. Pharmac.*).

Studies on *in vivo* effect of drugs are carried out in two stages. Platelet 5-HT uptake kinetics are determined as described before in PRP obtained from drug-free subjects initially to obtain a baseline response. The subjects are then treated with a drug for a desired period and the procedures are repeated to obtain the drug response. The inhibitory effect of drugs on platelet 5-HT kinetics can be expressed either as percentage difference from baseline response, or similarly as amine pressor response studies, and the decreased uptake can be defined as the ratio of drug response to that of baseline response.

Measurement of platelet uptake of DA The procedures are identical to 5-HT uptake studies except that incubations should be carried out for 10 min in labelled DA solutions. However, DA should always be freshly prepared and ascorbic acid (0.1 mg/ml) should be added to each solution to prevent oxidative decomposition.

Inhibition of labelled 5-HT/DA uptake by drugs

In vitro *studies* The inhibitory effects of some antidepressive drugs on *in vitro* uptake of 5-HT into human platelets are shown in Table 3. Clomipramine at 10^{-4} M concentration inhibits 5-HT uptake 92% and DA uptake 34%, whereas maprotiline (21% 5-HT and 56% DA) and tandamine (24% 5-HT and 49% DA) have different inhibitory effects at the same concentration (Turner & Eshanullah, 1977; Eshanullah, Ghose, Kirby, Turner & Witts, 1977). In other words, an *in vitro* uptake study is helpful to assess both qualitative and quantitative effects of a drug.

In vivo *effect of drugs on platelet uptake* This is the more desirable way to assess the effect of a drug on amine uptake kinetics in man than an *in vitro* study. Lack of effect of a drug as assessed by an *in vitro* experiment may not always necessarily mean that it

has no effect on the platelet amine uptake mechanism, as this effect could be due to one of its metabolites. Besides, a drug may possess uptake blocking effects in concentrations which are much higher than the blood levels usually achieved following oral administration of that drug at the recommended therapeutic dose, and probably will be only observed in relation to overdoses in man. The uptake of 5-HT/DA should preferably be calculated in K_m, $\bar{Y}$ and V_{max} (Figure 6) and the effect of a drug on these parameters ideally should be compared with the plasma drug levels to establish a relationship with the parent drug and (if possible) with its metabolites.

b. *Effect of antidepressive drugs on change in shape of human platelets*

TCA and related antidepressive drugs also possess some effect on 5-HT receptors. Recently, Laubscher & Pletscher (1979) observed that some antidepressive drugs acted as antagonists of the shape change mediated by the 5-HT receptor in blood platelets of man incubated in protein poor medium. They failed to observe any correlation between this effect with the 5-HT uptake inhibition, and suggested that human platelets may serve as models for the neuronal 5-HT receptors of some areas of the CNS. This method appears to be a promising one for the evaluation of a drug's effect on 5-HT receptors, but clearly requires further confirmation.

Comments

It will be seen from Table 3 that 5-HT and DA uptakes in human platelets are of a similar range as

Table 3 5-HT uptake inhibition by some antidepressive drugs in rat brain synaptosomal preparations and in human platelets (*in vitro*). Although the concentrations causing 50% inhibition appear to be different, the potency in relation to imipramine is within similar range.

Method	Drug	Concentration causing 50% inhibition (μM)	Potency in relation to imipramine	Reference
Rat brain synaptosomal preparations	Imipramine	0.24	1.0	Randrup & Braestrup (1977)
	Desmethylimipramine	2.0	0.12	
	Nortriptyline	0.42	0.57	
	Chlorimipramine	0.015	16.0	
	Maprotiline	12.0	0.02	
Human platelets (*in vitro*)	Imipramine	0.17	1.0	Wielosz et al. (1976)
	Chlorimipramine	0.016	10.65	
	Imipramine	0.01	1.0	Omenn & Smith (1978)
	Nortriptyline	0.10	0.10	
	Doxepine	0.4	0.025	
	Imipramine	0.0042	1.0	Laubscher & Pletscher (1979)
	Desmethylimipramine	0.052	0.08	
	Chlorimipramine	0.0005	8.4	

studied in crude synaptosomal preparations from rat brain (Randrup & Braestrup, 1977). Hence, undoubtedly platelets are an ideal model to study peripheral effects of a drug in man. However, although the platelet uptake mechanism has been shown to have kinetic constants similar to those reported for brain synaptosome preparations in animals (Shaskin & Snyder, 1970), it still remains inconclusive whether this is also applicable to man. Nevertheless, at present this is the best model available to study the uptake system in man, and probably reflects the central neuronal mechanism.

Biogenic amines and their metabolites: CSF and urinary concentrations of amines

It has been shown in animal studies that the antidepressive drugs which block the reuptake of biogenic amines and increase the functional amines at the receptor sites are also likely to inhibit the synthesis of their respective amines through a receptor mediated negative feedback mechanism (Neilsen, Eplov & Scheel-Krugger, 1975; Carlsson & Lindqvist, 1978). In addition, several investigators (Maas, Fawcett & Dekirmenjian, 1972; Schildraut, 1973; Asberg et al., 1977) observed a relationship between the concentrations of pretreatment urinary 3-methoxy-4-hydroxyphenylglycol (MHPG)/CSF 5-hydroxyindole acetic acid (5-HIAA) and the subsequent outcome of antidepressive drug therapy. For example, patients with low pre-treatment urinary MHPG levels are likely to respond to imipramine and fail to respond to amitriptyline. Hence, measurements of these amines and their metabolites before and during treatment with an antidepressive drug may be helpful. CSF and urinary amine concentrations may provide some information regarding a drug's effect on the synthesis and turnover of biogenic amines. They may also have predictive value in selecting a patient for a particular antidepressive drug. Biogenic amines which are commonly measured are NA, DA, 5-HT and their central metabolites. Amine concentrations can be estimated by a gas liquid chromatographic (Dekirmenjian & Maas, 1970) or a fluorometric (Korf, Ottema & Vanderveen, 1971) method. Recently a more sensitive massfragmentographic method has been introduced (Bertilsson, 1980).

NA is metabolised to MHPG in the CNS. This is highly lipid soluble and crosses the blood brain barrier readily and is subsequently excreted in the urine. In animals approximately 50% of urinary MHPG originates in brain. Hence, measurement of 24 h urinary excretion is likely to reflect CNS NA synthesis and turnover. Similarly, central DA and 5-HT are metabolised to homovanillic acid (HVA) and 5-HIAA respectively. However, 5-HIAA crosses

the CSF barrier poorly and is usually removed by an energy dependent transport system (which can be inhibited by probenecid).

In a double-blind study, although there was no significant change in urinary MHPG concentrations in patients treated with imipramine/amoxapine/placebo, a correlation was observed in the imipramine treated group between pre-treatment MHPG and response to treatment (Steinbook, Jacobson, Weiss & Goldstein, 1979). No such relationship or any other change was observed by Perry et al. (1978) in patients treated with imipramine/mianserin/placebo. However, CSF 5-HIAA and MHPG concentrations were reported to be reduced during chlorimipramine therapy, indicating decreased synthesis of biogenic amines (Asberg et al., 1977), and similar assessment during antidepressive drug treatment is likely to be more informative than measurements of amines in urine. Roccatagliata, Cociot & Maffini (1979) measured the concentrations of DA and 5-HT in CSF before and during treatment with various antidepressive drugs, and observed a reciprocal modification of their metabolites after treatment.

Other biochemical assessment

Of the various other biochemical changes, the activities of MAO and cyclic adenosine monophosphate (c-AMP) are of clinical interest in view of their probable role in the alleviation of depressive symptoms. However, apart from the MAO inhibitor group other antidepressive drugs are usually devoid of any effect on this enzyme and hence only c-AMP assessment is discussed below.

Cyclic adenosine monophosphate (c-AMP)

This nucleotide acts as the second messenger substance for many neurotransmitters and hormone induced responses. It is formed from adenosinetriphosphate by the action of the enzyme adenylcyclase and is degraded by the enzyme c-AMP phosphodiesterase; both of these occur in the brain. Although the role of c-AMP in the pathogenesis of affective disorders remains inconclusive (Abdulla & Hamadah, 1970; Eccleston, Loose, Puller and Sugden, 1970), it has been suggested that NA sensitive adenylcyclase in the brain may be involved in the mechanism of action of antidepressive drugs (Vetulani & Sulser, 1975). TCA antidepressive drugs inhibit phosphodiesterase (Janice, Korczak & Herman, 1971) and may increase the accumulation of c-AMP in brain (Huang & Daly, 1972). However, there is also controversy as to the action of antidepressive drugs on c-AMP and several animal studies have indicated that these drugs can inhibit the accumulation of c-AMP (Palmer, 1976). It has also been suggested that imipramine, amitriptyline and viloxazine stimulate c-AMP at low concentrations and inhibit c-AMP at high concentrations in rat cerebral cortex (Jones, 1978). In man, urinary excretion of c-AMP has been reported to be increased following ECT (Hamadah, Holmes, Barber, Hartman & Park, 1972) and antidepressive drug treatment (Ramsden, 1970), but these have not been confirmed by other investigators (Brown, Salway, Albano, Hullin & Ekins, 1972). These differences may be due to the fact that c-AMP has a wide distribution in brain and the urinary excretion or CSF concentration may not be a sensitive indicator for small changes occurring at certain parts of the CNS. In addition, c-AMP is also related to physical exercise (Eccleston *et al.*, 1970) and anxiety states (Moyes & Moyes, 1977). Hence, the methodologies used to measure c-AMP in urine (Abdulla & Hamadah, 1970) and in CSF (Robinson, Coppen, Whybrow & Prange, 1970) are unlikely to be helpful in the assessment of drug interactions in man.

Naylor and co-workers (Naylor, Buckley, Boardman, Smith & Moody, 1978) tried to evaluate the effect of mianserin on erythrocyte c-AMP concentrations in depressed patients, but no significant change was observed. These investigators have also failed to observe any effect of mianserin on erythrocyte $Na^+ - K^+$ ATPase activity. Since mianserin has no significant effect on the uptake mechanism (Ghose, 1980a), it may be possible that other drugs like imipramine may show some effects on these tests. Recently, Ridges & Goldberg (1980) have suggested that a c-AMP stimulation test may be of value in predicting individual responses to antidepressive therapy and obviously requires further evaluation.

Conclusions

The peripheral adrenergic interactions of antidepressive drugs in man can be assessed by using various sympathomimetic amines as pharmacological tools. TY, NA and PE pressor response tests are shown to be safe, reproducible and they provide reliable information regarding adrenergic interactions of drugs in man.

Human platelet is a convenient and satisfactory model to study the peripheral amine (5-HT and DA) uptake mechanisms in man. However, whether this peripheral effect correlates with the central neuronal amine reuptake pump in man has yet to be confirmed.

Measurement of biogenic amines and their metabolites in CSF appear to be helpful in the evaluation of a drug's effect on the synthesis of these amines in the CNS and may provide some guidance regarding outcome of treatment with a specific antidepressive drug in a particular patient. However, urinary excretion of these amines appears to have limited value probably because of the lack of a sensitive method to assay these amines in biological fluids.

There is some potential in assessing drug induced changes in the c-AMP generating system, but these changes are influenced by other physiological factors and at present there is no evidence that the techniques available to measure c-AMP in man are sensitive enough to demonstrate drug induced changes.

References

ABDULLA, Y.H. & HAMADAH, K. (1970). 3'5' cyclic adenosine monophosphate in depression and mania. *Lancet,* i, 378–381.

ASBERG, M., RINGBERGER, V.A. SJOQVIST, F., TOREN, P., TRASKMAN, L. & TUCK, J.R. (1977). Monoamine metabolites in cerebrospinal fluid and serotonin uptake inhibition during treatment with chlorimipramine. *Clin. Pharmac. Ther.,* **21,** 201–207.

ASBERG, M., THOREN, P., TRASKMAN, L. & BERTILSSON, L. (1975). Serotonin depression—a biochemical subgroup within the affective disorders. *Science,* **191,** 487.

BECKMANN, H. & GOODWIN, F.K. (1975). Antidepressant response to tricyclics and urinary MHPG in unipolar patients. *Arch. gen. Psychiat.,* **32,** 17–21.

BERTILSSON, L., (1980). Quantitative mass fragmentography—a valuable tool in clinical psychopharmacology: In *Clinical Pharmacology in Psychiatry,* eds. Davis, J. & Usdin, E. North-Holland, New York: Elsevier.

BRIANT, R.H., REID, J.L. & DOLLERY, C.T. (1973). Interaction between clonidine and despiramine in man. *Br. med. J.,* **1,** 522–523.

BROWN, B.L., SALWAY, J.G., ABANO, J.D.H., HULLIN, R.P. & EKINS, R.P. (1972). Urinary excretion of cyclic AMP and manic depressive psychosis. *Br. J. Psychiat.,* **120,** 405–408.

BURN, J.H. & RAND, M.J. (1958). The action of sympathomimetic amines in animals treated with reserpine. *J. Physiol. Lond.,* **144,** 314–316.

CARLSSON, A. & LINDQVIST, M. (1978). Effects of antidepressant agents on the synthesis of brain monoamines. *J. Neurol. Transmission,* **43,** 73–91.

COLBURN, R.W., GOODWIN, F.K., BUNNEY, W.E. & DAVIS, J.M. (1967). Effect of lithium on the uptake of noradrenaline by synaptosomes. *Nature,* **215,** 1395–1397.

COPPEN, A. (1970). The chemical pathology of the affective disorders. In *The Scientific Basis of Medicine,* Annual Reviews, pp. 189–210, London: Athlone Press.

COPPEN, A. & GHOSE, K. (1978). Peripheral α-adrenoceptor and central dopamine receptor activity in depressive patients. *Psychopharmacology,* **59,** 171–177.

COPPEN, A., GHOSE, K., SWADE, C. & WOOD, K. (1978). Effects of mianserin hydrochloride on peripheral uptake mechanisms for noradrenaline and 5-hydroxytryptamine in man. *Br. J. clin. Pharmac.,* **5,** 13s–17s.

COSTA, J.L. & MURPHY, D.L. (1965). Platelet 5-HT uptake and release stopped rapidly by formaldehyde. *Nature,* **255,** 407–408.

DAY, M.D. & RAND, M.J. (1963). Tachyphylaxis to some sympathomimetic amines in relation to monoamine oxidase. *Br. J. Pharmac.*, **21**, 84–96.

DEKIRMENJIAN, H. & MAAS, J. W. (1970). An improved procedure of 3-methoxy-4-hydroxyphenylethylene glycol determination by gas liquid chromatography. *Analyt. Biochem.*, **35**, 113–114.

ECCLESTON, D., LOOSE, R., PULLER, I.A. & SUGDEN, R.E. (1970). Exercise and urinary excretion of cyclic AMP. *Lancet*, **ii**, 25.

ESHANULLAH, R., GHOSE, K., KIRBY, M., WITTS, D. & TURNER, P. (1977). Clinical pharmacological studies of tandamine, a potential antidepressive drug. *Psychopharmacology*, **52**, 73–77.

FANN, W.E., DAVIS, J.M., JANOWSKY, D.S., KAUFMANN, J.S. CAVANAUGH, J.H. & OATES, J.A. (1974). Effect of antidepressant and antimanic drugs on amine uptake in man. *J. Nerv. Ment. Dis.*, **158**, 361–368.

FREYSCHUSS, U., SJÖQVIST, F. & TUCK D. (1970). Tyramine pressor effects in man before and during treatment with nortriptyline or ECT: Correlation between plasma level and effect of nortriptyline. *Pharmacologia Clin.*, **2**, 72–78.

GHOSE, K. (1976). Correlation of pupil reactivity to tyramine or hydroxyamphetamine and tyramine pressor responses in patients treated with amitriptyline or mianserin. *Br. J. clin. Pharmac.*, **3**, 666–667.

GHOSE, K. (1977). *Autonomic actions and interactions of some antidepressive drugs*. Ph.D. Thesis, University of London, pp. 68–69.

GHOSE, K. (1980a). Assessment of peripheral adrenergic activity and its interaction with drugs in man. *Eur. J. clin. Pharmac.*, **17**, 233–238.

GHOSE, K. (1980b). Decreased tyramine sensitivity following discontinuation of amitriptyline therapy. An index of pharmacodynamic half-life. *Eur. J. clin. Pharmac.*, **18**, 151–157.

GHOSE, K. (1980c). Sympathomimetic amines and tricyclic antidepressant drugs. *Neuropharmacology* (in press).

GHOSE, K. & COPPEN, A. (1977). Noradrenaline, depressive illness and the action of amitriptyline. *Psychopharmacology*, **54**, 57–60.

GHOSE, K., GIFFORD, L., TURNER, P. & LEIGHTON, M. (1976). Studies of the interaction of desmethylimipramine with tyramine in man after a single oral dose and its correlation with plasma concentration. *Br. J. clin. Pharmac.* **3**, 334–337.

GHOSE, K., RAO, V.A.R., BAILEY, J. & COPPEN, A. (1978). Antidepressant activity and pharmacological interactions of ciclazindol. *Psychopharmacology*, **57**, 109–114.

GLOWINSKI, J., HAMON, M., JAVOY, F. & MOROT GAUDRY, Y. (1972). Rapid effects of monoamine oxidase inhibitors on synthesis and release of central monoamines. In *Monoamine Oxidases—New Vistas. Advances in Biochemical Psychopharmacology*, **5**, 423–440. Eds. Costa, E. & Sandler, M., New York, Raven Press.

HAMADAH, K., HOLMES, H., BARKER, G.B., HARTMAN, G.C. & PARKE, D.V.W. (1972). Effect of electric convulsion therapy on urinary excretion of 3'5' cyclic adenosine monophosphate. *Br. med. J.*, **3**, 439.

HOLLISTER, L.E. (1978). Treatment of depression with drugs. *Ann. intern. Med.*, **89**, 78–84.

HUANG, H. & DALY, J.W. (1972). Accumulation of c-AMP in incubated slices of brain tissue—1. Structure activity relationships of agonists and antagonists of biogenic amines and of tricyclic tranquillizers and antidepressants. *J. med. Chem.*, **15**, 458–462.

IVERSEN, L.L. (1965). Inhibition of noradrenaline uptake by drugs. *J. Pharm. Pharmac.*, **17**, 62–64.

JANICE, W., KOREZAK, K. & HERMAN, Z.S. (1971). Effect of phenothiazine neuroleptic drugs and tricyclic antidepressants on phosphodiesterase activity in rat cerebral cortex. *Psychopharmacology*, **37**, 351–358.

JONES, R.S.G. (1978). Noradrenaline sensitive adenylate cyclase in rat cerebral cortex: Effects of antidepressant drugs. *Neuropharmacology*, **17**, 771–774.

KORF, J., OTTEMA, S. & VANDER VEEN, I. (1971). Fluorometric determination of homovanillic acid in biological material after isolation on sephadex G-10. *Analyt. Biochem.*, **40**, 187–191.

LAUBSCHER, A. & PLETSCHER, A. (1979). Shape change and uptake of 5-hydroxytryptamine in human blood platelets: Action of neuropsychotropic drugs. *Life Sci.*, **24**, 1833–1840.

LEONARD, B.E. (1980). Drug treatment of depression: a critical evaluation of the current situation. Roy. Soc. Med. International congress and symposium series no. 25, pp. 1–10. Eds Stonier, P.D. & Jenner, F.A.

LINEWEAVER, A. & BURK, D. (1934). The determination of enzyme dissociation constants. *J. Ann. Chem. Soc.*, **56**, 666–685.

LINGJAERDE, O. (1979). Inhibitory effect of clomipramine and related drugs on serotonin uptake in platelets: More complicated than previously thought. *Psychopharmacology*, **61**, 245–249.

MAAS, J.W. (1975). Biogenic amines and depression. *Arch. gen. Psychiat.*, **32**, 1357–1361.

MAAS, J.W., FAWCETT, J.A. & DEKIRMENJIAN, H. (1972). Catecholamine metabolism, depressive illness and drug response. *Arch. gen. Psychiat.*, **26**, 252–255.

MOYES, I.C.A. & MOYES, R.B. (1977). Urinary 3'5' cyclic adenosine monophosphate (c-AMP) as a measure of anxiety. *Postrgrad. med. J.*, **53**, Suppl. 4, 41–46.

MURPHY, D.L., COLBURN, R.W., DAVIS, J.M. & BUNNEY, W.E. (1969). Stimulation by lithium of monoamine uptake in human platelets. *Life Sci.*, **8**, 1187–1193.

NACHEV, C., COLLIER, J. & ROBINSON, B. (1971). Simplified method for measuring compliance of superficial veins. *Cardiovascular Res.*, **5**, 147–159.

NAYLOR, G.S., BUCKLEY, D.E., BOARDMAN, L.J., SMITH, A.H.W. & MOODY, J.P. (1978). Attempt to demonstrate an *in vivo* effect of mianserin hydrochloride on erythrocyte Na$^+$ − K$^+$ − ATPase activity and cyclic AMP concentration. *Br. J. clin. Pharmac.*, **5**, 49s–52s.

NIELSEN, M., EPLOV, L. & SCHEEL-KRUGER, J. (1975). The effect of amitriptyline, desipramine and imipramine on the *in vivo* brain synthesis of [^{3}H]-noradrenaline from [^{3}H]-L-Dopa in the rat. *Psychopharmacologia (Berl.)*, **41**, 249–254.

OMENN, G.S. & SMITH, L.T. (1978). A common uptake system for serotonin and dopamine in human platelets. *J. clin. Invest.* **62**, 235–240.

OSBORNE, M. & SIGG, E.B., (1960). Effects of imipramine on the peripheral autonomic system. *Arch. int. Pharmacodyn.*, **129**, 273–288.

PALMER, G.C. (1976). Influence of tricyclic antidepressants

on the adenylate cyclase-phosphodiesterase system in the rat cortex. *Neuropharmacology*, **15**, 1–7.

PERRY, G.T., FITZSIMMONS, G., SHAPIRO, L. & IRWIN, P. (1978). Clinical study of mianserin, imipramine and placebo in depression: blood level and MHPG correlations. *Br. J. clin. Pharmac.*, **5**, 35s–41s.

RAFTERY, E.B. (1979). The methodology of blood pressure recording. In *Methods in Clinical Pharmacology—Cardiovascular System.* pp. 20–28. Ed. Shanks, R.G. London: Macmillan Journals Ltd.

RAMSDEN, E. (1970). Cyclic AMP in depression and mania. *Lancet*, **ii**, 108.

RANDRUP, A. & BRAESTRUP, C. (1977). Uptake inhibition of biogenic amines by newer antidepressant drugs: Relevance to the dopamine hypothesis of depression. *Psychopharmacology*, **53**, 309–314.

RIDGES, A.P. & GOLDBERG, I.J.L. (1980). A possible cyclic adenosine monophosphate stimulation test in depression. *Postgrad. med. J.* **56**, Suppl. 1, 42–44.

ROCCATAGLIATA, G., ALBANO, C., COCITO, L. & MAFFINI, M. (1979). Interactions between central monoaminergic systems: dopamine-serotonin. *J. Neurol. Neurosurg. Psychiat.*, **42**, 1159–1162.

ROBINSON, G.A., COPPEN, A.J., WHYBROW, P.C. & PRANGE, A.J. (1970). Cyclic AMP in affective disorders. *Lancet*, **ii**, 1028–1029.

SCHILDKRAUT, J.J. (1965). The catecholamine hypothesis of affective disorders: A review of supporting evidence. *Am. J. Psychiat.*, **12**, 509–522.

SCHILDKRAUT, J.J. (1973). Norepinephrine metabolites as biochemical criteria for classifying depressive disorders and predicting responses to treatment: preliminary findings. *Am. J. Psychiat.*, **130**, 695–699.

SHASKIN, E.G. & SNYDER, S.J. (1970). Kinetics of serotonin accumulation into slices from rat brain. Relationship to catecholamine uptake. *J. Pharmac. exp. Ther.*, **175**, 404–418.

SHAW, D.M., MacSWEENEY, D.A., WOODCOCK, N. & BEVAN-JONES, A.B. (1971). Uptake and release of ^{14}C-5-hydroxytryptamine by platelets in affective illness. *J. Neurol. Neurosurg. Psychiat.*, **34**, 224–225.

SIWERS, B., TUCK, D., FREYSCHUSS, U., AZARNOFF, D. & SJÖQVIST, F. (1969). Abstract for Fourth International Congress of Pharmacology, July 14 to 18, Basel.

SJÖQVIST, B. & JOHANSSON, B. (1978). A comparison between flurometric and mass fragmentographic determination of homovanillic acid and 5-hydroxy-indoleacetic acid in human cerebrospinal fluid. *J. Neurochem.*, **31**, 621–625.

SNEDDON, J.M. (1973). Blood platelets as a model for monamine containing neurones. *Prog. Neurobiol. (N.Y.)*, **1**, 151–198.

STAHL, S.M. & MELTZER, H.Y. (1978). A kinetic and pharmacologic analysis of 5-hydroxytryptamine transport by human platelets and platelet storage granules: Comparison with central serotonergic neurones. *J. Pharmac. exp. Ther.*, **205**, 118–121.

STEINBOOK, R.M., JACOBSON, A.F., WEISS, B.L. & GOLDSTEIN, B.J. (1979). Amoxapine, imipramine and placebo: A double blind study with pre-therapy urinary 3-methoxy-4-hydroxyphenylglycol levels. *Curr Ther. Res. Opn.*, **26**, 490–496.

TRENCHARD, A., TURNER, P., PARE, C.M.B. & HILLS, M. (1975). The effects of protriptyline and clomipramine *in vitro* on the uptake of 5-hydroxytryptamine and dopamine in human platelet rich plasma. *Psychopharmacologia (Berl.)*, **43**, 89–93.

TODRICK, A. & TAIT, A.C. (1969). The inhibition of human platelet 5-hydroxytryptamine uptake by tricyclic antidepressive drugs. The relation between structure and potency. *J. Pharm. Pharmac.*, **21**, 751–762.

TURNER, P. (1975). Human pupil as a model for clinical pharmacological investigations. *J. Roy. Coll. Physcns. Lond.*, **9**, 165–171.

TURNER, P. & ESHANULLAH, R.S.B. (1977). Clomipramine and maprotiline on human platelet uptake of 5-hydroxytryptamine and dopamine *in vitro*: What relevance to their antidepressive and other central actions? *Postgrad. med. J.*, **53**, (Suppl. 4), 14–18.

VETULANI, J. & SULSER, F. (1975). Action of various antidepressant treatments reduces reactivity of noradrenergic cyclic AMP-generating system in limbic forebrain. *Nature*, **257**, 495–496.

WEISS, J.J. (1975). Platelet physiology and abnormalities of platelet function. *New Engl. J. Med.*, **293**, 531–541.

WIELOSZ, M., SALMONA, M., GAETANO, G.D.E. & GARATTINI, S. (1976). Uptake of ^{14}C-5-hydroxytryptamine by human and rat platelets and its pharmacological inhibition. A comparative kinetic analysis. *Naunyn-Schmiedeberg's Arch. Pharmac.*, **296**, 59–65.

THE CLINICAL ASSESSMENT OF DEPRESSION

MALCOLM LADER

Institute of Psychiatry,
de Crespigny Park, London SE5

Introduction

No laboratory tests can establish the diagnosis or quantify the severity of any functional psychiatric condition. Clinical interview, skilled observations and self-reports remain the standard ways of assessing psychiatric patients. Because many syndromes are complex and ill-defined, rational methods of assessing psychopathology in many areas of psychiatry are difficult to devise. For example, the concept of 'severity' in schizophrenia or in psychopathology is ambiguous and consequently difficult to assess rationally. Depression presents fewer problems, most of which are soluble. It thus provides a useful paradigm for the discussion of clinical ratings in psychiatry.

Some of the general principles and problems of clinical ratings will be discussed with particular reference to depressed patients. Then, currently available depression rating scales will be outlined with some suggestions for a choice of instrument. Future developments will be adumbrated. The principles described are similar for other psychiatric conditions and available scales are fully reviewed by Pichot & Olivier-Martin (1974) and by Guy (1976).

The purposes of clinical assessment

Accurate clinical assessment is a laudable aim in itself. Most natural laws have been developed as an intuitive appreciation of the relationship of observed phenomena, and the more clearly and precisely that relationship can be defined and measured, the wider the applicability of the natural law. Thus, precise measurement of any natural phenomenon will ultimately prove worthwhile. However, clinicians function in an imperfect world and their clinical assessments are made with more practical objects in mind.

Firstly, assessing a patient carefully is a prerequisite for an accurate diagnosis (Montgomery, 1980). By 'accurate' is meant reproducible, stable, generally accepted and heuristic. However, diagnostic schemata are usually unsatisfactory because the underlying relationships between syndromes and between conditions within syndromes are so poorly understood. For example, where do the schizoaffective disorders belong? Also, classifications within the general context of the depressive syndromes have been too Procrustean. Official lists of diagnoses reflect the most elaborate of such classifications (DSM III, 1979), and too often an elementary rule of classificatory systems is broken, namely, that all elements in a classification should be mutually exclusive. The use of rating scales to rationalise or at least to reduce the inchoate nature of these systems has not been taken very far (see reviews by Akiskal & Webb, 1978; Rakoff, Stancer & Kedward, 1977).

The basic problem with the use of rating scales in this context is that diagnosis may depend on more than psychopathology at the time of interview. The history of the illness, family history, previous episodes and many other factors are relevant. Also, statistics appropriate to analyse rating scales differ from those best suited to allocating to categories.

The second function of rating scales is to increase the precision of prognostic statements. Attempts to do this in depressed patients have not been very successful in the sense that formal predictors of outcome based on rating scales are not appreciably better than informal predictors based on clinical judgment and experience. Part of the problem stems from the difficulty, already stressed, of defining the population under study. Predictive indicators can only apply to patients drawn from the same population as the patients from which the predictors were derived: poorly defined populations will lead to prognostic imprecision as well. Another difficulty is in defining the end-point; different outcomes may be desired in different patients. Thus, return to work may be the goal in one patient, improved marital relationships in another, but disappearance of symptoms is a universal goal.

The widest application for rating scales is the assessment of response to medication. The general acceptance of controlled clinical trials with double-blind procedures as the ultimate arbiter of the effectiveness of drugs has also encouraged the use of rating scales to quantify drug actions. Some standardisation has been achieved with the bonus that comparisons can be made between trials.

Many depression scales are extant which implies that comparisons between them have been insufficient to uncover their relative advantages and disadvantages. Although some scales are designed for particular purposes, most are used to assess patients with primary depression presenting to the general practitioner or to the hospital psychiatrist. But there is no satisfactory scale to quantify depression in a schizophrenic or a psychopath: although the symptom patterns broadly resemble those of patients with primary depressive illnesses, certain features differ and may profoundly alter the assessment. Care is needed in borrowing a rating scale developed for one application and using it in another.

The use of rating scales has been overplayed at times. Some have hoped that the widespread use of rating scales might resolve many, if not all, of the major controversies in psychiatry. This is an elementary mistake. Rating scales increase the precision with which certain phenomena can be assessed but their prime function is to increase standardisation so that studies can be compared. Data from several studies can be pooled once the homogeneity of the data has been established. But controversies must be resolved before sensible rating scales can be developed. A good example concerns the attempts to distinguish clearly between endogenous and reactive depression. Drawing up a rating scale on the preconceived idea of two distinct syndromes resulted in rating scale data which, on analysis, yielded two distinct groups. Drawing up a rating scale on the null hypothesis that there were *not* two distinct syndromes generated data fitting a unimodal distribution. Rating scales are most useful when concepts have been clarified, syndromes delineated and psychopathology defined. Even then, rating scales should be devised for a particular purpose in a well-defined population.

Development of scales

Validity

Validity can be defined in various ways but for the purposes of the present discussion it means that the scores on a rating scale accurately reflect the degrees of severity of the phenomenon measured, in this case depression. The two most important methods of assessing validity are construct and concurrent validity.

Construct validity can be estimated by calculating the discriminability between groups provided by a particular scale. Schwab, Bialow & Holzer (1967) administered the Hamilton Depression Rating Scale to medical students and to depressives and found an acceptable separation of scores for the Hamilton Scale. The Beck self-rating scale showed a unimodal distribution. Very little overlap occurred in the scores on the Wakefield Self-Assessment Depression Scale of a group of normal subjects and a group of depressed patients (Snaith, Ahmed, Metha & Hamilton, 1971). Downing & Rickels (1972) administered some depression rating scales to a group of depressed patients and a group of non-depressed psychiatric

patients. They found few differences, which might indicate the low validity of these scales. However, it might suggest that the initial allocation to the groups on clinical grounds was unsound in that depression was being missed in some of the so-called 'non-depressive' group. Also scales devised to measure the severity of a condition along a continuum are usually unsuited to making diagnostic distinctions of an all-or-none nature.

Another popular method of establishing validity is to make a global judgment of the severity of the depression in each of a large group of patients. A scale can then be used to quantify the depression and the correlation to the global rating computed. This graded approach avoids the oversimplified judgment of whether a person is depressed or not. Zealley & Aitken (1969) used this method with the Hamilton Rating Scale for Depression and obtained the gratifyingly high correlation of 0.90 for patients on admission to hospital. Midway through the stay, the correlation fell to 0.76 and on discharge, to 0.55. Similarly, the visual analogue scale correlated 0.78 with global severity rating on patients when admitted but only 0.13 at the time of discharge.

Validities for self-rating of depression scales against global observer ratings of depression tend to be low. However, the rationale for self-ratings versus observer ratings is complex and will be discussed later.

Construct validity can also be determined by showing that the scores on a rating scale are affected by experimental factors. By far the most extensive examples involve the use of rating scales in clinical trials. By and large, the improvements associated with drug therapies assessed by rating scales accord with clinical experience although they can be greater.

Concurrent validity refers to the agreement between different scales all purporting to measure approximately the same phenomenon. Of course, all the scales might be measuring the wrong or irrelevant thing and concurrent validity is essentially an estimate of corporate judgment. It assesses whether different ways of making the same judgment accord. Concurrent validity is weaker evidence for a scale than is construct validity.

With respect to depression scales, the Hamilton Depression Rating Scale (HDRS) has become the yardstick by which other scales are judged. Bech, Gram, Dein, Jacobsen, Vitger & Bolwig (1975) found that the Beck depression inventory correlated 0.72 with the HDRS; a similar correlation was found by Schwab *et al.* (1967) but Tan (1969) found a lower value of 0.51. The Zung Depression Scale correlated 0.79 with the HDRS (Brown & Zung, 1972). Studying patients soon after admission, Zealley & Aitken (1969) obtained a correlation of 0.79 between the visual analogue scale and the Hamilton. The correlation was zero when the patients were retested midway through their stay and again on discharge. The reasons for this discrepancy are obscure but suggest caution in assessing the results of therapeutic trials which rely too heavily on one assessment instrument.

Self-assessment inventories tend not to correlate highly with observer rating scales. The Minnesota Multiphasic Personality Inventory (MMPI) depression scale correlated only 0.25 with the HDRS (Tan, 1969) although the neuroticism scale of the Maudsley Personality Inventory actually correlated 0.5 with the HDRS (Garside, Kay, Roy & Beamish, 1970). Thus, the items sampling neuroticism in the MPI bear more relationship to observer-rated depression than do the MMPI items purporting to measure depression as a personality dimension.

The Beck Depression Inventory has also been used as a standard with correlations of 0.40 to 0.66 with the Lubin Adjective Check List in various groups of patients (Lubin, 1965) and 0.53 with the MMPI depression scale (Tan, 1969). Other studies suggest that, in general, correlations among self-rating scales are lower than those among observer rating scales.

Reliability

The two most important types of reliability are inter-rater and test-retest. Inter-rater reliability poses no problems in calculation or interpretation. There are various ways of performing inter-rater reliability tests but raters must all have been trained to use the rating scale. One observer can conduct the interview while he and the other observer rate; or both can interview in the same session; or both can interview in succession. Another way is for an independent observer to interview with the two raters observing passively. Or the interview can be recorded on video-tape and the ratings made later. Inter-rater reliability for the Hamilton Depression Scale is around 0.90.

Test-retest reliability is more problematical. If the two interviews are too close together in time, some of the replies may be remembered and become stereotyped. If the two interviews are too far apart, the condition being rated may alter so that the correlation becomes diluted. This is probably the least useful manoeuvre during the development of a rating scale.

Inter-rater reliability cannot be used with self-rating scales. However, for both self- and observer-rating instruments, split-half reliability can help establish the consistency of the scale. In this technique, the scale is split randomly into two subscales and the correlation between them computed. It should be quite high if the scale is to be useful.

Types of rating scales

The most important operational distinction among rating scales concerns the method of administration. Scales can be administered by an observer, trained or untrained, or can be completed by the patient him-

self. Controversy has attended the rival claims of observer versus patient rating scales (see Table 1) (Kendell, 1975): A skilled observer can assess the intensity of any one symptom against the background of his experience. The more experience he has the less he rates towards the severe end of the scale. Patients may rate in quite an extreme way, either denying their symptoms or exaggerating them. Skilled observers should be able to detect these distortions and allow for them. Behaviour of the patient is the easiest for the observer to assess, the most difficult for the patient. The greatest difficulties occur with patients who lose insight; they cannot be expected to rate themselves. Such symptoms as mild retardation, delusions, agitation, hypochondriasis and depersonalisation are liable to be inaccurately rated by the patient. Observer ratings will be more reliable and valid although the rating of depersonalisation is a peculiarly difficult one. Finally, to fill in a questionnaire, a patient must be cooperative, attentive, able to concentrate and literate. Furthermore, the patient's usage of words such as 'anxiety' and 'depression' must accord with general professional usage.

The main drawback of observer rating scales is that most can be used only by trained and experienced personnel. They are also time-consuming. Another drawback with primarily symptomatic complaints such as mild anxiety and depression is that the interviewer merely retails the patient's account and further questioning adds little to the initial assessment.

On balance, observer- and self-rating scales are most apposite for rather different types of patient. Severely depressed patients especially those with impairment of insight require skilled observer rating. Patients with mild conditions, typically the majority of those in general practice, are suited to self-ratings. When repeated ratings at fairly short intervals are involved, self-ratings are usually the most cost-effective. A rough guide to which form of self-rating is most appropriate can be obtained by asking the simple question, 'Who is most concerned about this patient's condition, the patient himself or those about him?'. If self-concern is paramount, self-rating is almost always sufficient; if others are concerned, observer rating on its own, or in addition, will be needed.

In many studies, several instruments are used (e.g. Young, Lader & Hughes, 1979; Figure 1). This is a 'belt-and-braces' policy and is commendable. Occasionally, the different types of rating scales may differ in their conclusions and seeking the cause of such a discrepancy may lead to interesting studies.

Mechanics of rating scales

Items for rating scales are usually selected by considering the clinical features of the condition under

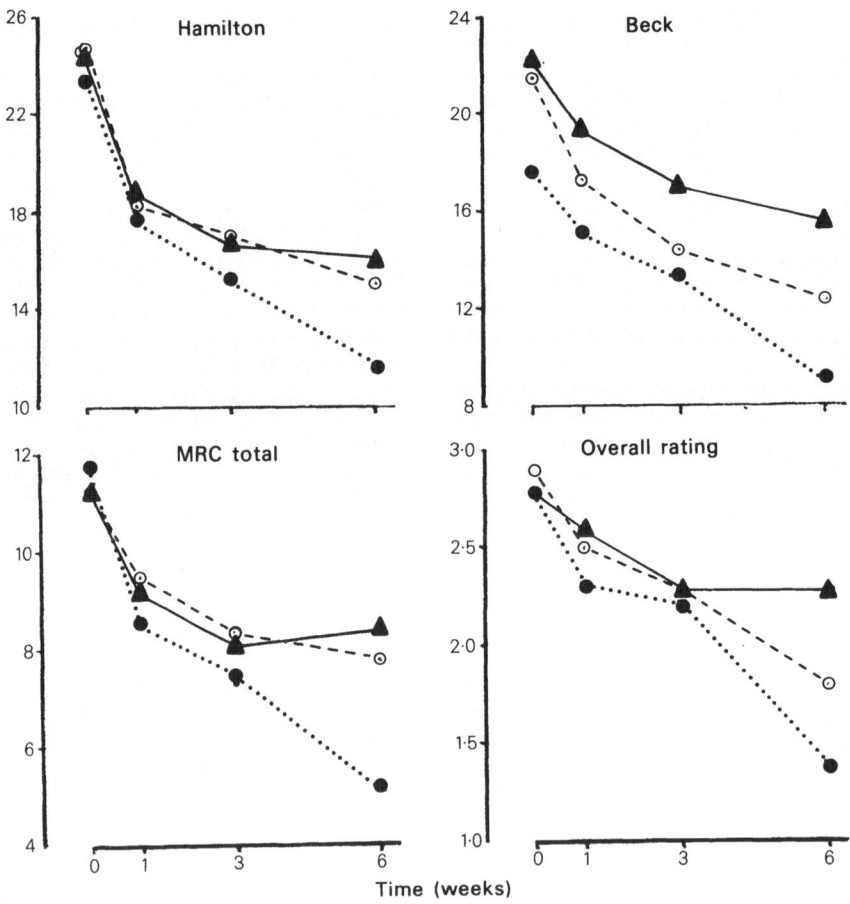

Figure 1 Mean scores for various ratings in groups of depressed patients treated with trimipramine (●········●), a monoamine oxidase inhibitor (O---O) or combined treatment (▲——▲) for 6 weeks.

Table 1 The main source of unreliability in clinical ratings

Source of unreliability	Rating scale	Structured interview	Self-assessment questionnaire
The interviewer's behaviour	May be limited to some extent	Limited by rules for interview	Eliminated
The interviewer's expectations	Largely unaffected	Limited by rules for interview	Eliminated
The interviewer's interpretation of the clinical terms involved	Providing definitions reduces this	Reduced by the provision of definitions	Problem transferred to the patient

analysis. As many psychiatric symptoms and signs cut across syndromes some items may appear on scales purporting to measure different conditions. For example, the Hamilton Depression Rating Scale contains an anxiety item, the Anxiety Scale a depression item. Care must be taken than such items are really appropriate. For example, items assessing depressive symptoms in a primary depressive illness may need modifying to evaluate depressive symptoms in schizophrenic patients. For example, apathy may be confused with retardation.

Care must be taken in drawing up the categories within each item. The grades of severity must follow logically from one to the next with no ambiguities, overlaps or gaps. In some items the severity domain is mixed up with frequency or with social consequences. It is better, despite practical problems, to rate frequency, severity and social effects separately even if a long questionnaire is generated. Preliminary administration of a new rating scale to a pilot sample of patients for whom the instrument was developed will uncover problems both in the item structure and in the logistics of administration.

One debate concerns the number of points which an answer rubric should contain. In general 3–5 points are preferred even for observer ratings; beyond 5, most observers and almost all patients have difficulty distinguishing among the possibilities. Another approach is a 100 mm line, pompously dubbed the visual analogue scale. Patients can usually rate themselves meaningfully on such a line. The advantages of such a line are most apparent with self-ratings of the *intensity* of a symptom. Its *frequency* can usually be rated using operationally defined points such as 'once-daily', etc. The other advantage of a 100 mm line is that it yields ostensibly parametric data. It is doubtful whether this is strictly true but in practice parametric statistics give credible results when used on such data.

Some clinicians are unhappy at the practice of taking scores on the individual items and computing a total score. However, clinicians are doing this intuitively all the time: they consider the various aspects of a patient's pathology but end up with a global assessment upon which they base diagnosis, prognosis and treatment.

Some detail can be retained by using some form of component analysis (Hamilton, 1967). This statistical technique elucidates the structure of the rating scale as it reduces the total number of items to a very few derived component (factor) scores which are sampling secondary factors of the main condition. For example, The Hamilton Anxiety Rating Scale yields a first component which reflects the severity of illness. The second component distinguishes between two different symptom patterns, the somatic and the psychological. These derived components can be useful for assessing treatment factors. Thus, β-adrenoceptor antagonists are more effective against the somatic symptoms of the bipolar second component than the psychological symptoms.

Measurement of improvement

The problem of appropriate statistics has been touched on above. The points on the scales used for each item follow a logical sequence but are not numerically unequal. It is impossible to say whether improvement from point 2 ('moderate') to point 1 ('mild') is the same as from point 3 ('severe') to point 2. Consequently, elaborate statistics on such data strain credulity. However, summing scores to give a total value and then taking difference scores is probably meaningful even if frowned upon by the purist statistician.

A second problem concerns the quantification of a response. Typically, two scores are obtained, before and after treatment. Is the response best measured as a simple difference score, or a percentage change; or by covariance statistics, the variate being the end-score, the covariate the initial score? If the initial scores are not statistically different between groups, analysis can be made on the final scores alone. This also reflects clinical reality. The operational outcome of a treatment e.g., whether a patient is discharged from hospital, returns to full-time work or engages in his hobbies depends on this final score rather than on the degree of improvement. A more sophisticated approach is to use trend analysis.

Observer scales

These are based on a clinical interview of the depressed patient and require skilled personnel. The patient must feel comfortable in the interview situation and not be misled into believing that his treatment or his staying in hospital is decided by his score on the rating scale. Good rapport should be established so that the patient volunteers information about his feelings and symptoms. The interview should be semistructured: if unstructured it tends to become prolix and inconsequential; if too structured the patient may feel restrained from volunteering useful information. Questions should not be asked in rapid-fire succession as this leads the patient to give stereotyped, ill-considered replies. Nor should questions be asked in a desultory way implying that the assessor has no real interest in the replies. And, of course, leading questions must not be asked nor questions phrased in such a way as to reflect any preconceived notions of the questioner nor the social desirability of the answers. During the interview the appearance and behaviour of the patient should be carefully noted. In particular, the form as well as the content of speech should be recorded as psychomotor retardation is often most apparent in speech. Depressed patients with definite retardation or who are deluded and have lost insight present particular problems, and patience and persistence are needed to elicit any worthwhile information.

The original Hamilton Depression Scale was designed for use by two raters simultaneously, the total score being the sum of the two ratings. This also provides a routine assessment of inter-rater reliability. Two statistics should be calculated as a check, the correlation between the two raters over a range of patients and some statistic such as the t-test to detect whether one observer is consistently rating higher or lower than the other. Any such biases should be identified and eradicated by careful discussions between the raters. Video-tapes of the interviews provide a useful technique here.

Rating scales in common use

Hamilton Rating Scale for Depression

This scale is the most widely used observer rating scale comprising 21 items of which 17 are used to calculate the total score (Hamilton, 1960; 1967). The responses are either three-point (absent, mild, severe) or five-point (absent, trivial, mild, moderate, severe), depending on the feasibility of grading the responses coarsely or finely. It is not intended as a diagnostic tool, that is, it should be used only to quantify depressive illnesses. The depressive symptoms are presumed to be part of a depressive syndrome and not secondary to some other condition such as schizophrenia or dementia. The ratings are made on the basis of a semi-structured psychiatric interview. This takes 30–45 minutes to complete on the first occasion but usually only about half this time on subsequent rating occasions when the patient's symptoms are known to the rater. The time span of the rating is the previous few days and care must be taken not to over-emphasize minor fluctuations in mood.

The Hamilton Depression Rating Scale contains many items pertaining to the somatic symptoms of depression and is therefore most appropriate for rating 'endogenous' depressives. Cognitive disturbances are represented but less so than are affective changes. Social malfunctioning is covered by an item relating directly to work and social activities. The last four items of the scale cover diurnal mood variation, derealization—depersonalisation, paranoid symptoms, and obsessive—compulsive phenomena. Hamilton excluded them from the total score because he regarded them either as too infrequent or as reflecting the type of the depression rather than its severity. These items are useful, however, in establishing the symptom profile of the depression for other purposes such as seeking prognostic indicators. Other items

reflecting the features of helplessness, worthlessness and hopelessness are available in some versions of the scale.

As described earlier, the Hamilton scale was originally intended for two raters with their scores totalled. This is not now generally followed because of the exigencies of finding trained personnel with available time. Also, somewhat different versions of the HDRS exist and it is imperative that users describe carefully the version they used in any particular trial. The validity and reliability of the scale has been outlined earlier: it is highly reliable and its validity is more than adequate. It is therefore not surprising that this scale has stood the test of time and remains so popular. It has been translated into many languages.

Other observer scales

Another observer rating scale which has been extant for 20 years is that or Cronholm & Ottosson (1960). It comprises five items concerned with depression, three with retardation, and one with ability for work. Psychological symptoms predominate but no items concern guilt and agitation. It has a high reliability and correlates fairly well with other established scales.

Two widely used scales for general psychopathology contain some items relating to depression. The Inpatient Multidimensional Psychiatric Scale (IMPS) (Lorr, 1974) is an interview-based rating scale consisting of 89 items, 68 on a yes-no basis, the remainder on a 5-point scale. It is designed to measure 12 psychiatric syndromes including anxious depression and motor retardation. It is not easy to apply to the syndromal clusters used in the U.K. The Brief Psychiatric Rating Scale (BPRS) (Overall & Gorham, 1962; Overall, 1974) provides a rapid assessment of a wide range of psychopathology including anxiety and depression. It is useful as an additional wide-range instrument in non-homogeneous groups of patients.

Self-rating scales

The advantages and disadvantages of self-rating scales as compared to observer rating scales have been discussed earlier. Self-rating scales are most useful in assessing patients with mild to moderate degree of depression, with retention of full insight. Patients in general practice are most appropriate especially where large numbers are involved as in large-scale surveys or extensive clinical trials of therapy.

Beck Depression Inventory (BDI)

This American inventory contains 21 items referring to symptoms and attitudes with four ranked statements to each item (Beck, 1967; Beck, Ward, Mendelson, Mock & Erbaugh, 1961). The patient chooses the response which most nearly matches his state at the time. The maximum total score is 62 with scores of 10 or less reflecting no significant clinical depression. The Inventory was originally intended to be read out aloud to the patient by a technician. Almost invariably now it is administered as a self-rating scale, the subject reading the question to himself (Bech et al., 1975).

The BDI has a fair validity (Metcalfe & Goldman, 1965) and acceptable reliability (Beck & Beamesderfer, 1974). However, it is not good at differentiating moderate from severe depression. Bailey & Coppen (1976) compared the Beck and the Hamilton in depressed inpatients. The scales tallied well in about two-thirds of patients but with low or negative relationship in the rest of the patients. The latter resembled their peers with respect to severity of depression, clinical features and personality. The BDI showed less percentage change over time than did the HRSD.

The Beck Depression Inventory, reflecting the country and time of its development, is more psychodynamically-oriented than the Hamilton Scale. Less than a third of the Beck items refer to somatic or behavioural features of depression.

Self-Rating Depression Scale

Zung's (1974) Self-Rating Depression Scale (SDS) is a slight modification of an earlier Zung (1965) scale. It contains 20 items dealing with a wide range of depressive features, rated on a 4-point scale of frequency of occurrence. The maximum total score is 80 which is multiplied by 1.25 to yield a standardised score ranging from 0–100. A score of 50 or more includes 80% of clinically diagnosed depressed patients and only 12% of normals.

Concurrent validity is good with mildly to moderately depressed patients but less impressive with the more severely ill. Thus, the SDS correlated 0.6 with the HRS with general practice depressed patients but only around 0.4 with depressed inpatients and day hospital patients (Carroll, Fielding & Blashki, 1973). The discrepancies were suggested as reflecting the lack of such items as retardation, guilt feelings and hypochondriasis in the Zung Scale, although it is doubtful whether patients with marked features of this kind are capable of rating themselves accurately. The authors criticise the utility of self-rating scales and regard them as mainly suitable for case-finding, i.e., as screening instruments.

Wakefield Self-assessment Depression Inventory

This scale comprises 10 of the 20 Zung scale items plus two concerned with psychological feelings of anxiety. Four-point scales are used (Snaith et al., 1971). It correlates 0.87 with the Hamilton Depression Rating Scale.

General self-rating scales

Several of the general rating scales for psychopathology contain sections pertaining to depressive symptoms. The Hopkins Symptom Check List (HSCL) is designed as a general scale for assessing symptoms in psychiatric outpatients (Derogatis, Lipman & Covi, 1973). It contains 58 items rated on 4-point scales of distress. Factor analyses suggest 5 main areas of psychopathology—somatic symptoms, obsessive-compulsive phenomena, interpersonal sensitivity, depression and anxiety. Test-retest reliability for the depression component was 0.81. The HSCL is sensitive to drug effects (Derogatis et al., 1973).

The Symptom Check List—90 items (SCL-90) is an extension of the Hopkins Scale designed to improve sensitivity to drug effects by including frequency and intensity dimensions (Derogatis, et al., 1973). Five-point scales are used. To the original five factors are added anger/hostility, phobic anxiety, paranoid ideation and psychoticism factors, together with 3 indices of global distress.

The Goldberg (1972) General Health Questionnaire is a screening device for detecting patients with minor psychiatric symptoms either presenting in general practice or in population surveys. Many of the items relate to depression. It is available as a long form (140 items), a shorter form (60 items) and abbreviated versions (12–, 20- and 30-item questionnaires).

Other scales

Other symptom scales include the Depression and Psychasthenia Scales of the Minnesota Multiphasic Personality Inventory (MMPI) (Graham, 1977) and the Depression Scale of the Middlesex Hospital Questionnaire (Crown & Crisp, 1966). The former is more appropriate for assessing personality depressive attributes and the latter is a useful symptomatic scale.

Adjective check lists are useful for assessing feelings and affects but, as these are only a part of morbid depressive phenomena, the checklists are rather restricted in the information obtained. The Depression Adjective Check List of Lubin (1965, 1967), assesses transient mood states as does the Bond & Lader (1974) mood rating scale which uses 100 mm visual analogue scales. Both are more appropriate for work with normal subjects than with depressed patients. The Profile of Mood States (POMS) is a 65-item adjective check-list which yields 6 factors, tension/anxiety, depression/dejection, anxiety/hostility, vigour, fatigue and confusion (McNair, Lorr & Droppleman, 1971). It is a useful screening device but is not very sensitive to change in psychopathology with treatment.

Visual analogue scales are becoming increasingly popular as instruments to measure many phenomena including depressive states. Often such scales are developed *ad hoc* but proper validation and estimation of reliability remains essential. They can be used for both self- and observer-ratings. One advantage with self-rating is that depressed patients, being typically indecisive, may have difficulty in allocating their symptoms to specific categories but can usually cope with an analogue line (Aitken, 1969). Problems with using the scales can usually be overcome by careful initial supervision of the patient. Later sessions are usually trouble-free. Correlations between 100 mm self-ratings of depression, the Zung SDS, the Hamilton Depression Scale and a psychiatrist's global rating are moderately high in newly admitted patients (Zeally & Aitken, 1969; Luria, 1975).

Ward behaviour rating scales are useful for assessing longitudinal changes in severely depressed hospitalized patients, especially those who are incapable of providing much information at interview. Ward ratings made by nurses from their sustained and close observation of the patient may differ substantially from assessments made by psychiatrists from a semi-structured interview. Various scales have been developed at various centres and comparisons between them are sketchy. It is unclear which is the most generally satisfactory scale nor whether any scale has a particular application (Burdock, Hakerem, Hardesty & Zubin, 1960; Green, Bigelow, O'Brien, Stahl & Wyatt, 1977; Hargreaves, 1968; Heninger, French, Slavinsky, Davis & Mueller, 1970; Honigfeld, 1974; Wyatt & Kupfer, 1968).

The Social Adjustment Scale was designed to evaluate social functioning in various treatment programmes (Weissman & Paykel, 1974). Work, family relationships, especially marital and parental roles, and social and leisure activities are covered by its 48 items. Its time-scale covers the previous two months. It has high inter-rater reliability and seems sensitive to change.

Future developments: Computer evaluation

The operational usefulness and practicability of employing rating scales can greatly facilitate the reliable assessment of the effects of medication. A depression self-relating scale is merely one method of helping the doctor to monitor the progress of his patient and to provide data to help him in his clinical management. Questionnaires have been used for many years in research projects but have not been widely employed in routine clinical care in psychiatric clinics or in general practice. Perhaps many doctors feel that the time it takes to rate their patients could be better employed, especially in the busy surgery. However, an automated system to assess the severity of depression, based on the now-ubiquitous and cheap microcomputer, has been developed by one of the author's research groups in the Institute of Psychiatry.

The questionnaire chosen was the Hamilton Depression Rating Scale but modified for self-rating. Existing self-rating scales tend to concentrate on mood disturbance whereas the Hamilton Depression Rating Scale is widely based. Thus, the computer uses the questions asked by the doctor by displaying them on a visual display unit with 3–5 possible answers. Using a computer enabled the inclusion of additional questions on delicate topics such as suicide; similar work in America (Greist, Gustafson, Stauss, Rowse, Laughren & Chiles, 1973) suggests that at initial interview patients more readily admit to symptoms and feelings that they otherwise deny to their doctor. Our preliminary data in general practice confirm this observation.

The results so far obtained on several hundred patients tested in a wide variety of clinical settings, including general practice, are encouraging. Only about 3% of depressed patients were misclassified as not depressed and in all cases these patients were very severely disturbed and self-rating is known to be unreliable. A high and significant positive correlation (0.8) was found between computer-administered self-ratings and global ratings of depression made by doctors.

Using this sort of system which now costs under £2000, the doctor is able to monitor large numbers of patients reliably and accurately and with little expenditure of time. The system is simple enough for untrained staff to operate and supervise and patients appear to enjoy the experience. Because a microcomputer storing data on small discs is used, no distant computer extracts the information and thus confidentiality is maintained.

The most important development of this application of the microcomputer is that large number of patients can be assessed and their data stored, so that new scales can be quickly evaluated. The subsequent improvement in the sensitivity of assessing depression and other psychiatric syndromes should lead to its routine use in clinics and surgeries. Then, optimal treatments based on data gathered in routine clinical situations can be established—something that has been absent from the bulk of psychiatric practice.

Conclusions

The widest application for rating scales is in clinical trials both to categorise the patients studied and to chart their progress. For an all-round observer rating scale for depression, the Hamilton Scale remains the 'best-buy'. The choice for self-rating scales is less satisfactory with the Beck or the Zung Scales probably being the best available. The administration of self-rating scales by microcomputer is a potentially useful development.

I am grateful to Dr. J. Leff and Dr. R. Ancill for helpful comments and discussion.

References

AITKEN, R.C.B. (1969). Measurement of feelings using visual analogue scales. *Proc. Roy. Soc. Med.*, **62**, 989–993.

AKISKAL, H.S. & WEBB, W.L. (1978). *Psychiatric Diagnosis. Exploration of Biological Predictors*, SP Medical and Scientific Books, New York.

BAILEY, J. & COPPEN, A. (1976). A comparison between the Hamilton Rating Scale and the Beck Inventory in the measurement of depression, *Br. J. Psychiatry*, **128**, 486–489.

BECH, P., GRAM, L.F., DEIN, E., JACOBSEN, O., VITGER, J. & BOLWIG, T.G. (1975). Quantitative rating of depressive states. *Acta Psychiat. Scand.*, **51**, 161–170.

BECK, A.T. (1967). Measure of depression: the Depression Inventory. In *Depression: Clinical, Experimental and Theoretical Aspects*. Harper and Row, New York.

BECK, A.T., WARD, C.H., MENDELSON, M., MOCK, J. & ERBAUGH, J. (1961). An inventory for measuring depression. *Arch. gen. Psychiat.*, **4**, 561–571.

BECK, A.T., & BEAMESDERFER, A. (1974). Assessment of depression: the Depression Inventory. *Mod. Probl. Pharmacopsychiatry* **7**, 151–169.

BOND, A. & LADER, M. (1974). The use of analogue scales in rating subjective feelings. *Br. J. med. Psychol.*, **47**, 211–218.

BROWN, G.L. & ZUNG, W.W.K. (1972). Depression scales: self or physician rating? A validation of certain clinically observable phenomena. *Compr. Psychiat.*, **13**, 361–367.

BURDOCK, E.I., HAKEREM, G., HARDESTY, A.S. & ZUBIN, J. (1960). A ward behaviour rating scale for mental hospital patients. *J. clin. Psychol.*, **16**, 246–247.

CARROLL, B.J., FIELDING, J., & BLASHKI, T.G. (1973). Depression rating scales. *Arch. gen. Psychiat.*, **28**, 361–366.

CRONHOLM, B. & OTTOSSON, J.O. (1960). Experimental studies of the therapeutic action of electroconvulsive therapy in endogenous depression. *Acta Psychiat. Scand.*, suppl. **145**, 69–101.

CROWN, S. & CRISP, A.H. (1966). A short clinical diagnostic self-rating scale for psycho-neurotic patients. *Br. J. Psychiat.*, **112**, 917–921.

DEROGATIS, L.R., LIPMAN, R.S. & COVI, L. (1973). SCL-90 an outpatient psychiatric rating scale—preliminary report. *Psychopharmac. Bull.*, **9**, 13–28.

DOWNING, R.W. & RICKELS, K. (1972). Some properties of the Popoff index. *Clin. Med.*, **79**, 11–18.

DSM III (1979). *Diagnostic and Statistical Manual of Mental Disorders*. Third Edition. American Psychiatric Association, 1700 Eighteenth Street, N.W., Washington, D.C. 20009, USA.

GARSIDE, R.F., KAY, D.W.K., ROY, J.R. & BEAMISH, P. (1970). M.P.I. scores and depression. *Br. J. Psychiat.*, **116**, 429–432.

GOLDBERG, D.P. (1972). *The Detection of Psychiatric Illness by Questionnaire. A Technique for the Identification and Assessment of Non-psychotic Psychiatric Illness*. Oxford University Press, London.

GRAHAM, J.R. (1977). *The MMPI: a Practical Guide*. Oxford University Press, New York.

GREEN, R.A., BIGELOW, L., O'BRIEN, P., STAHL, D. & WYATT, R.J. (1977). The Inpatient Behavioural Rating Scale: a 26-item scale for recording nursing observations of patients' mood and behaviour. *Psychol. Rep.*, **40**, 543–549.

GREIST, J.J., GUSTAFSON, D.H., STAUSS, F.F., ROWSE, G.L., LAUGHREN, T.P. & CHILES, J.A. (1973). A computer interview for suicide-risk prediction. *Am. J. Psychiat.* **130**, 1327–1332.

GUY, W. (1976). *ECDEU Assessment Manual for Psychopharmacology*. DHEW Publication No. (ADM) 76–338.

HAMILTON, M. (1960). A rating scale for depression. *J. Neurol. Neurosurg. Psychiat.*, **23**, 56–61.

HAMILTON, M. (1967). Development of a rating scale for primary depressive illness. *Br. J. Soc. clin. Psychol.*, **6**, 278–296.

HARGREAVES, W.A. (1968). Methods for large scale recording of clinical ratings. *J. Psychiatr. Res.*, **6**, 169–174.

HENINGER, G.R., FRENCH, N.H., SLAVINSKY, A.T., DAVIS, L. & MUELLER, P.S. (1970). A short clinical rating scale for use by nursing personnel. II. Reliability, validity, and application. *Arch. gen. Psychiat.*, **23**, 241–248.

HONIGFELD, G. (1974). NOSIE-30: History and current status of its use in pharmacopsychiatric research. *Mod. Probl. Pharmacopsychiatry*, **7**, 238–263.

KENDELL, R.E. (1975). Defining diagnostic criteria for research purposes. In *Methods of Psychiatric Research*, pp. 101–119, eds Sainsbury, P. & Kreitman, N. Second Edition, London: Oxford University Press.

LORR, M. (1974). Assessing psychotic behaviour by the IMPS. *Mod. Probl. Pharmacopsychiatry*, **7**, 50–63.

LUBIN, B. (1965). Adjective checklists for measurement of depression. *Arch. gen. Psychiat.*, **12**, 57–62.

LUBIN, B. (1967). *Depression Adjective Checklists*. Educational and Industrial Testing Service, San Diego.

LURIA, R.E. (1975). The validity and reliability of the visual analogue mood scale. *J. Psychiatr. Res.*, **12**, 51–57.

McNAIR, D.M., LORR, M. & DROPPLEMAN, L.F. (1971). *Profile of Mood States*. Educational and Industrial Testing Services, San Diego.

METCALFE, M. & GOLDMAN, E. (1965). Validation of an inventory for measuring depression. *Br. J. Psychiat.*, **111**, 240–242.

MONTGOMERY, S.A. (1980). Measurement of serum drug levels in the assessment of antidepressants. *Br. J. clin. Pharmac.*, **10**, 411–416.

OVERALL, J.E. (1974). The Brief Psychiatric Rating Scale in psychopharmacology research. *Mod. Probl. Pharmacopsychiatry*, **7**, 67–78.

OVERALL, J.E. & GORHAM, D.R. (1962). The Brief Psychiatric Rating Scale. *Psychol. Rep.*, **10**, 799–812.

PICHOT, P. & OLIVIER-MARTIN, R. (Eds.) (1974). Psychological measurements in psychopharmacology. *Mod. Probl. Pharmacopsychiatry*, **7**.

RAKOFF, V.M., STANCER, H.C. & KEDWARD, H.B. (1977). *Psychiatric Diagnosis*. New York: Brunner/Mazel.

SCHWAB, J.J., BARLOW, M.R. & HOLZER, C.G. (1967). A comparison of two rating scales for depression. *J. clin. Psychol.*, **23**, 94–96.

SNAITH, R.P., AHMED, S.N., METHA, S. & HAMILTON, M. (1971). The assessment of the severity of primary depressive illness. *Psychol. Med.*, **1**, 143–149.

TAN, B.K. (1969). Ein voorlopig onderzoek naar da praktische brulkberheid van drie vertaalde depressieschalen.

Bull. Coord. Comm. Biochem. Onderzooch, **3**, 49–57.

WEISSMAN, M.M. & PAYKEL, E.S. (1974). *The Depressed Woman: A Study of Social Relationships.* University of Chicago Press, Chicago: pp. 234–266.

WYATT, R.J. & KUPFER, D.J. (1968). A fourteen-symptom behavior and mood rating scale for longitudinal patient evaluation by nurses. *Psychol. Rep.,* **23**, 1331–1334.

YOUNG, J.P.R., LADER, M.H. & HUGHES, W.C. (1979). Controlled trial of trimipramine, monoamine oxidase inhibitors, and combined treatment in depressed outpatients. *Br. med. J.,* **2**, 1315–1317.

ZEALLEY, A.K. & AITKEN, R.C.B. (1969). Measurement of mood. *Proc. Roy. Soc. Med.,* **62**, 993–996.

ZUNG, W.W.K. (1965). A self-rating depression scale. *Arch. gen. Psychiat.,* **12**, 63–70.

ZUNG, W.W.K. (1974). The measurement of affects: depression and anxiety. *Mod. Probl. Pharmacopsychiatry,* **7**, 170–188.

ASSESSMENT OF EXTRAPYRAMIDAL DISORDERS

C.D. MARSDEN & M. SCHACHTER

University Department of Neurology,
Institute of Psychiatry and King's
College Hospital Medical School,
Denmark Hill, London SE5

Introduction

In the last twenty years the accurate evaluation of extrapyramidal disorders has become essential to assess the efficacy of an increasing number of potentially useful drugs. Not surprisingly, since the introduction of levodopa, Parkinson's disease has attracted the most attention for developing assessment techniques. It is a common condition, producing a complex and varying pattern of disabilities, and effective treatment is available with which new drugs may be compared. Techniques suitable for use in patients with Parkinson's disease are applicable also to patients with other akinetic-rigid syndromes, but different methods have to be employed to assess the severity and impact of other extrapyramidal diseases which cause abnormal involuntary movements (dyskinesias). The many types and causes of the extrapyramidal disorders under consideration are shown in Table 1.

The problem with all these conditions is that there is no simple sensitive technique for quantifying their severity. This is not surprising, for all the diseases in question are characterised primarily by difficulty in movement, which inevitably interferes with a wide range of bodily actions and activities of daily living. To judge the impact of such disorders on function requires a battery of observations or tests. Such an approach gives a satisfactory global impression of the severity of an extrapyramidal disorder, but inevitably it restricts the scope of each individual observation. The time available and the patient's resilience puts a limit on how long a reasonable assessment may take. Many sophisticated techniques have been derived for quantifying individual items of extrapyramidal disorders, for example tremor or rigidity, but frequently the time involved is too great to allow such methods to be included within a general battery of observations designed to obtain a global impression of disease severity.

For these and other reasons, clinical pharmacologists have approached extrapyramidal diseases in two different ways, depending upon the particular questions being asked. On the one hand, simple, rapid clinical scoring systems of symptoms, signs and dis-ability are employed to establish whether a new pharmacological agent is of value in the treatment of a disease. On the other hand, the more sophisticated quantitative techniques are suitable for studies where more specific problems of pharmacology or pathophysiology are to be examined.

This review will attempt a comprehensive summary of existing methods for the assessment of extrapyramidal diseases. The emphasis throughout will be on the applicability of these techniques to the investigation of new forms of treatment for these disorders.

Parkinson's disease

Introduction

There is a very large and growing literature on the assessment of Parkinsonism. Two approaches have been employed:

(a) subjective assessment, generally based on rating scales of symptoms and signs, or of functional disability, or both;

(b) objective methods of two types: relatively simple tests, most often based on the timing of specific tasks, and more complex neurophysiological investigations designed to measure particular motor abnormalities (Table 2).

Many investigators have used a combination of subjective and simple objective tests, and it is logical to consider these together. Neurophysiological techniques, on the other hand, usually have been developed independently.

Subjective assessment

Table 3 lists the principal subjective rating systems described in studies on Parkinson's disease. Most were developed when levodopa was introduced and the need for such techniques become a matter of urgency.

Assessment systems which concentrated on functional disability usually were developed separately.

Table 1 Extrapyramidal disorders and their causes

A. Kinetic-rigid syndromes
'Pure Parkinsonism
  Idiopathic Parkinson's disease
  Post-encephalitic Parkinsonism
  Drug-induced Parkinsonism
Parkinsonism of early onset, with other signs
  Wilson's disease
  Huntington's disease (rigid type)
  Hallervorden-Spatz disease
  Progressive pallidal atrophy
Parkinsonism of late onset, with other signs
  Progressive supranuclear palsy
  Strio-nigral degeneration   ⎫
  Shy-Drager syndrome   ⎬ Multi-system
  Olivo-ponto-cerebellar degeneration ⎭ degenerations

Parkinsonism of late onset, due to diffuse brain disease
  Alzheimer's disease
  Pick's disease
  Multi-infarct dementia
  Creutzfeldt-Jakob disease
Parkinsonism, onset at any age, with diffuse brain damage
  Trauma
  Cerebral anoxia (including carbon monoxide poisioning)
  Manganese poisoning
  Neurosyphilis

B. Dyskinesias
1. *Chorea*
  Huntington's disease
  Senile chorea
  Sydenham's chorea
  Chorea gravidarum
  Thyrotoxicosis
  Systemic lupus erythematosus
  Polycythaemia rubra vera
  Encephalitis lethargica
  Drugs (neuroleptics, phenytoin, contraceptive pill)

2. *Dystonia*
  Idiopathic dystonia musculorum deformans
  Paroxysmal dystonia (paroxysmal choreoathetosis)
  Dystonia with marked diurnal variation
  Wilson's disease
  Huntington's disease (juvenile type)
  Lesch-Nyhan syndrome
  Athetoid cerebral palsy
  Hallervorden-Spatz disease
  Drugs (neuroleptics, metoclopramide)

3. *Tremor*
  Rest tremor
  Parkinsonism (idiopathic, post-encephalitic, drug-
    induced)
  Postural tremor
  Physiological (exaggerated in thyrotoxicosis and anxiety
    states, and by alcohol and drugs)
  Benign essential (familial) tremor
  Wilson's disease
  Severe cerebellar lesions
  Neurosyphilis
  Intention (action) tremor
  Brain stem or cerebellar disease (multiple sclerosis,
    spinocerebellar degenerations, vascular disease,
    tumours)

4. *Myoclonus*
  Idiopathic benign essential (familial) myoclonus
  Idiopathic epilepsy
  Progressive myoclonic epilepsy (familial, Lafora body
    disease, lipidoses, spinocerebellar degenerations)
  Metabolic disturbances (with or without seizures) (renal
    failure, hepatic failure, respiratory failure)
  Drug withdrawal (alcohol, barbiturates)
  Structural brain disease (without seizures) (post-anoxic,
    subacute sclerosing panencephalitis, Creutzfeldt-
    Jakob disease, encephalitis lethargica)

5. *Tics*
  Simple benign tics of childhood
  Simple persisting tics
  Complex tics
  Complex tics with vocalisation ⎫
  Complex with coprolalia   ⎬ Gilles de la Tourette's syndrome

C. Drug-induced syndromes
  Parkinsonism
  Reserpine and tetrabenazine; phenothiazines and other
    neuroleptics
  Tremor
  As for Parkinsonism, and β-adrenergic receptor
    agonists, tricyclic anti-depressants, lithium
  Akathisia
  Reserpine and tetrabenazine; neuroleptics
  Acute dystonia
  Neuroleptics, metoclopramide, diazoxide
  Tardive dyskinesia
  Neuroleptics

Table 2 Features of Parkinson's disease and appropriate modes of assessment

	Subjective assessment	Simple objective assessment[1]	Complex objective assessment[2]
Major motor signs and symptoms			
Tremor	+		+
Rigidity	+		+
Akinesia	+	+	+
Postural abnormalities	+		+
Other motor signs and symptoms			
Dysarthria	+	+	
Dysphagia	+		
Autonomic signs and symptoms			
Hypersalivation	+		+
Seborrhoea	+		
Postural hypotension		+	
Constipation	+		
Urinary frequency/ incontinence	+	+	

[1] Simple objective assessment requiring no specialised apparatus beyond stopwatch, tape-measure, pegboard, sphygmomanometer, tape-recorder, etc.
[2] Complex methods requiring specialised mechanical, electrical or electronic devices and sometimes requiring computing facilities for analysis.

Karnofsky's scale (Karnofsky, Burchenal, Armistead, Southam, Bernstein, Craver & Rhoads, 1951), originally used in evaluating the response to cancer chemotherapy, rated normality as 100% with proportional decrements for increasing disability. Riklan & Diller (1956) described a 98-item scale listing various activities of daily living, but this did not prove reliable, or feasible. By contrast the North-Western University Disability Scale (Canter, de la Torre & Mier, 1961) has been used very widely; it consists of 5 or 10 point rating scales for walking, dressing, hygiene, feeding and speech, based on clearly defined criteria (Appendix 3). A popular and very simple method of staging Parkinson's disease was described by Hoehn & Yahr (1967) (Appendix 1). The scale provides a generally accepted basis for assessing the severity of Parkinsonism, and Lieberman, Dziatolowki, Gopinathan, Kopersmith, Neophytides & Korein (1980) have noted a good correlation between Hoehn & Yahr's (1967) staging and more detailed scoring systems. However, such staging is relatively insensitive to changes in the patient's clinical state. McDowell, Lee, Swift, Sweet, Ogsbury & Tessler (1970) described a combined rating scale for symptoms and signs and for functional disability which was unusual in assigning weighting factors for each item in the scale; for instance, akinesia was given a weighting of 9, seborrhoea 2, walking difficulties 10, and difficulty in bathing 5. Treciokas, Ansel & Markham (1971) also employed weighting, but the concept has not been adopted widely.

Some investigators developed combined subjective rating scales with simple objective tests of motor function (for example, Godwin-Austen, Tomlinson, Frears & Kok, 1969; Parkes, Zilkha, Marsden, Baxter

Table 3 Rating scales in Parkinson's disease

	Subjective rating		Objective assessment	
	Symptoms and signs	Functional disability	Simple	Complex
Webster (1968)	+			
Alba *et al.* (1968)[1]	+			
Duvoisin (1969)[2]	+			
Klawans & Garvin (1969)	+			
Parkes *et al.* (1970a,b)[3]	+	+		
Cotzias *et al.* (1970)	+			
Rinne *et al.* (1970)	+	+		
McDowell *et al.* (1970)	+	+		
Anden *et al.* (1970)	+	+	+	+
Treciokas *et al.* (1971)	+	+		
Birkmayer & Neumayer (1972)	+	+		
Lhermitte *et al.* (1978)	+	+		
Lieberman *et al.* (1980)	+	+	+	

[1] New York University Rating Scale, but may be superseded by Lieberman *et al.* (1980) rating system from the same institution.
[2] Columbia University Rating Scale.
[3] King's College Hospital Rating Scale.

& Knill-Jones, 1970b). The most frequently used tests involved peg-boards, the measurement of walking speed and of the time taken to put on mittens or socks. In a series of papers Schwab and his colleagues (Schwab & Prichard, 1951; England & Schwab, 1956; Schwab, 1960) described a similar approach, and also used a rating scale for functional disability but not for symptoms and signs.

Others have been even more ambitious. Anden, Carlsson, Kerstell, Magnusson, Olsson, Roos, Steen, Steg, Svanborg, Thieme & Werdinius (1970) used a wide-ranging scheme of assessment, intended to evaluate the effects of treatment on severely disabled in-patients. While noting changes in tremor, rigidity and functional disability as well as the time taken to perform specific tasks, these workers recorded standardised movement patterns on cine film, and a tracking device was used to quantify akinesia. Probably the most elaborated combination of objective tests, both simple and complex, was that described by Potvin & Tourtelotte (1975). This was designed for general neurological assessment, rather than specifically for evaluating Parkinsonism. The full examination was said to take 2.5 h for a moderately disabled patient, and it has not been considered suitable for routine use.

Most of the methods described so far were applied successfully to demonstrate the therapeutic action of levodopa and other anti-Parkinsonian drugs in the late 1960s and early 1970s. At that time it was sufficient to assess a patient at any time of day, at infrequent intervals during therapy. Benefit was more or less sustained, so the timing of assessment was not particularly critical. Long-term treatment with levodopa, however, has led to a problem that was not foreseen when these techniques were devised. An increasing number of patients on levodopa have developed 'on-off' phenomena of 'swinging', terms which refer to fluctuations in response (Marsden & Parkes, 1976). Periods of normal mobility often with dyskinesia ('on'), alternate with periods of severe akinesia ('off'). The timing of each of these phases may be related to when the drugs are administered, but is often random and unpredictable; in the most extreme cases these fluctuations can occur within minutes or even seconds. This phenomenon must be distinguished from the well-known variation in Parkinsonian symptoms with emotion, and from the sudden 'freezing episodes' (akinesia paradoxica) which Parkinson described in his original account. To assess new drugs it is now essential to quantify 'on-off' effects. Several methods have been devised in an attempt to do this.

Frequent ratings by a doctor can be used, but these necessarily give only a general impression of the patient's clinical state, and are exceptionally time-consuming. The alternative is to ask the patient, with the help of his family if necessary, to score their own mobility and side-effects. This is done either at fixed intervals throughout the day, or when the patient detects some change in his own condition. Several similar self-rating scales have now been described (Kartzinel & Calne, 1976; Lees, Shaw, Kohout, Stern, Elsworth, Sandler & Youdim, 1977; Lieberman et al., 1980; Schachter, Marsden, Parkes, Jenner & Testa 1980). Kartzinel & Calne (1976) calculated mean daily Parkinsonism and dyskinesia scores, while Lees et al. (1977) and Schachter et al. (1980) used mean hourly mobility and dyskinesia scores. Lieberman et al. (1980) and Schachter et al. (1980) both emphasised the importance of the total time each day occupied by 'off' periods, that is, the time spent immobile during the average day.

Objective and neurophysiological methods

Techniques have been developed for the assessment of each of the major clinical features of Parkinsonism.

(a) *Tremor* The earliest devices for the recording and measurement of tremor were designed in the 1880s by Charcot and several German neurologists (reviewed by Boshes, Wachs, Brumlik, Mier & Petrovick, 1960). The apparatus, known as a tambour, transmitted tremor in one plane to a recording device through a number of pneumatic and mechanical components. Optical recording systems were developed some forty years later (Beall, 1925). These techniques have been largely superseded in recent years by methods based on EMG recordings and accelerometry, frequently combined with computer analysis such as Fourier frequency analysis. For example, Schwab & Prichard (1951) and Burns & de Jong (1960) used EMG recordings, while Calne & Lader (1969) analysed similar recordings with a computer, as more recently did Teravainen & Calne (1979). The latter, however, commented that this approach was better suited to the analysis of neurophysiological problems than to the evaluation of drug therapy.

Accelerometry was introduced by Agate, Doshay & Curtis (1956), and has been employed frequently since then (Wachs & Boshes, 1961; Owen & Marsden, 1965; Velasco & Velasco, 1973; Potvin & Tourtelotte, 1975; Oppel & Umbach, 1977). Accelerometry is relatively simple, it is reliable, and causes little inconvenience to the patient. However, the method as originally described has two major limitations. Firstly, tremor is only measured in a single plane, and the 'total' tremor therefore can be considerably underestimated. Clarke, Hay & Vas (1966) and Salzer (1972) described methods for recording tremor in three dimensions, but their techniques have not been used widely. More recently, several investigators have devised apparatus for computerised triaxial accelerometry (Dietrichson, Langbretson & Houland, 1978; Teravainen & Calne, 1979; Stuart, Gopinathan,

Teravainen, Dambrosia, Ward, Sanes, Evarts & Calne, 1980; Jankovic & Frost, 1980). Secondly, there is considerably variability of all types of tremor, and particularly that of Parkinson's disease which is notoriously susceptible to stress and to other emotional influences. Prolonged recording therefore is desirable, but difficult to achieve with most of the systems mentioned. Owen & Marsden (1965) and also Cowall, Marsden & Owen (1965) used single-plane accelerometry combined with telemetry to obtain several hours of recording from each patient so as to assess the effect of β-adrenoceptor blockers on tremor. Although triaxial accelerometry and telemetry have not yet been combined, advances in electronics now make such studies feasible.

(b) *Rigidity* The earliest methods measured the force required to flex a voluntarily relaxed limb through a fixed distance (Boshes *et al.*, 1960). Measurements usually were made in the horizontal rather than the vertical plane (la Joie & Gersten, 1956). A constant velocity of limb movement was employed subsequently to eliminate inertial factors. Thus, Agate *et al.* (1956) measured the torque by which the patient passively resisted a constant-velocity extension of the elbow joint. Boshes *et al.* (1960) and Brumlik & Boshes (1960) used an electric motor to move the forearm alternately through a fixed distance of flexion and extension. Webster refined this technique by designing a servo-controlled electronic device to perform this manoeuvre at a constant angular velocity (Webster, 1959, 1964, 1966). His studies also established that the area of the hysteresis loop of torque versus displacement of the forearm, averaged over several cycles of flexion and extension, was a more accurate measure of rigidity than the torque required to extend the arm. Webster & Mortimer (1977) used this method, with computer analysis, to evaluate the effect of levodopa on rigidity. A somewhat similar approach, with passive movement of the finger rather than the forearm, was described in the early 1960s (Wright & Johns, 1960; Long, Thomas & Crochetiere, 1964), but apparently has not been developed further.

There has been considerable interest in the relationship between Parkinsonian rigidity and stretch-reflex responses, especially those of long latency (Marsden *et al.*, 1978). Lee & Tatton (1975) and Tatton & Lee (1975) reported that the long latency responses to sudden stretch of the wrist flexors and extensors of Parkinsonian patients were increased in amplitude. Mortimer & Webster (1979) have reported similar findings in the biceps and triceps brachii. They also demonstrated a linear relationship between the magnitude of the biceps long-latency response and the degree of activated rigidity (that is, rigidity measured while the limb was performing a voluntary movement). Lee & Tatton (1978) showed that the amplitude of the reflex diminished when rigidity was

alleviated by levodopa. However, Teravainen & Calne (1980) found considerable overlap between responses in normal and Parkinsonian subjects on testing the biceps reflex, and Marsden, Merton, Morton & Adam (1978) were unable to find any change in the long latency responses evoked by fast stretching of the long thumb flexor of Parkinsonian patients. It is clear that long-latency responses to stretch, while of great neurophysiological interest, are not a substitute for more direct measurements of rigidity.

(c) *Akinesia and hypokinesia* Tremor and rigidity are relatively easy to assess and quantify, since each is essentially a single variable. This is not true of akinesia and hypokinesia, which are difficult even to define precisely. Several components of akinesia can be measured separately: (i) reaction time (the interval between a stimulus and a motor response), (ii) movement time (the time taken to complete a movement), (iii) the rate of repetition of alternating movements, and (iv) the speed and precision of complex movements using one or both hands. Some of the tests are easy to devise and standardise, while others pose greater difficulties.

Although most studies agree that reaction time is prolonged by 25–30% in Parkinsonian patients, there is an overlap with that of normal subjects. Both visual (Barbeau, 1966; Potvin & Tourtelotte, 1975; Heilman, Bowers, Watson & Greer, 1976) and auditory stimuli (Velasco & Velasco, 1973) have been employed as cues for releasing a switch. More commonly a tracking task is used. Moving targets on an oscilloscope screen are followed by using the arm or hand to manipulate a lever or joy-stick (Anden *et al.*, 1970; Angel, Alston & Higgins, 1970; Cassell, Shaw & Stern, 1973; Flowers, 1975, 1976; Potvin & Tourtelotte, 1975). A few studies have compared reaction times in Parkinsonian patients before and after treatment (Draper & Johns, 1960; Angel *et al.*, 1971; Velasco & Velasco, 1973). There was a tendency for reaction times to diminish with levodopa therapy in the last two papers cited, but the differences were not statistically significant.

Movement times have been studied by many investigators using the same apparatus as employed to measure reaction times (Barbeau, 1966; Flowers, 1975, 1976). Flowers (1976) noted that movement time in Parkinson's disease is almost always longer than reaction time in individual subjects, that movement velocity is reduced for all amplitudes of movement, and that tracking error increases disproportionately as the velocity of the target is increased. As might be expected, movement time is more abnormal when the amplitude of movement is large. Velasco & Velasco (1973) reported marked improvement in movement time in some, but not all, patients after levodopa therapy. Teravainen & Calne (1980) confirmed these findings, using a test-system which involved greater use of proximal shoulder-girdle muscles (the hand had to be moved between two targets 32 cm apart), and noted little change in reaction time. They found good correlation between movement time and clinical estimates of akinesia, and conclude that proximal movement time was the best index of this feature of Parkinsonism.

Several subjective rating scales include a score of the ease and speed of rapid alternate movements, especially pronation-supination (Webster, 1968; Parkes, Zilkha, Calver & Knill-Jones, 1970a). Pronation-supination has also been timed (Draper & Johns, 1964; Parkes *et al.*, 1970b; Knutson & Mortenson, 1971; Evarts, Teravainen, Beuchart & Calne, 1979; Teravainen & Calne, 1980). Parkinsonian patients generally were slower than normal controls, and the speed of movement increased with treatment. This improvement did not always correlate well with the observer's subjective assessment. Nor is there necessarily a close correlation between the time taken for single movements and that taken for alternating movements (Flowers, 1976; Teravainen & Calne, 1980).

Tests involving rapid tapping also have been used as estimates of alternating movement speed (Velasco & Velasco, 1973; Cassell *et al.*, 1973; Potvin & Tourtelotte, 1975), but are considered less satisfactory indicators of clinical state than those involving pronation-supination. More complex tapping tasks have been employed to assess the precision of movements rather than their speed (Perret, 1968; Perret, Eggensberger & Siegfried, 1970; Cassel *et al.*, 1973). Peg-board tests have been devised for the same purpose (Godwin-Austen *et al.*, 1969; Parkes *et al.*, 1970b; Cassell *et al.*, 1973; Velasco & Velasco, 1973). The use of timed tasks such as putting on socks and drawing circles, has been described in the previous section. The time taken to walk a set distance, and the number of steps taken, also appear to be accurate indices of hypokinesia; Stuart *et al.* (1980) have automated this test by using a mat with sensors on which the patient walks.

It is reasonable to ask to what extent these ingenious procedures provide a helpful estimate of functional disability, superior to that obtained by simpler methods. In general, they offer few advantages from this point of view, and most are likely to remain within the scope of investigative neurophysiology rather than clinical pharmacology. Nevertheless, a battery of simple largely automated tests, such as that describe by Jankovic & Frost (1980) may become more widely used, though even this was employed in conjunction with subjective scoring methods.

Conclusion

In designing a protocol for the evaluation of an anti-Parkinsonian drug, we recommend the following methods of assessment:

(a) The Hoehn & Yahr (1967) staging system (Appendix 1)

(b) The Webster rating scale for symptoms and signs (Appendix 2)

(c) The North-Western University Disability Scale (Appendix 3)

It may also be necessary to use one of the 'on-off' self-rating schemes (for example, that of Lees *et al.*, 1977) and a dyskinesia rating scale (to be discussed below). A small number of simple objective tests also may be added; for example, the time taken to walk a measured distance; the time to sit down and stand up a number of times, and a pegboard-test. As a simpler alternative to the latter, the patient may be asked to pile plastic counters on top of one another in a measured period. Taken together, the above procedures give a very comprehensive estimate of the severity and impact of Parkinsonism.

Dyskinesias

Introduction

Less attention has been given to the development of techniques for assessing the various dyskinesis encountered as a result of extrapyramidal disease. This reflects the great difficulty in characterising the many bizarre abnormal movements encountered in these conditions, and lack of knowledge as to their basic pathophysiology. In general, two approaches have been adopted. On the one hand, some workers have utilised subjective assessment of the intensity and distribution of the dyskinesias. Others, in contrast, have concentrated on more objective methods of recording abnormal movements.

Subjective techniques

The severity of a dyskinesia may be expressed in very simple terms, for example as mild, moderate or severe, or may be defined by more extensive and complex rating scales. The latter can take into account not only the severity of the abnormal movement at a given site, but can also document the movements at various sites throughout the body. Both approaches have been used to rate a number of dyskinesias, but there is no general agreement as to whether complex rating scales are more efficient or sensitive than simpler techniques. However, our own experience would suggest that rating dyskinesias at different body sites (face, neck, trunk, each arm and each leg) on a simple 0–3 scale (nil, mild, moderate and severe) is the most satisfactory way of approaching the problem. Such subjective rating takes little time and is relatively easily accomplished.

Such a simple subjective rating scale, however, does not take into account one of the major difficulties in assessing dyskinesias, namely the fact that they may occur intermittently. This problem may be approached by rating dyskinesias at each body site not only for their severity, but also for the frequency (occasional, frequent or continuous). Multiplication of the severity factor by the frequency factor gives a score for overall dyskinesias at each body site, which may be summed for all the sites examined to give a global subjective rating score for the severity of a given abnormal movement.

Another question to be considered is whether to rate abnormal movements with the patient in front of one, or whether to take a filmed or videotaped record of the patient for subsequent analysis. Both techniques have advantages and disadvantages. To have the patient in view makes it easier to decide on the significance of the given abnormal movement, and enables the observer to prolong the interview or instruct the patient to undertake certain acts which may resolve ambiguity as to whether a movement is abnormal or not. Unfortunately, it is often difficult to avoid picking up clues as to what treatment a patient may be taking in the course of such a live subjective assessment. Even the timing of the assessment in the course of a known clinical trial may give some clue as to the nature of the treatment being administered at that instant.

Filming or videotaping avoids many of these problems but introduces others (see Table 4). It is much easier to ensure that the raters are quite 'blind' as to treatment at the time when they undertake their assessment, and of course it is possible for a number of raters to examine a given patient's filmed or videotaped record on a number of occasions. The difficulty, however, is in deciding from film or videotape alone whether a given movement really is abnormal or not! Unless a sound-track is available, impromptu speech closely resembles oro-facial dyskinesias, and expressive gesticulation may be misinterpreted as abnormal movements of the limbs. Even with a sound-track it is often difficult to be certain as to the nature of what one witnesses.

Unfortunately, as yet there have been few useful studies comparing the various techniques of rating dyskinesias for inter-rater reliability, reproducibility, and sensitivity to change. Until such information is available, it is impossible to decide on whether to rely on live interview or videotaped recording.

Functional assessment

As in the case of Parkinson's disease, subjective, or even objective assessment of the incidence, frequency and severity of abnormal movements may give little information on their functional impact. This is what disturbs the patient, in terms of therapeutic gain, and changes in functional disability produced by treatment are much more significant than changes in the intensity of abnormal movements. For this reason, most investigators are now supplementing assessments of the dyskinesias with functional assessments of disability. By analogy with Parkinson's disease, rating scales of function have been developed for Huntington's disease and dystonia. Furthermore, again akin to Parkinson's disease, simple systems of staging the severity of illness have been developed for these two conditions.

A more accurate picture of the severity of diseases causing dyskinesias is obtained by rating the abnormal movements themselves, the functional disability they produce, and the stage of severity of the disease.

Objective assessment

Many dyskinesias interfere with manual dexterity and gait, so simple objective timed tests of motor acts

Table 4   Audiovisual recordings in the assessment of dyskinesias

Advantages	Disadvantages
Permanent record	Cost of apparatus
Opportunity for repeated assessment by several observers	Time needed to set up apparatus and record
Observers can be truly ignorant of treatment and side-effects	Difficulty in distinguishing normal from abnormal movements or speech
Sequences can be randomised to ensure blind rating	Impossible to prolong observation period in case of doubt
Sequences can be used to train raters and validate rating scales	Impossible to ask patient to undertake tasks which may resolve ambiguities or provoke dyskinesias
	Visual recording in two dimensions only

such as finger tapping, performance on a peg board, and walking have been employed.

More complex methods of objectively recording dyskinesias have not been developed to any great extent. The tambours used to record tremor (described above) also were employed to record abnormal movements of other kinds, and subsequently accelerometers have been employed for the same purpose. Unfortunately, the unpredictability of most dyskinesias and their considerable variability from moment to moment have not encouraged extensive use of techniques such as these for pharmacological research. Nor have other methods such as the use of flash lights attached to the body combined with time lapse photography, or electromyographic recording of individual muscle contractions responsible for abnormal movements, gained widespread favour. Technical advances in the future may improve the reliability and sensitivity of objective methods of recording abnormal involuntary movements, but at present clinical pharmacologists rely mainly upon subjective assessment perhaps coupled with very simple timing tests.

Huntington's disease

Introduction

The concept of neurotransmitter imbalance, which has proved so rewarding in the treatment of Parkinsonism, has greatly encouraged therapeutic research in Huntington's disease (Urquhart, Perry & Hansen, 1975; Enna, Stern, Wastek & Yamamura, 1977). Only the motor aspects of the disease will be considered here; the neuropsychiatric manifestations have been reviewed recently elsewhere (see Chase, Wexler & Barbeau, 1979).

Assessment

The simplest assessments have been by rating scales. A relatively crude global rating of the characteristic movements as worse, unchanged, moderately improved and/or markedly improved in response to treatment has been used by some workers (Swash, Roberts, Zakko & Heathfield, 1972; Perry, Wright, Hansen & Macleod, 1979), supplemented by film and videotape recordings in other studies (Barr, Heinze, Mendoza & Perlik, 1978). Most investigators, however, have preferred more elaborate assessment schemes. Shoulson, Goldblatt, Charlton & Joynt (1978) recorded chorea on a 5-point scale and also scored activities of daily living—eating, dressing, bathing, sleeping and speech to establish the degree of disability. Of course, the latter is influenced by both neuropsychiatric and purely motor problems. Shoulson et al. (1978) also counted the number of finger taps performed in a set time, and the time taken to walk a fixed distance. McLellan, Chalmers & Johnson (1974) supplemented global and regional rating scales with tests of manual dexterity (such as handwriting, a peg-board test, and the time taken to pile up a given number of counters).

In the study of Barr et al. (1978), elements of all these approaches were combined. The patients' movements were filmed and rated 'double-blind'. Handwriting, a peg-board test, finger tapping and bead-stringing were used to assess aspects of manual dexterity. The degree of disability in walking and bathing were also noted. Shoulson & Fahn (1979) have proposed a scheme for staging the severity of Huntington's disease based upon functional disability (Appendix 4). By allocating scores to the individual items of functional capacity in everyday affairs, the same authors have provided a functional disability scale for Huntington's disease (Appendix 5).

Fahn & Lhermitte (unpublished observations) also have devised a scoring scale for the severity of chorea in Huntington's disease, a scale which we have modified in the light of our own experience (Appendix 6). While this scale will give a reasonable estimate of the severity of chorea, other psychological tests are required to estimate the severity of associated personality change and cognitive impairment in Huntington's disease.

Klawans, Rubovits, Ringel & Weiner (1972) employed a very different approach to assessment, which Klawans & Rubovits (1974) have also used in tardive dyskinesia research (see below). The duration of sustained tongue protrusion and eye closure were recorded. The patient was asked to draw an Archimedes screw, and time-lapse photographs were taken in a darkened room, with flashlights attached to the patient's hands. However, it is difficult to present such photographic records in quantitive terms.

Instrumental methods have played little part in the assessment of Huntington's chorea. Petajan, Jarcho & Thurman (1979) have recently suggested that the degree of control of single motor unit activity, using an audiovisual feedback technique, may be a predictive test in Huntington's disease. However, this claim has not been substantiated by adequate follow-up, and the advisability of predictive tests in this disease, at the present time, is questionable. Witzman et al. (1976) quantified abnormal movements in Huntington's disease by power spectrum analysis of the EMG. There appear to be no tracking studies in this disease, analogous to those in Parkinsonism, and very little use of accelerometry (Falek, 1969).

Conclusion

Shoulson & Fahn's (1979) staging system (Appendix 4) and the disability scale derived from it (Appendix 5) are sensitive indicators of functional impairment, while Marsden and Quinn's chorea rating (Appendix 6) is a reasonable estimate of the severity. A simple timed test, such as the duration of tongue protrusion, may be added to the evaluation. Separate tests for personality and cognitive change also are required to assess the full severity of the illness.

Torsion dystonia

Introduction

Torsion dystonia presents in many ways. In children the disease frequently is hereditary, especially among Ashkenazim Jews. When the illness begins in early life it commonly spreads to involve most parts of the body to produce the disabling generalised torsion dystonia known as dystonia musculorum deformans. In adults, the illness usually is sporadic and remains localised to one particular body part. Such focal dystonias include spasmodic torticollis, writer's cramp, and cranial dystonia in the form of blepharospasm and oro-mandibular dystonia.

All types of this illness are difficult to treat. The problem is that drugs have a very variable effect, and no particular therapeutic agent can be relied upon to be of benefit in an individual patient (Marsden & Harrison, 1974). It is necessary to try a range of drugs in sequence to discover which, if any, may help. Frequently, such drug trials are confused by the great tendency for the severity of this disease to wax and wane spontaneously. The intensity of dystonic muscle spasms is very variable, and is influenced considerably by the emotional state of the patient. This introduces considerable difficulty in assessment of any new form of treatment. In fact, there has been little formal clinical pharmacological study of this group of illnesses, and as a result there have been few attempts to develop standardised, reliable means of assessment.

Assessment

Marsden & Fahn (unpublished observations) have developed a staging system, and a rating scale for assessing the severity of generalised dystonia and its functional impact (see Appendix 7, 8 and 9). Like other rating scales for assessing extrapyramidal disease, this is based on scoring the severity of movement at different sites of the body, severity being judged on the basis of the product of the intensity of the movement and the circumstances in which it occurs. In addition, functional capacity is rated subjectively. We have found this scoring system reasonably reliable and sensitive in the assessment of drugs in generalised dystonia, although modification with future experience may become necessary.

With regard to the various focal dystonias, even less information is available on their assessment.

Couch (1976) has described a simple arbitrary rating scale for the frequency and severity of spasmodic torticollis, grading frequency as absent (0), occasional (1), intermittent, occurring less than 50% of the time (2), intermittent, occurring 50–80% of the time (3) and continuous (4). Severity was graded as absent (0), mild (1), moderate (2), severe (3), and very severe and incapacitating (4). Such rating was undertaken during a 10–15 minute interview, and subsequently was supplemented by similar rating of filmed records. Korein, Brodny, Grynbaum, Sachs-Frankel, Weisinger & Levidow (1976) have been one of the few groups to explore objective electromyographic techniques for the measurement (and treatment) of spasmodic torticollis. However, they too relied upon rating of videotape recordings for evaluating the response to therapy.

Recently Marsden, Sheehy & Lang (unpublished observations) have introduced subjective assessment scales for rating two other focal dystonias, namely cranial dystonia (Brueghel's syndrome or Meige's disease) (Appendix 10) and dystonic writer's cramp (Appendix 11).

There have been few other studies of the objective measurement of torsion dystonia, and further work is necessary to explore such methods.

Myoclonus

Myoclonus is a feature of many neurological conditions. It is characterised by generalised or localised, involuntary, very brief muscular contractions. Relatively successful treatment is now available for some forms of myoclonus and has stimulated further therapeutic interest. Electrophysiological techniques have been employed more frequently than in most other extrapyramidal disorders, but rating scales have usually been used in parallel. Chadwick, Harris, Jenner, Reynolds & Marsden (1975) rated co-ordination, speech, gait and handwriting on four-point scales. Van Woert, Rosenbaum, Howieson & Bowers (1977) scored myoclonic jerks on a five-point scale, according to their severity and frequency, and rated speech, handwriting, walking and dressing on similar scales. The patient's movements and speech were recorded on film and tape. Growdon, Young & Shahari (1976) rated the severity of the myoclonus observed when the patient performed certain set movements, such as standing with the arms outstretched, and also used films, surface EMG and accelerometric recordings.

The most comprehensive assessment protocol in myoclonus was described by Chadwick, Hallett, Harris, Jenner, Reynolds & Marsden (1977) (Appendix 12). The ability to sustain a posture (for example, standing with arms outstretched, or on one leg) was assessed. A series of tests of dynamic motor function also were performed (for example, finger-nose movements, rapid tapping and rising from a recumbent position). All these were rated on a four-point scale. Finally, several electrophysiological recording techniques were employed, including simultaneous EEG and polygraphic EMG studies, as well as somatosensory evoked potentials.

Tics

Gilles de la Tourette's syndrome has attracted much attention from both neurologists and psychiatrists. It is the most complex of the tic syndromes and includes both bodily and vocal tics, the latter often obscene in character (coprolalia) (Fernando, 1967). It is generally believed to have an organic basis (Shapiro, Shapiro & Wayne, 1973a). Assessment has been based on counting the number of bodily tics and vocalisations in a given period (Shapiro, Shapiro & Wayne, 1973b; Feinberg & Carroll, 1979). Sweet, Bruun, Shapiro & Shapiro (1974) converted these counts into scores. Motor tics in each region of the body were counted over a five minute period, with particular emphasis on facial movements. Vocalisations also were counted, with words (obscene or otherwise) and sounds such as grunts and barks being recorded separately. Based on the observed frequency, results were expressed on a scale from 0 to 4.

Tardive dyskinesia

Introduction

Over twenty years ago a syndrome of abnormal involuntary movements associated with prolonged phenothiazine therapy was described (Hall, Jackson & Swain 1956; Sigwald et al., 1959). This is now known as tardive dyskinesia and is recognised as a major hazard of chronic antipsychotic therapy. Estimates of its prevalence in patients at risk range from 4 to 46% (Fann, Davis & Janowsky, 1972; Jus, Pineau & Lachange, 1976; Kane, Wegner, Stenzlek & Ramsey, 1980), although many of the higher figures undoubtedly include patients with minimal or doubtful symptoms. In some cases the syndrome appears irreversible (Crane, 1971). Clinically the condition is characterised by involuntary movements of the limbs, especially the hands. However, any part of the body may be affected (Marsden, Tarsy & Baldessarini, 1975) and in young patients a dystonic picture often occurs. The list of drugs used to treat this syndrome is very long, illustrating that there is considerable individual variation in response to any particular drug (Mackay & Sheppard, 1979). Approaches to assessment have been reviewed by Gardos, Cole & La Brie (1977).

Subjective assessment

Many rating scales have been devised for tardive dyskinesia research. Crude overall assessments indicating an impression of 'better', 'worse' and 'unchanged' have been used (Laterre & Fontetemps, 1975), but more complex rating scales are now more popular, either global (Pryce & Edwards, 1966; Crane & Smeets, 1974), or specific by rating movements of different types at different sites. Villeneuve & Boszormenyi (1970), for example, differentiated between choreiform, buccolingual and buccofaciomandibular dyskinesias and rated the severity of each type, while Gerlach, Reisby & Randrup (1974) divided the body into five areas and ascribed a combined severity/frequency rating to the movements in each area.

Such an anatomical approach to the analysis of dyskinesias has been widely accepted. As early as 1969 Crane, Ruiz & Kernohan devised an 11-item scale in which each symptom was scored on a five-point rating. This method was shown to have high inter-observer reliability and was used by other investigators (for example, Decker, Davis & Janowsky, 1971). An expanded version of this scale was developed by Smith, Tamminga & Haraszti (1977) to include 27 items, combined with a global assessment. More elaborate schemes, also based on anatomical regions, have been developed by others including up to 47 items (Hippius & Logemann, 1970; Simpson, Zoubok & Lee, 1976; Simpson, Lee, Zoubok & Gardos, 1979). Reda, Escobar & Scanlan (1975) used a simpler, 14-item scale, rated according to severity or frequency, as appropriate. Barnes & Kidger (1979) have described a similar system.

The Abnormal Involuntary Movements Scale (1976) (AIMS) devised at the U.S. National Institute of Mental Health, seems likely to gain wide acceptance. It is fairly simple to apply, the terms used are clearly defined, and there is a standardised examination procedure. The scale includes global assessments of severity (both by the patient and the observer) and dyskinesia scores for the face, lips, jaw, tongue and limbs, as well as a functional disability score (see also Kennedy, Hershon & McGuire, 1971).

Audiovisual recordings, especially videotape, have proved very popular in studies of tardive dyskinesia therapy (Reda et al., 1975; Gerlach & Thorsen, 1976; Fann, Stafford, Malone, Frost & Richman, 1977). Since the recordings are themselves rated, this technique is really an extension of those described above (the advantages and disadvantages of recording systems were discussed above).

A different development of the concept of rating has been the use of frequency counts and related techniques. Kazamatsuri, Chien & Colt (1972) counted all orofacial dyskinetic movements for three separate one-minute periods at a fixed time and place during several drug trials. The patients were unaware that they were being observed. Other investigators have counted lip, tongue and jaw movements separately (Fann & Lake, 1974; Davis, Berger & Hollister, 1975). These methods are simple and objective, but results are subject to rapid fluctuations in the patient's condition and not all patients with tardive dyskinesia have movements that are counted easily. The tongue protrusion test, where the patient protrudes his tongue as long as he can and the duration is noted, avoids the latter disadvantage and may be more widely applicable (Klawans & Rubovits, 1974; Gerlach & Thorsen, 1976).

Objective assessment

Objective assessment methods have not been used extensively in tardive dyskinesia research. EMG recordings have been obtained from facial and buccal muscle groups (Jus, Jus & Villeneuve, 1973), from the limbs (Crayton, Smith & Klass, 1977), or from several anatomical sites (Lonowski, Sterling & King, 1979). Accelerometry of the upper limbs also has been employed in drug evaluation (Alpert et al., 1976; Gardos et al., 1977; Fann et al., 1977).

Since buccofacial dyskinesias are so prominent a feature of tardive dyskinesia, Denny & Casey (1975) designed a pneumatic transducer which was placed in the patient's mouth to record many movements that were not clinically detectable. A similar device was placed between the third and fourth fingers of each hand. Using this system the effects of several drugs were documented. Chien, Chung & Ross-Townsend (1977) found that clinical ratings correlated well with results obtained by this technique.

Finally, Klawans & Rubovits (1974) used a recording method also employed in patients with Huntington's chorea, and first described by Holmes in 1938. The patient was seated in a darkened room and a flashlight was attached to each hand. Time-lapse photographs were then taken at intervals. As noted in the section on chorea, the results obtained cannot easily be quantified.

Summary

Rating scales of tardive dyskinesia, such as the AIMS (Appendix 13) are accurately defined, relatively simple, sensitive and reliable. The tongue protrusion test may be used to supplement any rating scale. Videotape and other audiovisual recording methods are certainly not essential. At present, objective instrumental techniques have no clear advantages in assessing drug responses in tardive dyskinesia.

Other drug-induced syndromes

Two conditions will be considered under this heading, namely dopamine agonist-induced dyskinesia and neuroleptic-induced Parkinsonism.

The occurrence of levodopa-induced involuntary movements was described very soon after the introduction of the drug (Cotzias, van Woert & Schiffer, 1967). Bromocriptine produces similar dyskinesias (Parkes, 1979). Any part of the body may be affected by dystonic or choreiform movements, although orofacial dyskinesia is probably the most common finding (Klawans & Garvin, 1969). Assessment of dyskinesia is now part of the evaluation of all anti-Parkinsonian drugs and there have been increasing efforts to find agents that alleviate dyskinesia without impairing anti-Parkinsonian efficacy of levodopa therapy (Tarsy, Parkes & Marsden, 1975; Miller, 1976; Price, Parkes & Marsden, 1978; Bedard, Parkes & Marsden, 1978; Lees, Lander & Stern, 1979; Lieberman et al., 1980). In all cases subjective four or five-point rating scales were used, with severity of movements scored for each region of the body. The AIMS (see section on tardive dyskinesia) also appears to be suitable for the assessment of dopamine agonist induced dyskinesias, and is being used in some current trials.

Neuroleptic-induced Parkinsonism is common; the lowest estimate is 23% (Ayd, 1961), but Kennedy et al. (1971) found that 88% of chronic schizophrenics after at least three months of treatment with a phenothiazine had tremor, and 68% had rigidity. Many studies of drug-induced Parkinsonism have employed techniques somewhat different from those in idiopathic Parkinson's disease. Simpson & Angus (1970) developed subjective rating scales for tremor, rigidity and hypersalivation, noted the glabellar tap, and observed changes in the size and form of handwriting. Mindham (1976) described a rating scale in which facial expression, rigidity of the neck and limbs, tremor of the face and limbs, associated movements on walking and a global rating were all scored on a four-point scale. Mindham, Lamb & Bradley (1977) used this scale, together with simple timing tests, and commented that the subjective assessment of clinical signs appeared to show differences between treatments more clearly than the timing tests. It is arguable whether specific rating systems are necessary for drug-induced, as opposed to idiopathic Parkinsonism. Though the pattern of symptoms is somewhat different in the drug-induced disease, the Webster scale (see section on Parkinson's disease) can still be applied. Alternatively, Mindham's (1976) simpler system appears to be suitable.

Design of clinical trials in extrapyramidal disorders

The particular problems involved in the design of therapeutic trials in extrapyramidal disease are worthy of discussion. Most extrapyramidal disorders are chronic and many are progressive. In addition, there may be considerable variation in the severity of symptoms over hours or even minutes. This is evident most spectacularly in the 'on-off' phenomena occurring in levodopa-treated Parkinson's disease. These problems can be overcome by careful design of the assessment protocol, but otherwise can lead to misleading conclusions.

An important consideration arises from the variable rate of progression of many extrapyramidal diseases. In any population of patients with, say, Parkinson's disease, there will be a very wide range of severity of symptoms and of disability. This makes parallel drug trials at best difficult, and for the rarer conditions quite impracticable; adequate stratification and randomisation will be impossible without unreasonably large populations. This implies that trials of cross-over design almost always will be needed. The disadvantages of such trials, recently examined in detail elsewhere (Vere, 1979; Hills & Armitage, 1979), must be borne in mind in interpreting any such study, but they remain the most practical means of evaluating new therapeutic agents in this group of neurological disorders.

Since these diseases tend to progress, there is always the possibility that drug-induced improvements, particularly small ones, may be masked. Drug trials in extrapyramidal conditions often need to be prolonged for it may take weeks or months for a drug to produce significant benefit even at optimal dosage, and it may require a similar period before that dose is reached. Gradual introduction of new drugs principally is aimed at minimising side-effects. A protracted trial introduces further problems. It must be remembered that many of the patients involved may be severely disabled, and may need to be transported to a hospital or other centre for frequent assessments. Furthermore, the longer the trial lasts the greater is the possibility of intercurrent disease, with consequent clinical deterioration. It is clearly not possible to completely eliminate these problems.

An important concept in the treatment of extrapyramidal disease is that of individualising the dose of the drug for each patient. Frequently there is a large variation in the optimal dose required, as for example with levodopa in Parkinson's disease and haloperidol in Gilles de la Tourette's syndrome. With many new therapeutic agents it is necessary to find the optimal dose for each patient by trial and error, being aware that the tolerated dose may vary tenfold or even more between individual subjects. As a consequence, initial evaluation of most drugs includes an open 'dose-finding' phase.

The individualisation of the drug used is a more recent concept. Mackay & Sheppard (1979) emphasised the value of single-dose drug challenge in an individual patient with tardive dyskinesia, as a guide to which drug would be most likely to be useful in long-term therapy. This can obviously save both the patient and the investigator time and disappointment.

To summarise, the following sequential stages are generally needed in a drug trial in extrapyramidal disease:

(a) If possible, a single-dose drug challenge to establish the most suitable drug for an individual patient

(b) An open, dose-finding study to establish possible efficacy and toxicity

(c) A randomised, double-blind cross-over trial against placebo and/or a standard drug, with appropriate wash-out periods if required, to confirm efficacy. Ideally, the time of cross-over should be randomised from patient to patient so that it is unknown by either the investigator or the patient, but this is rarely achieved in practice.

(d) A large scale multi-centre trial to establish practicability and long-term toxicity. This may provide a large enough population for a parallel study to be carried out, but obviously suffers from the organisational difficulties of any trial where many investigators are involved, and inter-observer reliability of assessment may not prove adequate. In fact, such studies are relatively rare in this field.

(e) Post-marketing surveillance.

Appendix 1

Hoehn & Yahr's (1967) staging for Parkinson's disease

Stage I
  Unilateral involvement, usually minimal or no functional impairment
Stage II
  Bilateral or mid-line involvement, without impairment of balance
Stage III
  First signs of impaired righting reflexes: evident in unsteadiness as the patient turns or demonstrated when he is pushed from standing equilibrium with feet together and eyes closed. Functionally somewhat restricted, but may be able to work, depending on nature of employment. Capable of independent living, with mild to moderate overall disability

Stage IV
  Fully developed, severely disabling disease. Can stand and walk unaided, but is markedly incapacitated
Stage V
  Confined to wheel-chair or bed without assistance

Appendix 2

Webster's Parkinson's disease rating scale
Directions
Apply a gross clinical rating to each of the 10 listed items, assigning value ratings of 0–3 for each item, where (0) = no

involvement and (1), (2) and (3) are equated to early, moderate and severe disease respectively.

Bradykinesia of hands (including handwriting)

(0) No involvement

(1) Detectable lowering of the pronation-supination rate, evidenced by beginning of difficulty in handling tools, buttoning clothes, and with handwriting.

(2) Moderate slowing of supination-pronation rate, one or both sides, evidenced by moderate impairment of hand function. Handwriting is greatly impaired, micrographia is present

(3) Severe slowing of supination-pronation rate. Unable to write or button clothes. Marked difficulty in handling utensils.

Rigidity

(0) None detectable

(1) Detectable rigidity in neck and shoulders. Activation[1] phenomenon is present. One or both arms show mild, negative[2], resting rigidity.

(2) Moderate rigidity in neck and shoulders. Resting rigidity is positive[2] when patient not on medication

(3) Severe rigidity in neck and shoulders. Resting rigidity cannot be reversed by medication

Posture

(0) Normal posture. Head flexed forward less than 4 inches

(1) Beginning 'poker' spine. Head flexed forward up to 5 inches

(2) Beginning arm flexion. Head flexed forward up to 6 inches. One or both arms raised but still below waist.

(3) Onset of simian posture. Head flexed forward more than 6 inches. One or both hands elevated above waist. Sharp flexion of hand, beginning interphalangeal extension. Beginning flexion of knees.

Upper extremity swing

(0) Swings both arms well

(1) One arm definitely decreased in amount of swing

(2) One arm fails to swing

(3) Both arms fail to swing

Gait

(0) Steps out well with 18–30 inch stride. Turns about effortlessly.

(1) Gait shortened to 12–18 inch stride. Beginning to strike one heel. Turn around time slowing. Requires several steps.

(2) Stride moderately shortened—now 6–12 inches. Both heels beginning to strike floor forcefully.

(3) Onset of shuffling gait, steps less than 3 inches. Occasional stuttering type of blocking gait. Walks on toes—turns around very slowly.

Tremor

(0) None detectable

(1) Less than 1 inch of peak-to-peak tremor movement observed in limbs or head at rest or in either hand while walking or during finger to nose testing

(2) Maximum tremor envelope fails to exceed 4 inches. Tremor is severe but not constant and patient retains some control of hands

(3) Tremor envelope exceeds 4 inches. Tremor is constant and severe. Patient cannot get free of tremor while awake. Writing and feeding are impossible

Facies

(0) Normal. Full animation. No stare

(1) Detectable immobility. Mouth remains closed. Beginning features of anxiety and depression

(2) Moderate immobility. Emotion breaks through at markedly increased threshold. Lips parted some of the time. Moderate appearance of anxiety or depression. Drooling may be present

(3) Frozen facies. Mouth open ¼ inch or more. Drooling may be severe

Seborrhea

(0) None

(1) Increased perspiration, secretion remaining thin

(2) Obvious oiliness present. Secretion much thicker

(3) Marked seborrhoea, entire face and head covered by thick secretion

Speech

(0) Loud, clear, resonant, easily understood

(1) Beginning of hoarseness with loss of inflection and resonance. Good volume and still easily understood

(2) Moderate hoarseness and weakness. Constant monotone, unvaried pitch. Beginning of dysarthria, hesitancy, stuttering, difficult to understand

(3) Marked harshness and weakness. Very difficult to hear and understand

Self-care

(0) No impairment

(1) Still provides full self-care but rate of dressing definitely impaired

(2) Requires help in certain critical areas, such as turning in bed, rising from chairs etc. Very slow in performing most activities, but manages by taking more time

(3) Continuously disabled. Unable to dress, feed or walk alone

[1] Activation phenomenon is an increase in rigidity in involved limb evoked by voluntary movement of contralateral limb

[2] Negative rigidity indicates that the patient aids passive movements performed by the observer, to a greater or lesser extent. Positive rigidity implies involuntary resistance associated with increased tone.

Appendix 3

North-Western University Disability Scale

Scale A: Walking

Never walks alone

    0 Cannot walk at all, even with maximum assistance

    1 Needs considerable help, even for short distances; cannot walk outdoors with help

    2 Requires moderate help indoors; walks outdoors with considerable help

    3 Requires potential help indoors and active help outdoors

Sometimes walks alone

    4 Walks from room to room without assistance, but moves slowly and uses external support; never walks alone outdoors

    5 Walks from room to room with only moderate difficulty; may occasionally walk outdoors without assistance

    6 Walks short distances with ease; walking outdoors is difficult but often accomplished without help

Always walk alone

    7 Gait is extremely abnormal; very slow and shuffling; posture grossly affected; there may be propulsion

    8 Quality of gait is poor and rate is slow; posture

moderately affected; there may be a tendency towards mild propulsion; turning is difficult

9 Gait only slightly deviant from normal in quality and speed; turning is the most difficult task; posture essentially normal

10 Normal

Scale B: Dressing

Requires complete assistance

0 Patient is a hindrance rather than a help to assistant

1 Movements of patient neither help nor hinder assistant

2 Can give some help through bodily movements

3 Gives considerable help through bodily movements

Requires partial assistance

4 Performs only gross dressing activities alone (hat, coat)

5 Performs about half of dressing activities independently

6 Performs more than half of dressing activities alone, with considerable effort and slowness

7 Handles all dressing alone with the exception of fine activities (tie, buttons)

Complete self-help

8 Dresses self completely with slowness and great effort

9 Dresses self completely with only slightly more time and effort than normal

10 Normal

Scale C: Hygiene

Requires complete assistance

0 Unable to maintain proper hygiene even with maximum help

1 Reasonably good hygiene with assistance, but does not provide assistant with significant help

2 Hygiene maintained well; gives aid to assistant

Requires partial assistance

3 Performs a few tasks alone with assistant nearby

4 Requires assistance for half of toilet needs

5 Requires assistance for some tasks not difficult in terms of co-ordination

6 Manages most of personal needs alone; has substituted methods for accomplishing difficult tasks

Complete self-help

7 Hygiene maintained independently, but with effort and slowness; accidents are not infrequent; may employ substitute methods

8 Hygiene activities are moderately time-consuming; no substitute methods; few accidents

9 Hygiene maintained normally, with exception of slight slowness

10 Normal

Scale D: Eating and feeding (scored separately)

Eating

0 Eating is so impaired that a hospital setting is required to get adequate nutrition

1 Eats only soft foods and liquids; these are consumed very slowly

2 Liquids and soft foods handled with ease; hard foods occasionally eaten, but require great effort and much time

3 Eats some hard foods routinely, but these require time and effort

4 Follows a normal diet, but chewing and swallowing are laboured

5 Normal

Feeding

0 Requires complete assistance

1 Performs only a few feeding tasks independently

2 Performs most feeding activities alone, slowly and with effort; requires help with feeding

3 Handles all feeding alone with moderate slowness; still may get assistance in specific situation (e.g. cutting meat in restaurant); accidents not infrequent

4 Fully feeds self with rare accidents; slower than normal

5 Normal

Scale E: Speech

0 Does not vocalise at all

1 Vocalises, but rarely for communicative purposes

2 Vocalises to call attention to self

3 Attempts to use speech for communication, but has difficulty in initiating vocalisation; may stop speaking in middle of phrase and be unable to continue

4 Uses speech in most communication, but articulation is highly unintelligible; may have occasional difficulty in initiating speech; usually speaks in single words or short phrases

5 Speech always employed for communication, but articulation is still very poor; usually uses complete sentences

6 Speech can always be understood if listener pays close attention; both articulation and voice may be defective

7 Communication accomplished with ease, although speech impairment detracts from content

8 Speech easily understood, but voice or speech rhythm may be disturbed

9 Speech entirely adequate; minor voice disturbances present

10 Normal

Appendix 4   Shoulson & Fahn's (1979) Staging of Huntington's Disease

	Engagement in occupation	*Capacity to handle financial affairs*	*Capacity to manage domestic responsibilities*	*Capacity to perform activities of daily living*	*Care can be provided at*
Stage 1	Usual level	Full	Full	Full	Home
Stage 2	Lower level	Requires slight assistance	Full	Full	Home
Stage 3	Marginal	Requires major assistance	Impaired	Mildly impaired	Home
Stage 4	Unable	Unable	Unable	Moderately impaired	Home or extended care facility
Stage 5	Unable	Unable	Unable	Severely impaired	Total care facility only

Appendix 5   Shoulson & Fahn's (1979) functional disability scale for Huntington's Chorea

A. *Engagement in occupation*

3 Usual level: refers to full-time salaried employment, actual or potential (e.g. job offer or qualified) with normal work expectations and satisfactory performance.

2 Lower level: refers to full or part-time salaried employment, actual or potential, with a lower than usual expectation or performance relative to patient's training and education.

1 Marginal level: refers to part-time voluntary or salaried employment, actual or potential, with less than satisfactory work performance.

0 Unable: indicates patient is totally unable to engage in voluntary or salaried employment.

B. *Capacity to handle financial affairs*

3 Full: refers to normal capacity to handle personal and family finances (income tax, balancing cheque book, paying bills).

2 Requires assistance: refers to decline in ability to handle financial affairs such that accustomed routine responsibilities (budgeting, shopping, maintaining chequing account) now require organisation and assistance from family member or financial advisor.

1 Limited: handles pocket money only.

0 Unable: indicates patient is unable to comprehend the financial process and is unable to perform tasks related to routine financial procedures.

C. *Capacity to manage domestic responsibilities*

2 Full: no impairment in performance of routine domestic tasks (cleaning, laundering, dishwashing, table setting, recipes, answering mail, civic responsibilities).

1 Impaired: refers to decline in performance of routine domestic tasks such that patient requires some assistance carrying out these tasks.

0 Unable: indicates marked decline in function with marginal performance requiring major assistance.

D. *Capacity to perform activities of daily living*

3 Full: refers to complete independence in eating, dressing and bathing activities.

2 Mildly impaired: refers to somewhat laboured performance in eating (avoids certain foods which cause chewing/swallowing problems), in dressing (difficulty in fine tasks only, e.g. buttoning, tying shoes), in bathing (difficulty in fine performance only, e.g. brushing teeth); requires only slight assistance.

1 Moderately impaired: refers to substantial difficulty in eating (swallows only liquid or soft foods and requires considerable assistance), in dressing (performs only gross dressing activities and requires assistance with everything else), in bathing (performs only gross bathing tasks, otherwise requiring assistance).

0 Severely impaired: indicates that patient requires total care in activities of daily living.

E. *Care can be provided*

2 Home: patient living at home and family readily able to meet care needs.

1 Home or extended care facility: patient may be living at home but care needs would be better and more easily provided at an extended care facility.

0 Total care facility only: patient requires full-time skilled nursing care.

Appendix 6   Marsden & Quinn's chorea severity evaluation scale

1. *Speech*
   0 Normal
   1 Slight dysarthria
   2 Slurred but understandable
   3 Considerable dysarthria, with interruptions in flow
   4 Dysarthria with considerable 'interruption' in flow
   5 Unintelligible

3. *Gait*
   0 Normal
   1 Increase in choreic movements
   2 Definite 'stuttering, dancing' gait
   3 Pronounced 'stuttering and dancing' gait; tends to be thrown off balance
   4 Walks only with assistance
   5 Unable to walk, even with assistance

3. *Postural stability*
   0 Normal
   1 Decreased postural reflexes
   2 Would fall if not caught, after marked pulls
   3 Would fall if not caught, after mild pulls
   4 Tends to fall spontaneously
   5 Cannot stand alone

4. *Manual Dexterity*
   0 Normal
   1 Occasionally fumbles or drops objects
   2 Difficulty in dressing and/or eating
   3 Requires some help dressing and/or eating
   4 Requires to be dressed and/or fed

5. *Severity of Chorea*
   0 None
   1 Rare to slight
   2 Mild
   3 Moderate
   4 Severe; interferes with some functions
   5 Very severe; unable to function

Face	Upper	____
	Lower	____
Neck		____
Trunk		____
Limbs	R	L
Arms	____	____
Legs	____	____

Appendix 7   Fahn & Marsden's staging of torsion dystonia

Stage

I   Focal: a single segment (e.g. 1 limb; torticollis; blepharospasm; dysphonia; both arms or both legs).

II Segmental: 2–3 continuous (e.g. Meige syndrome, torticollis plus shoulder)

III Unilateral arm and leg

IV Bilateral generalised

Appendix 8 Fahn & Marsden's functional disability scale for torsion dystonia

A. *Speech*
  0 Normal
  1 Slightly involved; easily understood
  2 Some difficulty to understand
  3 Marked difficulty to understand
  4 Completely or almost completely aphonic or anarthric

B. *Handwriting (tremor or dystonia)*
  0 Normal
  1 Slight difficulty; legible
  2 Almost illegible
  3 Illegible
  4 Unable to grasp or maintain hold on pen

C. *Feeding*
  0 Normal
  1 Uses 'tricks'; independent
  2 Can feed, but not cut
  3 Finger food only
  4 Completely dependent

D. *Eating*
  0 Normal
  1 Occasional choking
  2 Chokes frequently; difficulty swallowing
  3 Unable to swallow firm foods
  4 Marked difficulty swallowing soft foods and liquids

E. *Hygiene*
  0 Normal
  1 Clumsy; independent
  2 Needs help with some activities
  3 Needs help with most activities
  4 Needs help with all activities

Dressing
  0 Normal
  1 Clumsy; independent
  2 Needs help with some
  3 Needs help with most
  4 Helpless

G. *Walking*
  0 Normal
  1 Slightly abnormal; hardly noticeable
  2 Moderately abnormal; obvious to naive observer
  3 Considerably abnormal
  4 Needs assistance to walk
  5 Wheel-chair bound

Appendix 9 Fahn & Marsden's dystonia severity evaluation scale

Segments	Provoking factor	Severity factor	(Product)
Eyes			
Mouth			
Speech and swallowing			
Neck			
Right arm			
Left arm			
Trunk			
Right leg			
Left leg			

Total

Provoking factor
  0 No dystonia at rest or action
  1 Dystonia on particular action
  2 Dystonia on many actions
  3 Dystonia on action of distant part of body
  4 Dystonia present at rest

Speech and swallowing
  1 Occasional either or both
  2 Frequent either
  3 Frequent one and occasional other
  4 Frequent both

Severity factor
  0 No dystonia present
  1 Slight dystonia, but not causing impairment. Clinically insignificant
  2 Mild. Impairment but not disabling
  3 Moderate. Disabling, but not eliminating basic function
  4 Severe. Preventing basic functions

Appendix 10   Marsden & Lang's cranial dystonia evaluation scale

Rate: *Severity*   and   *Provoking factor*

0 nil	0 nil
1 slight	1 reading and viewing, or talking and eating
2 mild (or not interfering with basic function)	2 movement of distant parts
3 moderate (disabling but not eliminating basic function)	3 at rest
4 severe (prevents basic function)	

For: Upper face

      Lips

      Jaws

      Tongue

Also score: *Vision*

Vision	*Speech*	*Swallowing*
0 normal	0 normal	0 normal
1 rarely troubled	1 slurred	1 occasionally chokes
2 cannot drive or read	2 dysarthric but intelligible	2 frequently chokes but can feed
3 cannot cross roads or leave house	3 dysarthric and difficult to understand	3 significant difficulty in feeding
4 Functionally blind	4 Unintelligible	4 Cannot feed

Appendix 11   Marsden & Sheehy's writer's cramp evaluation scale

Subjective (observe while writing)

0 Normal

1 Curious hand posture which could be interpreted as normal

2 Obviously abnormal hand posture, but abnormalities confined to wrist and/or fingers

3 Abnormal posture involves elbow and/or shoulder as well

4 Abnormal posture involves other distant body parts, for example the neck (specify)

Objective (using affected limb)

1 Gibson's maze traced as accurately and rapidly as possible

2 Number of times the word "sunshine" can be written completely in one minute

3 Number of counters piled on top of one another in one minute

4 Ability to hold a full cup of water with arm outstretched (measured as the percentage of water spilt in one minute)

5 Handwriting sample compared with script prior to illness, using for example the signature, and rated

0 no change

1 slight, uncertain deterioration

2 mild but definite deterioration

3 moderate deterioration, difficult to read

4 severe deterioration, very difficult to read

5 illegible

Appendix 12   Chadwick & Marsden's myoclonus evaluation scale

(a) *Score[1] sustained posture[2]*

1 Of outstretched arm

2 Of flexed arm in front of face

3 Of leg elevated from bed while lying

4 Of body while standing on one leg

5 Of face while pursing lips

(b) *Score[1] dynamic function[2]*

1 Finger-nose test

2 Rapid hand tapping

3 Rapid pronation-supination hand movements

4 Heel-shin test

5 Gait

6 Speech

7 Handwriting

8 Drawing of Archimedes spiral

[1] Score as 0 = normal

          1 = mild abnormality

          2 = moderate abnormality

          3 = severe abnormality

[2] Where appropriate, an individual score was given for each limb tested

Appendix 13a The abnormal involuntary movement scale (AIMS, 1976): examination procedure

Either before or after completing the examination procedure observe the patient unobtrusively, at rest (e.g. in waiting room). The chair to be used in this examination should be a hard, firm one without arms.

1. Ask patient whether there is anything in his/her mouth (i.e. gum, candy, etc) and if there is, to remove it.

2. Ask patient about the current condition of his/her teeth. Ask patient if he/she wears dentures. Do teeth or dentures bother patient now?

3. Ask patient whether he/she notices any movements in mouth, face, hands, or feet. If yes, ask to describe and to what extent they currently bother patients or interfere with his/her activities.

4. Have patient sit in chair with hands on knees, legs slightly apart, and feet flat on floor. (Look at entire body for movements while in this position).

5. Ask patient to sit with hands hanging unsupported. If male, between legs, if female and wearing a dress, hanging over knees. (Observe hands and other body areas).

6. Ask patient to open mouth. (Observe tongue at rest within mouth). Do this twice.

7. Ask patient to protrude tongue. (Observe abnormalities of tongue movement). Do this twice.

8. Ask patient to tap thumb, with each finger, as rapidly as possible for 10–15 seconds; separately with right hand, then with left hand. (Observe facial and leg movements).

9. Flex and extend patient's left and right arm (one at a time).

10. Ask patient to stand up. (Observe in profile. Observe all body areas again, hips included).

11. Ask patient to extend both arms outstretched in front with palms down. (Observe trunk, legs and mouth).

12. Have patient walk a few paces, turn and walk back to chair. (Observe hands and gait). Do this twice.

Appendix 13b The abnormal involuntary movements scale (AIMS, 1976): Scoring system

Instructions: Complete examination procedure before making ratings
Movement ratings: Rate highest severity observed. Rate movements that occur upon activation one less than those observed spontaneously.

Code: 0 = none
1 = minimal may be extreme normal
2 = mild
3 = moderate
4 = severe

		(Circle one)			
1. Muscles of facial expression e.g. movements of forehead, eyebrows, periorbital area, cheeks; include frowning, blinking, smiling, grimacing	0	1	2	3	4
Facial and oral movements 2. Lips and perioral area e.g. puckering, pouting, smacking	0	1	2	3	4
3. Jaw e.g. biting, clenching, chewing, mouth opening, lateral movement	0	1	2	3	4
4. Tongue Rate only increase in movement both in and out of mouth, *not* inability to sustain movement	0	1	2	3	4
5. Upper (arms, wrist, hands, fingers) Include choreic movements (i.e. rapid, objectively purposeless, irregular, spontaneous), athetoid movements (i.e. slow, irregular, complex, serpentine) Do *not* include tremor (i.e. repetitive, regular, rhythmic)	0	1	2	3	4
Extremity movements 6. Lower (legs, knees, ankles, toes) e.g. lateral knee movement, foot tapping, heel dropping, foot squirming, inversion and eversion of foot	0	1	2	3	4

Trunk movements	7. Neck, shoulders, hips e.g. rocking, twisting, squirming, pelvic gyrations	0	1	2	3	4

	8. Severity of abnormal movements	None, normal	0
		Minimal	1
		Mild	2
		Moderate	3
		Severe	4
Global judgements	9. Incapacitation due to abnormal movements	None, normal	0
		Minimal	1
		Mild	2
		Moderate	3
		Severe	4
	10. Patient's awareness of abnormal movements	No awareness	0
		Aware, no distress	1
		Aware, mild distress	2
		Aware, moderate distress	3
		Aware, severe distress	*l*

	11. Current problems with teeth and/or dentures	No	0
Dental status		Yes	1
	12. Does patient usually wear dentures?	No	0
		Yes	1

References

AGATE, F.J., DOSHAY, L.J. & CURTIS, F.K. (1956). Quantitative measurement of therapy in paralysis agitans. *J. Am. med. Ass.,* **160**, 352–354.

AIMS (1976). In *ECDEU Assessment Manual,* ed. Guy, W., pp. 534–537. Rockville, Maryland: US Department of Health, Education and Welfare.

ALBA, A., TRAINOR, F.S., RITTER, W. & DACSO, M.M. (1968). A clinical disability rating for Parkinsonian patients. *J. chron. Dis.,* **21**, 507–522.

ALPERT, M., DIAMOND, F. & FRIEDHOFF, A. (1976). Tremographic studies in tardive dyskinesia. *Psychopharmac. Bull.,* **12**, 5–7.

ANDEN, N-E., CARLSSON, A., KERSTELL, J., MAGNUSSON, T., OLSSON, R., ROOSE, B-B., STEEN, B., STEG, G., SVANBORG, A., THIEME, G. & WERDINIUS, B. (1970). Oral L-dopa treatment of Parkinsonism. *Acta med. Scand.,* **187**, 247–255.

ANGEL, R.W., ALSTON, W. & HIGGINS, J.R. (1970). Control of movement in Parkinson's disease. *Brain,* **93**, 1–14.

ANGEL, R.W., ALSTON, W. & GARLAND, H. (1971). L-dopa and error correction time in Parkinson's disease. *Neurology,* **21**, 1255–1260.

AYD, F.J. (1961). A survey of drug-induced extrapyramidal reactions. *J. Am. med. Ass.,* **175**, 1054–1060.

BARBEAU, A. (1966). The problem of measurement of akinesia. *J. Neurosurg.,* **24** (suppl. I, part II), 331–334.

BARBEAU, A. (1969). L-dopa therapy in Parkinson's disease—a critical review of nine years experience. *Can. med. Ass. J.,* **101**, 791–797.

BARNES, T.R.E. & KIDGER, T. (1979). Tardive dyskinesia and the problems of assessment. In *Current Themes in Psychiatry,* vol. 2, eds. Gaind, R. & Hudson, B.L., pp. 145–162. London: Macmillan.

BARR, A.N., HEINZE, W., MENDOZA, J.E. & PERLIK, S. (1978). Long-term treatment of Huntington disease with L-glutamate and pyridoxine. *Neurology,* **28**, 1280–1282.

BEALL, C.G. (1925). New method of recording muscular tremors. *Arch. Neurol. Psychiat.,* **14**, 751–755.

BEDARD, P., PARKES, J.D. & MARSDEN, C.D. (1978). Effect of new dopamine-blocking agent (oxiperomide) on drug-induced dyskinesias in Parkinson's disease and spontaneous dyskinesias. *Br. med. J.,* **1**, 954–956.

BIRKMAYER, W. & NIEMAYER, E. (1972). Die moderne medikamentose Behandlung des Parkinsonismus. *Z. Neurol.,* **202**, 257–264.

BOSHES, B., WACHS, H., BRUMLIK, J., MIER, M. & PETROVICK, M. (1960). Studies of tone, tremor and speech in normal persons and Parkinsonian patients. I. Methodology. *Neurology,* **10**, 805–813.

BRUMLIK, J. & BOSHES, B. (1960). Quantitation of muscle tone in normals and in Parkinsonians. *Arch. Neurol.,* **4**, 399–406.

BURNS, B.D. & DE JONG, J.D. (1960). A preliminary report on the measurement of Parkinson's disease. *Neurology,* **10**, 1096–1102.

CALNE, D.B. & LADER, M.H. (1969). Electromyographic studies of tremor using an averaging computer. *Electroencephal. clin. Neurophysiol.,* **26**, 86–92.

CANTER, C.J. de la TORRE, R. & MIER, M. (1961). A method of evaluating disability in patients with Parkinson's disease. *J. nerv. mental. Dis.,* **133**, 143–147.

CASSELL, K., SHAW, K. & STERN, G. (1973). A computerised tracking technique for the assessment of Parkinsonian motor disabilities. *Brain,* **96**, 815–826.

CHADWICK, D., HARRIS, R., JENNER, P., REYNOLDS, E.H. & MARSDEN, C.D. (1975). Manipulation of brain serotonin in the treatment of myoclonus. *Lancet,* **ii**, 434–435.

CHADWICK, D., HALLETT, M., HARRIS, R., JENNER, P., REYNOLDS, E.H. & MARSDEN, C.D. (1977). Clinical, biochemical and physiological factors distinguishing myoclonus responsive to 5-hydroxytryptophan, tryptophan with a monoamine oxidase inhibitor and clonazepam. *Brain*, **100**, 455–487.

CHASE, T.N., WEXLER, N.S. & BARBEAU, A. (1979). Huntington's Disease. In *Advances in Neurology*, vol. **23**, New York: Raven Press.

CHIEN, C.-P., CHUNG, K. & ROSS-TOWNSEND, A. (1977). The measurement of persistent dyskinesia by piezoelectric recording and clinical rating scales. *Psycho-pharmac. Bull.*, **13**, 34–36.

CLARKE, S., HAY, G.A. & VAS, C.J. (1966). Therapeutic action of methixene hydrochloride on parkinsonian tremor and a description of a new tremor recording transducer. *Br. J. Pharmac.*, **26**, 345–350.

COTZIAS, G.C., PAPAVASILIOU, P.S., FEHLING, C., KAUFMAN, B. & MENA, I. (1970). Similarities between neurologic effects of L-Dopa and apomorphine. *New Engl. J. Med.*, **282**, 31–33.

COTZIAS, C.G., van WOERT, M.M. & SCHIFFER, L.M. (1967). Aromatic aminoacids and modification of Parkinsonism. *New Engl. J. Med.*, **276**, 374–378.

COUCH, J.R. (1976). Dystonia and tremor in spasmodic torticollis. In *Advances in Neurology*, vol. **14**, 'Dystonia', eds. Eldridge, R. & Fahn, S., pp. 245–258. New York: Raven Press.

COWELL, T.K., MARSDEN, C.D. & OWEN, D.A.L. (1965). Objective measurement of Parkinsonian tremor. *Lancet*, **ii**, 1278–1279.

CRANE, G.E., RUIZ, P. & KERNOHAN, W.J. (1969). Effects of drug withdrawal on tardive dyskinesia. *Activ. Nerv. Super.*, **11**, 30–35.

CRANE, G.E. (1971). Persistence of neurological symptoms due to neuroleptic drugs. *Am. J. Psychiat.*, **127**, 1407–1410.

CRANE, G.E. & SMEETS, R.A. (1974). Tardive dyskinesia and drug therapy in geriatric patients. *Arch. Gen. Psychiat.*, **30**, 341–343.

CRAYTON, J.W., SMITH, R.C. & KLASS, D. (1977). Electrophysiological (H-reflex) studies of patients with tardive dyskinesias. *Am. J. Psychiat.*, **134**, 775–781.

DAVIS, K.L., BERGER, P.A. & HOLLISTER, L.E. (1975). Choline for tardive dyskinesia. *New Engl. J. Med.*, **293**, 152.

DECKER, B.L., DAVIS, J.M. & JANOWSKY, D.S. (1971). Amantadine hydrochloride treatment of tardive dyskinesia. *New Engl. J. Med.*, **289**, 860.

DENNY, D. & CASEY, D.E. (1975). An objective method for measuring dyskinetic movements in tardive dyskinesia. *Electroencephal. clin. Neurophysiol.*, **38**, 645–646.

DIETRICHSON, P., LANGBRETSON, O.F. & HOULAND, J. (1978). Quantitation of tremor in man. In *Prog. Clin. Neurophysiol.*, vol. **5**, ed. Desmedt, J.E., pp. 90–94. Basel: Karger.

DRAPER, I.T. & JOHNS, R.J. (1964). The disordered movement in Parkinsonism and the effect of drug treatment. *Bull. Johns Hopkins Hosp.*, **115**, 465–480.

DUVOISON, R.C. (1970). The evaluation of extrapyramidal disease. In *Monoamines, noyaux gris centraux et syndrome de Parkinson*, ed. de Ajuriagerra, J., pp. 313–325. Paris: Masson.

ENGLAND, A.C. & SCHWAB, R.S. (1956). Postoperative evaluation of 26 selected patients with Parkinson's disease. *J. Am. geriat. Soc.*, **4**, 1219–1232.

ENNA, S.J., STERN, L.Z., WASTEK, G.J. & YAMAMURA, H.I. (1977). Neurobiology and pharmacology of Huntington's disease. *Life Sci.*, **20**, 205–212.

EVARTS, E., TERAVAINEN, H., BEUCHERT, D. & CALNE, D. (1979). Pathophysiology of motor performance in Parkinson's disease. In *Dopaminergic ergot derivatives and motor functions*. eds. Fuxe, F. & Calne, D., pp. 45–59. London: Pergamon Press.

FALEK, A. (1976). Predictive detection of Huntington's chorea. In *Progress in neurogenetics*, eds. Barbeau, A. & Brunette, J.R., pp. 529–533. Amsterdam: Excerpta Medica Foundation.

FANN, W.E., DAVIS, J.M. & JANOWSKY, D.S. (1972). The prevalence of tardive dyskinesias in mental hospital patients. *Dis. Nerv. Syst.*, **33**, 182–186.

FANN, W.E. & LAKE, R. (1974). On the coexistence of Parkinsonism and tardive dyskinesia. *Dis. Nerv. Syst.*, **35**, 324–326.

FANN, W.E., STAFFORD, J.R., MALONE, R.L., FROST, J.D. & RICHMAN, B.W. (1977). Clinical research techniques in tardive dyskinesia. *Am. J. Psychiat.*, **134**, 759–762.

FEINBERG, M. & CARROLL, B.J. (1979). Effects of dopamine agonists and antagonists in Tourette's disease. *Arch. gen. Psychiat.*, **36**, 979–985.

FERNANDO, S.J.M. (1967). Gilles de la Tourette's syndrome. *Br. J. Psychiat.*, **113**, 606–617.

FLOWERS, K.A. (1975). Ballistic and corrective movements in an aiming task: intention tremor and parkinsonian movement disorder compared. *Neurology*, **25**, 413–421.

FLOWERS, K.A. (1976). Visual 'closed-loop' and 'open-loop' characteristics of voluntary movements in patients with Parkinsonism and intention tremor. *Brain*, **99**, 261–310.

GARDOS, G., COLE, J.O. & La BRIE, R. (1977). The assessment of tardive dyskinesia. *Arch. gen. Psychiat.*, **34**, 1206–1212.

GERLACH, J., REISBY, N. & RANDRUP, A. (1974). Dopaminergic hyperactivity and cholinergic hypofunction in the pathophysiology of tardive dyskinesia. *Psychopharmac.*, **34**, 21–35.

GERLACH, J. & THORSEN, K. (1976). The movement pattern of oral tardive dyskinesia in relation to anticholinergic and antidopaminergic treatment. *Int. Pharmacopsychiat.*, **11**, 1–7.

GODWIN-AUSTEN, R.B., TOMLINSON, E.B., FREARS, C.C. & KOK, H.W.L. (1969). Effects of L-dopa in Parkinson's disease. *Lancet*, **ii**, 165–168.

GROWDON, J.H., YOUNG, R.R. & SHAHANI, B.T. (1976). L-5-hydroxytryptophan in treatment of several different syndromes in which myoclonus is present *Neurology*, **26**, 1135–1140.

HALL, R.A., JACKSON, R.B. & SWAIN, J.M. (1956). Neurotoxic reactions resulting from chlorpromazine administration. *J. Am. med. Ass.*, **161**, 214–218.

HEILMAN, K.M., BOWERS, D., WATSON, R.T. & GREER, M. (1976). Reaction times in Parkinson disease. *Arch. Neurol.*, **33**, 139–140.

HILLS, M. & ARMITAGE, P. (1979). The two-period crossover clinical trial. *Br. J. clin. Pharmac.*, **8**, 7–20.

HIPPIUS, H. & LOGEMANN, G. (1970). Zur Wirkung von Dioxyphenylalanin (L-Dopa) auf extrapyramidalische

Hyperkinesien nach langzeitingen neuroleptische Therapie. *Arzneim. Forsch., 20,* 894–895.

HOEHN, M.M. & YAHR, M.D. (1967). Parkinsonism: onset, progression and mortality. *Neurology, 17,* 427–442.

HOLMES, G. (1938). The cerebellum of man. 10th Hughlings Jackson Memorial Lecture at the Royal Society of Medicine. In *Selected Papers of Gordon Holmes* (1979), ed. Phillips, C.G., pp. 248–277. Oxford: Oxford University Press.

JANKOVIC, J. & FROST, J.D. (1980). Quantitative assessment of Parkinsonism and essential tremor: clinical application of triaxial accelerometry. *Neurology, 30,* 393.

JUS, K., JUS, A. & VILLENEUVE, A. (1973). Polygraphic profile of oral tardive dyskinesia and of rabbit syndrome. *Dis. Nerv. Syst., 34,* 27–32.

JUS, A., PINEAU, R. & LACHANGE, R. (1976). Epidemiology of tardive dyskinesia. Part II. *Dis. Nerv. Syst., 37,* 257–261.

KANE, J., WEGNER, J., STENZLEK, S. & RAMSEY, P. (1980). The prevalence of presumed tardive dyskinesia in psychiatric in-patients and out-patients. *Psychopharmac., 69,* 247–252.

KARNOFSKY, D.A., BURCHENAL, J.H., ARMISTEAD, G.C., SOUTHAM, C.M., BERNSTEIN, J.L., CRAVER, L.F. & RHOADS, C.P. (1951). Triethylene melamine in the treatment of neoplastic disease. *Arch. int. Med., 87,* 477–516.

KARTZINEL, R. & CALNE, D.B. (1976). Studies with bromocriptine. Part I. 'On-off' phenomena. *Neurology, 26,* 508–510.

KAZAMATSURI, H. CHIEN, C-P. & COLE, J.O. (1972). Treatment of tardive dyskinesia: I. Clinical efficacy of a dopamine-depleting agent, tetrabenazine. *Arch. gen. Psychiat., 27,* 95–99.

KENNEDY, P.F., HERSHON, H.I. & McGUIRE, R.J. (1971). Extrapyramidal disorders after prolonged phenothiazine therapy. *Br. J. Psychiat., 118,* 509–518.

KLAWANS, H.L. & GARVIN, J.S. (1969). Treatment of Parkinsonism with L-dopa. *Dis. Nerv. Syst., 30,* 737–746.

KLAWANS, H.L., RUBOVITS, R., RINGEL, S.P. & WEINER, W.J. (1972). Observations on the use of methysergide in Huntington's chorea. *Neurology, 22,* 929–933.

KLAWANS, H.L. & RUBOVITS, R. (1974). Effects of cholinergic and anticholinergic agents on tardive dyskinesia. *J. Neurol. Neurosurg. Psychiat., 37,* 941–947.

KNUTSSON, E. & MARTENSON, A. (1971). Quantitative effects of L-Dopa on different types of movements and muscle tone in Parkinsonian patients. *Scand. J. Rehab. Med., 3,* 121–124.

KOREIN, J., BRODNY, T., GRYNBAUM, B., SACHS-FRANKEL, C., WEISINGER, M. & LEVIDOW, L. (1976). Sensory feedback therapy on spasmodic torticollis and dystonia: results in treatment of 55 patients. In *Advances in Neurology,* vol. 14. Dystonia, eds. Eldridge, R. & Fahn, S., pp. 375–402. New York: Raven Press.

LA JOIE, W.J. & GERSTEIN, J.N. (1956). An objective method of evaluating muscle tightness. *Arch. Phys. Med., 33,* 595–600.

LATERRE, E.C. & FONTETEMPS, E. (1975). Deanol in spontaneous and induced dyskinesias. *Lancet, i,* 1301.

LEE, R.G. & TATTON, W.G. (1975). Motor responses to sudden limb displacements in primates with specific CNS lesions and in human patients with motor system disorders. *Can. J. Neurol. Sci., 2,* 285–293.

LEE, R.G. & TATTON, W.G. (1978). Long-loop reflexes in man: clinical applications. In *Progr. Clin. Neurophysiol.,* vol. 4, ed. Desmedt, J.E., pp. 342–360. Basel: Karger.

LEES, A.J., SHAW, K.M., KOHOUT, L.J., STERN, G.M., ELSWORTH, J.D., SANDLER, M. & YOUDIM, M.B.H. (1977). Deprenyl in Parkinson's disease. *Lancet, ii,* 791–795.

LEES, A.J., LANDER, C.M. & STERN, G.M. (1979). Triapride in levodopa-induced involuntary movements. *J. Neurol. Neurosurg. Psychiat., 42,* 380–383.

LHERMITTE, F., AGID, Y. & SIGNORET, J.L. (1978). Onset and end-of-dose levodopa-induced dyskinesia. Possible treatment by increasing the daily dose of levodopa. *Arch. Neurol., 35,* 261–263.

LIEBERMAN, A., DZIATOLOWKI, M., GOPINATHAN, G., KOPERSMITH, M., NEOPHYTIDES, A. & KOREIN, J. (1980). Evaluation of Parkinson's disease. In *Ergot compounds and brain function: neuroendocrine and neuropsychiatric aspects,* ed. Goldstein, M., pp. 277–286. New York: Raven Press.

LONG, C., THOMAS, D. & CROCHETIERE, W.J. (1964). Objective measurement of muscle tone in the hand. *Clin. Pharmac. Ther., 5,* 909–917.

LONOWSKI, D.J., STERLING, F.E. & KING, H.A. (1979). Electromyographic assessment of dimethylaminoethanol (deanol) in treatment of tardive dyskinesia. *Psychiat. Rep., 45,* 415–419.

MACKAY, A.V.P. & SHEPPARD, G.P. (1979). Pharmacotherapeutic trials in tardive dyskinesia. *Br. J. Psychiat., 135,* 489–499.

McDOWELL, F., LEE, J.E., SWIFT, T., SWEET, R.D., OGSBURY, J.S. & TESSLER, J.T. (1970). Treatment of Parkinson's syndrome with dihydroxyphenylalanine (levodopa). *Ann. int. Med., 72,* 29–35.

McLELLAN, D.L., CHALMERS, R.J. & JOHNSON, R.H. (1974). A double-blind trial of tetrabenazine, thiopropazate and placebo in patients with chorea. *Lancet, i,* 104–107.

MARSDEN, C.D. & HARRISON, M.J.G. (1974). Idiopathic torsion dystonia (dystonia musculorum deformans): a review of forty-two patients. *Brain, 97,* 793–810.

MARSDEN, C.D., TARSY, D. & BALDESSARINI, R.J. (1975). Spontaneous and drug-induced movement disorders in psychiatric patients. In *Psychiatric aspects of neurological disease,* eds. Benson, D.F. & Blummer, D., pp. 219–226. New York: Grune & Stratton.

MARSDEN, C.D. & PARKES, J.D. (1976). 'On-off' effects in patients with Parkinson's disease on chronic levodopa therapy. *Lancet, i,* 292–296.

MARSDEN, C.D., MERTON, P.A., MORTON, H.B. & ADAM, J. (1978). The effect of lesions of the central nervous system on long-latency stretch reflexes in the human thumb. In *Progr. Clin. Neurophysiol.,* vol. 4, ed., Desmedt, J.E., pp. 342–360. Basel: Karger.

MILLER, E.M. (1976). Effectiveness of deanol on L-dopa induced dyskinesias: a placebo-controlled double-blind study. In *Advances in Parkinsonism,* eds Birkmayer, W. & Hornykiewicz, O., pp. 582–590. Basel: Editiones Roche.

MINDHAM, R.H.S. (1976). Assessment of drug-induced extrapyramidal reactions and of drugs given for their control. *Br. J. clin. Pharmac., 3,* 395–400.

MINDHAM, R.H.S., LAMB, P. & BRADLEY, R. (1977). A comparison of piribedil, procyclidine and placebo in the control of phenothiazine-induced Parkinsonism. *Br. J. Psychiat.*, **130**, 581–585.

MORTIMER, J.A. & WEBSTER, D.D. (1979). Evidence for a quantitative association between EMG stretch responses and Parkinsonian rigidity. *Brain Res.*, **162**, 169–173.

NUTT, J.G., ROBIN, A. & CHASE, T.N. (1978). Treatment of Huntington disease with a cholinergic agonist. *Neurology*, **28**, 1061–1064.

OPPEL, I. & UMBACH, W.U. (1977). A quantitative measurement of tremor. *Electroenceph. clin. Neurophysiol.*, **43**, 885–888.

OWEN, D.A.L. & MARSDEN, C.D. (1965). Effect of adrenergic β-blockers on Parkinsonian tremor. *Lancet*, **ii**, 1259–1262.

PARKES, J.D. (1979). Bromocriptine in the treatment of Parkinsonism. *Drugs*, **17**, 365–382.

PARKES, J.D., ZILKHA, K.J., CALVER, D.M. & KNILL-JONES, R.P. (1970a). Controlled trial of amantadine hydrochloride in Parkinson's disease. *Lancet*, **i**, 259–262.

PARKES, J.D., ZILKHA, K.J., MARSDEN, P., BAXTER, R.C.H. & KNIL-JONES, R.P. (1970b). Amantadine dosage in the treatment of Parkinson's disease. *Lancet*, **i**, 1130–1133.

PERRET, E. (1968). Simple motor performance of patients with Parkinson's disease before and after surgical lesion in the thalamus. *J. Neurol. Neurosurg. Psychiat.*, **31**, 284–290.

PERRET, E., EGGENSBERGER, E. & SIEGFRIED, J. (1970). Simple and complex finger movements of patients with Parkinsonism before and after controlled stereotaxic thalamotomy. *J. Neurol. Neurosurg. Psychiat.*, **33**, 16–21.

PERRY, T.L., WRIGHT, J.M., HANSEN, S. & MACLEOD, P.M. (1979). Isoniazid therapy of Huntington disease. *Neurology*, **29**, 370–375.

PETAJAN, J.H., JARCHO, L.W. & THURMAN, D.J. (1979). Motor unit control in Huntington's disease: a possible presymptomatic test. In *Advances in Neurology*, vol. 23. Huntington's Disease, eds. Chase, T.N., Wexler, N.S. & Barbeau, A., pp. 163–175. New York: Raven Press.

POTVIN, A.R. & TOURTELOTTE, W.W. (1975). The neurological examination: advancements in its quantification. *Arch. Phys. Med. Rehab.*, **56**, 425–437.

PRICE, P.A., PARKES, J.D. & MARSDEN, C.D. (1978). Sodium valproate in the treatment of levodopa-induced dyskinesia. *J. Neurol. Neurosurg. Psychiat.*, **41**, 702–706.

PRYCE, I.G. & EDWARDS, H. (1966). Persistent oral dyskinesia in female mental hospital patients. *Br. J. Psychiat.*, **112**, 983–987.

READ, F.A., ESCOBAR, J.I. & SCANLAN, J.M. (1975). Lithium carbonate in the treatment of tardive dyskinesia. *Am. J. Psychiat.*, **132**, 560–562.

RIKLAN, M. & DILLER, L. (1956). Certain psychomotor aspects of subtemporal pallidectomy for Parkinson's disease. *J. Am. Geriat. Soc.*, **4**, 1258–1265.

RINNE, U.K., SONNINEN, V. & SIIRTOLA, T. (1970). L-dopa treatment in Parkinson's disease. *Eur. Neurol.*, **4**, 348–369.

SALZER, M. (1972). Three-dimensional tremor assessments of hand. *J. Biomech.*, **6**, 217–221.

SCHACHTER, M., MARSDEN, C.D., PARKES, J.D., JENNER, P. & TESTA, B. (1980). Deprenyl in the management of response fluctuation in patients with Parkinson's disease on levodopa. *J. Neurol. Neurosurg. Psychiat.*, **43**, 1016–1021.

SCHWAB, R.S. (1960). Progression and progress in Parkinson's disease. *J. nerv. ment. Dis.*, **130**, 556–566.

SCHWAB, R.S. & PRICHARD, J.S. (1951). An assessment of therapy in Parkinson's disease. *Arch. Neurol. Psychiat.*, **65**, 489–501.

SHAPIRO, A.K., SHAPIRO, E. & WAYNE, H. (1973a). Organic factors in Gilles de la Tourette's syndrome. *Br. J. Psychiat.*, **122**. 659–664.

SHAPIRO, A.K., SHAPIRO, E. & WAYNE, H. (1973b). Treatment of Tourette's syndrome with haloperidol: review of 34 cases. *Arch. gen. Psychiat.*, **28**, 92–97.

SHOULSON, I. & FAHN, S. (1979). Huntington disease: clinical care and evaluation. *Neurology*, **29**, 1–3.

SHOULSON, I., GOLDBATT, D., CHARLTON, M. & JOYNT, R.J. (1978). Huntington's disease: treatment with muscimol, a GABA-mimetic drug. *Ann. Neurol.*, **4**, 279–284.

SIGWALD, J., BOUTTIER, D. & COURVOISIER, S. (1959). Les accidents neurologiques des medications neuroleptiques. *Rev. Neurol.*, **100**, 553–595.

SIMPSON, G.M. & ANGUS, J.W.S. (1970). Drug-induced extrapyramidal disorders. *Acta. Psychiat. Scand.*, **45**, (suppl. 212), 11–19.

SIMPSON, G.M., ZOUBOK, B. & LEE, H.J. (1976). An early clinical and toxicity trial of Ex11-582A in chronic schizophrenia. *Curr. Ther. Res.*, **19**, 87–93.

SIMPSON, G.M., LEE, J.H., ZOUBOK, B. & GARDOS, G. (1979). A rating scale for tardive dyskinesia. *Psychopharmac.*, **64**, 171–179.

SMITH, R.C., TAMMINGA, C.A. & HARASZTI, J. (1977). Effects of dopamine agonists in tardive dyskinesia. *Am. J. Psychiat.*, **134**, 763–768.

STUART, W., GOPINATHAN, G., TERAVAINEN, H., DAMBROSIA, J., WARD, C., SANES, J., EVARTS, E. & CALNE, D. (1980). Studies on Parkinson disease: I. Tests of motor function. *Neurology*, **30**, 415.

SWASH, M., ROBERTS, A.H., ZAKKO, H. & HEATHFIELD, K.W. (1972). Treatment of involuntary movement disorders with tetrabenazine. *J. Neurol. Neurosurg. Psychiat.*, **35**, 186–191.

SWEET, R.D., BRUUN, R., SHAPIRO, E. & SHAPIRO, A.K. (1974). Presynaptic catecholamine antagonists in treatment for Tourette syndrome. *Arch. gen. Psychiat.*, **31**, 857–861.

TARSY, D., PARKES, J.D. & MARSDEN, C.D. (1975). Metoclopramide and pimozide in Parkinson's disease and levodopa-induced dyskinesias. *J. Neurol. Neurosurg. Psychiat.*, **38**, 331–335.

TATTON, W.G. & LEE, R.G. (1975). Evidence for abnormal long-loop reflexes in rigid Parkinsonian patients. *Brain Res.*, **100**, 671–676.

TERAVAINEN, H. & CALNE, D. (1980). Quantitative assessment of Parkinsonian deficits. In *Parkinson's disease. Current progress, problems and management.* eds Rinne, U.K., Klingler, M. & Stamm, G. Amsterdam: Elsevier.

TRECIOKAS, L.J., ANSEL, R.D. & MARKHAM, C.H. (1971). One to two years treatment of Parkinson's disease with levodopa. *Calif. Med.*, **114**, 7–16.

URQUHART, N., PERRY, T.L. & HANSEN, S. (1975). GABA content and glutamic acid decarboxylase activity in brain of Huntington's chorea patients and control subjects. *J. Neurochem.* **24**, 1071–1075.

VAN WOERT, M.H., ROSENBAUM, D., HOWIESON, J. & BOWERS, M.P. (1977). Long-term therapy of myoclonus and other neurological disorders with hydroxytryptophan and carbidopa. *New Engl. J. Med.*, **296**, 70–75.

VELASCO, F. & VELASCO, M. (1973). A quantitative evaluation of the effects of L-dopa on Parkinson's disease. *Neuropharmac.*, **12**, 89–99.

VERE, D.W. (1979). Validity of cross-over trials. *Br. J. clin. Pharmac.*, **8**, 5–6.

VILLENEUVE, A. & BOSZORMENYI, Z. (1970). Treatment of drug-induced dyskinesias. *Lancet*, **i**, 353–354.

WACHS, H. & BOSHES, B. (1961). Tremor studies in normals and in Parkinsonians. *Arch. Neurol.*, **4**, 66–82.

WEBSTER, D.D. (1959). A method of measuring the dynamic characteristics of muscle rigidity, strength and tremor in the upper extremity. *IRE Tans. Med. Electr.*, **6**, 159–164.

WEBSTER, D.D. (1964). The dynamic quantitation of spasticity with automated integrals of passive motor resistance. *Clin. Pharmac. Ther.*, **5**, 900–908.

WEBSTER, D.D. (1966). Rigidity in extrapyramidal disease. *J. Neurosurg.*, **24** (suppl. I, part III), 299–309.

WEBSTER, D.D. (1968). Clinical analysis of the disability in Parkinson's disease. *Mod. Treat.*, **5**, 257–282.

WEBSTER, D.D. & MORTIMER, J.A. (1977). Failure of L-dopa to relieve activated rigidity in Parkinson's disease. In *Parkinson's disease: neurophysiological, clinical and related aspects*, eds. Messiha, F.S. & Kenny, A.D., pp. 297–313. New York: Plenum.

WEITZMAN, D.O., ROSENFELD, C. & KORENYI, C. (1976). Quantification of chorea in Huntington's disease by power spectral analysis. *Dis. Nerv. Syst.*, **37**, 264–268.

WRIGHT, V. & JOHNS, R.J. (1960). Physical factors concerned with the stiffness of normal and diseased joints. *Bull. Johns Hopkins Hosp.*, **106**, 215–231.

YAHR, M.D., DUVOISIN, R.C., SCHEAR, M.J., BARRETT, R.E. & HOEHN, M.M. (1969). Treatment of Parkinsonism with levodopa. *Arch. Neurol.*, **21**, 343–354.

ASSESSMENT OF ANTI-PSYCHOTIC DRUGS

A. V. P. MACKAY

Argyll and Bute Hospital, Argyllshire.

Introduction

The last thirty years have witnessed intense activity in the field of clinical psychopharmacology, since the birth of contemporary psychopharmacology in Paris in 1952 with the production and clinical evaluation of chlorpromazine. That original evaluation of chlorpromazine was relatively straightforward (Delay & Deniker, 1952). Its efficacy in controlling psychotic manifestations was so clearly superior to existing means at that time that no subtle clinical rating scale or statistical device was required to throw the observed benefit into relief. Since that time there have been many developments in the field of psychopharmacology and several new families of anti-schizophrenic drugs have appeared. During this process certain rules of clinical assessment have evolved and have become incorporated into a research and development ritual which now tends to be applied to any new anti-schizophrenic candidate. There is no doubt that real evolution has taken place in the technology of clinical assessment and that experimenters are more aware of the basic requirements needed to arrive at some scientific conclusion. However, it is arguable that there has been no substantial improvement in either the clinical efficacy or the safety of anti-psychotic drugs in the twenty-eight years since the introduction of chlorpromazine. Rational research and development seems, not unusually, to have been a rather poor substitute for accidental discovery. The failure to develop anything that is more than a trivial extension of existing pharmacia may have its roots in the earliest stages of pharmacological definition—in the pre-clinical screening procedures which fall outside the remit of this review. Nonetheless, the clinical experimenter has a responsibility to scrutinise the existing methodological habits of clinical assessment and enquire whether current approaches might hamper the search for more successful antipsychotic agents.

Most of this review will be devoted to the now well-established methodological rules for clinical assessment and to the tools available for assessing and predicting both the desired and undesired effects of a new drug. Attention will also be devoted to more fundamental questions of therapeutic goals in the context of schizophrenic illness.

The most economical approach to the subject is perhaps to trace the steps of development of a theoretically novel anti-schizophrenic compound from the point at which it has emerged from pre-clinical trials and is about to embark upon the lengthy process of clinical evaluation. It will be assumed that by this stage the requisite pre-clinical toxicity trials will have been completed to the satisfaction of the drug company and of the Committee on Safety of Medicines.

Volunteer studies

The first phase of clinical screening for a new drug is frequently the assessment in healthy volunteers. Indeed, a postal ballot of academic and industrial clinicians revealed that the vast majority felt that the first stage of screening should be a healthy volunteer population (Blackwell, 1972). However, it must be self-evident that such procedures are of limited value in screening for anti-schizophrenic properties (Hollister, 1972). Unlike simple sedatives where the observed action in volunteers may correlate with desired effect in anxious patients (Hollister, 1962), anti-schizophrenic agents can only be properly assessed in patients suffering from schizophrenia. The effects of chlorpromazine and thioridazine in volunteers were found to be generally sedative and equivalent to those of meprobamate (Hollister, Kanter & Wright, 1968), but this is trivial information. The problem is of course that we have no experimental model of schizophrenia which can be reproduced in the clinical laboratory. Despite this, volunteer studies have been cited as evidence for and against anti-schizophrenic properties of a new drug. A recent example is the selective D_2-dopamine receptor antagonist metoclopramide. Nakra, Bond & Lader (1975) reported a well-executed study in which metoclopramide, prochlorperazine and placebo were each given to ten healthy volunteers in a double-blind design and fourteen different measures of mental state and autonomic function were administered. The active drugs proved effective in altering only one physiological index, derived from analysis of EEG wavebands, in a manner previously documented for chlorpromazine. Of the psychological measures, the active drugs again affected only one, primarily a test of motor function. On the basis of these results, the authors concluded that 'neither metoclopromide nor prochlorperazine produce marked psychotropic effects' (Nakra *et al.*, 1975). While some useful conclusion could be drawn from this study concerning freedom from acute toxicity at the doses used, the conclusion that neither drug had marked psychotropic effects is potentially misleading. If taken as presumably intended—that neither drug produced psychological disturbance in healthy volunteers—then the results may have relevance for medical use in a non-psychiatric population. However this paper has been interpreted by others as support for the conclusion that metoclopramide is devoid of anti-schizophrenic activity (see, for example Robinson, Berney, Mishra & Sulser, 1979).

While little useful comment can be made about anti-schizophrenic actions from healthy volunteer studies, such studies are of some use in providing information about acute toxicity and pharmacokinetics (Tyrer, 1976).

Acute toxicity

For our new drug to have been labelled as a putative anti-schizophrenic agent it would probably have demonstrated some anti-dopaminergic activity in pre-clinical screening. Thus scrutiny for acute extrapyramidal disturbance in volunteers would be appropriate. Absence of overt neurological signs of pseudo-Parkinsonism or acute dystonia need not, of course, necessarily imply lack of substantial blockade of dopamine receptors in the basal ganglia since any coincidental atropinic activity of the drug would tend to mask such blockade (Marsden, Mindham & Mackay, 1981).

It is probably only justifiable to administer the test drug to volunteers as single doses, or at most, for very limited periods (Tyrer, 1976). Thus the sort of relevant information about acute toxicity which might usefully be collected is restricted largely to acute extrapyramidal effects and autonomic responses (including pulse rate, blood pressure and pupil diameter).

The rating of volunteer responses in the early evaluation of such a new drug must be flexible—in addition to the predictable range of side-effect items there should be ample opportunity for the reporting and recording of unexpected effects by means of open-ended questions or self-report options.

Pharmacokinetics

Given reliable methods for assaying the drug and its metabolites in plasma, certain basic pharmacokinetic variables may be assessed in acute studies in healthy volunteers. The theoretical basis of such pharmacokinetic variables is often opaque to the clinical experimenter but lucid accounts are available (Atkinson & Kushner, 1979; Tucker, 1980).

Estimates of the sustained-dosage concentrations likely to be achieved in plasma following prolonged use can often be made but these may have a wide margin of error (Greenblatt, 1979). Thus, although some basic practical information such as dose and dosage interval may be derived from volunteer studies, only approximate guidelines can be expected. While it may be possible to arrive at a reasonable prediction of the dosage schedule required to achieve a given range of plasma drug concentrations, the choice of a potentially therapeutic plasma concentration is largely a matter of guess work. It is usually impossible to identify a therapeutic range of sustained-dose plasma concentrations for an anti-schizophrenic compound, even with the benefit of full clinical trials (for example Johnstone, Bourne, Cotes, Crow, Ferrier, Owen & Robinson, 1980) and this is clearly impossible in volunteer studies. In the absence of a therapeutic index with which to identify potentially effective plasma concentrations, some independent biological reflection of the presumed pharmacodynamic effect of the drug (likely to be a dopamine receptor antagonist) in the CNS, such as hyperprolactinaemia or extrapyramidal impairment, might be used at the volunteer stage. Potent DA receptor antagonist drugs tend to provoke Parkinsonian signs and it has been suggested that such signs might provide a useful biological monitor for penetration of such a drug into brain. Wode-Helgodt, Borg, Fijro & Sedvall (1978) have shown a good correlation between plasma levels of chlorpromazine and extrapyramidal dysfunction.

Another major limitation of the healthy volunteer study is the lack of information about potential interaction of the drug under investigation with other drugs likely to be exhibited in parallel. This is particularly true of the conventional anti-schizophrenic agents where anti-Parkinson medication is a frequent accompaniment. This combination has been reported to cause significant reductions in the plasma concentration of the neuroleptic agent (Rivera-Calimlim, Nasrallah & Strauss, 1976; Gautier, Jus & Villeneuve, 1977), although this issue is controversial (Simpson, Cooper, Bark, Sud & Lee, 1980).

Clinical assessment proper

Having derived limited but useful information from volunteer studies, the investigator may be ready to assess the new drug against target aspects of psychopathology in patients suffering from schizophrenic illness. A fundamental aspect of this problem is the use of clinical rating scales, all of which address the question of reliably quantifying relatively intangible aspects of psychopathology. The well established strategies of trial design will not be reviewed here, only certain issues relating to actual clinical assessment. For useful texts on study design, Sainsbury & Kreitman (1975) can be recommended.

Clinical rating scales

The rating scale is a technique for recording judgements (by patient or observer) of a dimension, a trait, or a behaviour along some continuum. In the last century Galton introduced the idea by developing a crude scale for rating the subjective response of human subjects to physical discomfort and this century has seen a profusion of scales (see Spitzer & Endicott, 1975; Lyerly, 1973: ECDEU Assessment Manual, 1976). Before a brief consideration of which scales to use where, it is appropriate to restate two fundamental properties of any clinical rating scale about which information should be available.

Knowing your instrument

Often a particular scale is adopted simply because it is available and easy to use rather than appropriate for the illness or for the environmental context in question. For example, the target symptoms against which a new anti-schizophrenic drug must be judged are often quite different in the acute and chronic forms of schizophrenia.

The property of *validity* varies with the extent to which any scale is useful for the job intended. 'Content' validity is perhaps the most readily appreciated component of overall validity. It refers to the extent to which items on a scale are relevant, and this usually involves a highly subjective evaluation. 'Concurrent' validity allows objective assessment of the property of validity by comparing the performance of the scale against some independent external measure. In the context of a drug trial, the ability of an instrument to evaluate change in clinical state is a form of concurrent validity. 'Predictive' validity refers to the ability of the instrument to predict some measure, external to the scale, at a later time. Thus the only distinction between concurrent and predictive validity is the time point at which the external independent measure is obtained. Finally, 'construct' validity seeks to satisfy the question 'what does the rating scale really measure?' and when applied to the use of rating scales in evaluating treatment, construct validity addresses the question 'In what way have the patients really changed?' Construct validity is crucial to the extent that the investigator is more interested in inferred processes rather than in the actual behaviour from which ratings are made and which may have face (or 'content') validity. All the other forms of validity can be used to demonstrate construct validity. While many people believe that content validity answers the questions posed above, it is really only by examining all the other kinds of validity information that construct validity can be determined (Spitzer & Endicott, 1975).

The other fundamental property of the rating instrument to which attention must be paid is *reliability*, or in other words, the consistency with which subjects are discriminated one from the other. For observer ratings, reliability may be assessed by inter-rater correlation. Test-retest reliability (or stability) is another facet and seeks to evaluate constancy of ratings over time. However test-retest reliability assumes theoretical constancy in the observed subject population over time and this may only be assumed with taped material. There is a fundamental distinction, often missed, between inter-rater agreement and inter-rater reliability. For example if two observers agree on a rating of x for 100% of a patient sample then there may be perfect agreement, but reliability is unmeasurable. Reliability represents shared discrimination between subjects and can therefore only be measured when subjects vary in their scale ratings and are rated as different by different observers. Correlational measures are the best way to express inter-rater reliability, the data correlated being the raters' judgements for a series of subjects. Thus, strictly speaking, reliability is not a property of a rating instrument but rather of the rating scale applied to a particular sample of subjects by particular raters in a particular setting. The minimum number of patients with which inter-rater reliability should be assessed is fifteen and an acceptable reliability correlation coefficient would be anything greater than 0.7 (Spitzer & Endicott, 1975).

Diagnosis before severity rating

The importance of a valid and reliable diagnostic filter with which to define the study population cannot be over-emphasised (Strauss & Gift, 1977). If sufficient care is taken over the application of a rigorous set of diagnostic criteria to the task of case identification, then once the study population has satisfied these criteria the scale used to rate the severity of illness need not be very detailed. Various sets of reliable diagnostic criteria for schizophrenic illness are available. In the United States, the system of Feighner, Robins, Guze, Woodruff, Winokur & Munoz (1972), or the Research Diagnostic Criteria (RDC) of Spitzer, Endicott & Robins (1975) which were derived from it, are currently popular examples. Both embody present state phenomenological items such as delusions, hallucinations and thought disorder, and they also require the illness to have been present for a specified minimum time. This temporal requirement is an acknowledgement of the original Kraepelinian concept that chronicity is a diagnostically imperative facet of schizophrenic illness—although in the case of Feighner *et al.* (1972)

the minimum time requirement is 6 months and for the RDC only 2 weeks. In the U.K. the criteria contained in the Wing Present State Examination (PSE) have become popular for reasons of clarity of definition and excellent reliability in the hands of suitably trained observers. The results of this detailed mental state examination can be computer-processed to allocate a case into one of five categories relevant to the diagnosis of a schizophrenic psychosis (Wing, Cooper & Sartorius, 1974). The nuclear schizophrenic syndrome defined by the PSE relies heavily on the presence of Schneiderian first-rank phenomena (Schneider, 1959) within 4 weeks of the diagnostic interview but requires no minimum duration of symptoms.

The current fashion is to filter patients largely according to the presence of a set of florid or 'positive' symptoms and then, in the context of the drug trial, to apply ratings of severity at various times before, during and after treatment with the test drug.

Diagnostic definition in a chronic schizophrenic population is difficult since florid positive symptoms are frequently lacking and patients may only display the negative features of the schizophrenic defect state. Such negative features are difficult to identify with reasonable reliability and thus the applicability of a diagnosis of schizophrenia is often determined by retrospective assessment of case-records made at the time of the most recent florid breakdown. Such a retrospective diagnostic filter is clearly less than ideal, but if unavoidable then the Case Record Rating Scale or the New Haven Schizophrenia Index can be used for rating symptoms, selected psychiatric history and social function criteria from hospital records (Strauss & Gift, 1977).

Severity rating scales

Of the severity rating scales applicable to a diagnostically defined study population, the Brief Psychiatric Rating Scale (BPRS) of Overall & Gorham (1962) is a widely-used example. Developed from the lengthier Lorr Multidimensional Scale for Rating Psychiatric Patients (MSRPP) and the Lorr Inpatient Multidimentional Psychiatric Scale (IMPS), it comprises 18 items, each rated on a 7-point scale and was intended primarily for use with in-patients. It can provide a rapid evaluation of treatment response in clinical drug trials.

In most clinical research applications the BPRS is completed immediately prior to the start of drug treatment and again after fixed periods—say 4 to 6 weeks. Ratings are based on a clinical interview lasting about twenty minutes and are derived both from observations of the patient and from verbal report. It is recommended that each patient be interviewed and rated independently by two professional observers in order to enhance the reliability of ratings (Overall, 1976).

The Krawiecka scale was devised for rating schizophrenic psychopathology (Krawiecka, Goldberg & Vaughan, 1977) and has been used quite widely in psychopharmacological research. The scale was developed in order to provide a short, manageable instrument that could be used to screen and rate large numbers of chronic psychotic patients. Eight items are rated on 5-point scales and broadly cover disturbances of affect, thought content and form, and perception. Half of the items are rated according to replies to questions in a short clinical interview, the other half are rated according to observed abnormalities. The rater is expected to have the benefit of additional historical information derived from case-notes, etc. The Krawiecka scale is considered to be sensitive to change, and therefore an appropriate instrument to use in a drug trial (Krawiecka *et al.*, 1977). Inter-rater agreement on most items is good, but rather poor on the item 'flattened, incongruous affect'—a typically difficult phenomenon to rate. In a recent clinical trial of anti-schizophrenic medication in a sample of acutely ill patients, incongruity of affect and flattening of affect were rated separately to yield a total of nine items and this seems to represent a useful modification, although no report of inter-rater reliability was provided (Johnstone, Crow, Frith, Carney & Price, 1978). While the question of the validity of the Krawiecka scale remains open it does seem to represent a quickly administered severity scale, of reasonable reliability, for use in a diagnostically defined sample. More emphasis is given to negative psychotic features in this scale than in the BPRS, which would make it preferable for drug trials with chronic schizophrenic patients.

The benefit of observer ratings by members of the nursing staff should not be missed. Nursing staff are those most familiar with the patient in the ward environment and the Nurses' Observation Scale for In-Patient Evaluation (aptly abbreviated to NOSIE) was designed for the assessment of ward behaviour by nursing personnel (Honigfeldt & Klett, 1965). Using a 5-point scale, thirty items are presented in simple language and ask for ratings based on direct observation. The patient's strengths as well as pathology are recorded in areas such as personal hygiene, social interaction and manifest psychosis. Inter-rater reliability has been reported to be high— in a study by Lentz, Paul & Calhoun (1971), inter-rater correlation co-efficients varied between 0.82 and 0.95 over a series of seven factors derived from the thirty-item scale. Although NOSIE was designed with the long-stay patient in mind, the range of items would make it suitable for nurse ratings in the context of most drug trials. Content validity appears to be adequate—the scale covers a wide range of possible behaviours. However, construct validity (what the scale really measures) should be accepted with caution when, as in this case, the majority of items are derived from observed behaviour and where psycho-pathology is inferred.

Global ratings of change

In simplest form, the observer is asked to rate the patient as either the same, worse, or better as a result of the treatment under investigation. It is an attempt to allow the clinician to use all available cues in coming to the sort of decision which is made every day in normal clinical practice. The level of judgement is one of high complexity and although reliability might be expected to suffer, construct validity should be high in that the rater can take account of everything which he feels is important in coming to a single summary judgement. In particular, he can pay attention to change in target symptoms in response to a test drug. In fact, global judgement scales have been found to be surprisingly reliable and sensitive, particularly in drug studies (McGlashan, 1973; McNair, 1973).

Every drug study should include a global impression of change—it provides easy and useful information. The Clinical Global Impressions (CGI) and Nurses' Global Impressions are scales available in the ECDEU manual (ECDEU Assessment Manual, 1976). The CGI was developed during the Psychopharmacology Research Branch (of NIMH) collaborative studies of anti-schizophrenic medi-cation and in fact consists of three global scales; severity of illness, global improvement, and efficacy index. The efficacy index is in the form of a 4 x 4 matrix in which global change is related to severity of side-effects. If therapeutic effect is regarded as gross gain and side-effects as gross loss, then the index can be.regarded crudely as the net therapeutic gain. It is derived simply by dividing the therapeutic effect score by the side-effect score.

The chronic illness: special issues

Assessing long-term prophylaxis

While the majority of new anti-schizophrenic drugs are tested for their effectiveness at suppressing symptoms of the acute psychosis, if a clear anti-psychotic action is established then a reasonable extrapolation would be to ask whether the drug has the ability to protect against the re-emergence of symptoms in the recovered patient. The assessment of 'protective' pharmacology has been the subject of many recent studies. The usual setting is the maintenance of schizophrenic patients in the community, and the main criterion of success in the prevention of relapse over a specified, relatively lengthy period. The first definitive placebo-controlled trial of this nature (Leff & Wing, 1971)

judged relapse to have occurred if the clinician looking after the patient in the community was sufficiently concerned about the patient's clinical state to want to ascertain whether the patient was receiving active drug. If this happened, a patient would automatically be withdrawn from the trial and a detailed mental state examination would subsequently be performed. The trial by Hirsch, Gaind, Rhode, Stevens & Wing (1973) of depot neuroleptic medication also used a single first-line criterion of relapse; a decision by the hospital clinical team that a patient's schizophrenic symptoms had so deteriorated that he or she must be taken out of the trial and active medication ensured. The extensive studies of Hogarty and his colleagues on maintenance phenothiazine treatment used 'clinical deterioration of such magnitude that rehospitalisation was imminent' (Hogarty & Goldberg, 1973; Hogarty, Goldberg, Schooler & Ulrich, 1974). Similar global primary indices of drug failure have been used in other well-designed trials (Falloon, Watt & Shepherd, 1978; Quitkin, Rifkin, Kane, Ramos-Lorenzi & Klein, 1978), with detailed secondary assessments providing additional information. Thus the type of measure required to assess long-term success of a new agent is defined in terms of global clinical concern for the patient's condition. This is to be contrasted with the more usual acute situation in which the effect of the drug is judged against a base-line of florid symptomatology in a hospital setting and progress is judged by a reduction in the intensity or presence of a specified list of symptoms.

A particular methodological problem in such studies is that in order to create a placebo-treated control group, these patients are usually withdrawn from the sort of psychoactive medication which has helped resolution of their most recent acute illness. What is therefore being compared is a drug con-tinuation group with a drug-withdrawal group. In interpreting relapse rates in this latter group it is important to draw a distinction between the effects of absence of active drug and of sudden withdrawal from active drug. Such a distinction is, in practice, extremely difficult to make but clearly very important in evaluating any positive prophylactic action of the drug under test. Perhaps the only way of achieving this is to take a group of schizophrenic patients who have been well and without psychoactive drugs for a minimum period of three months and to introduce active medication or placebo at that stage, with the usual long term follow-up evaluation.

Drug-environment interactions

Any long term evaluation study of anti-schizophrenic drug which involves treatment in a domestic setting must take account of the informative studies of Brown, Wing, Leff and their colleagues into the potent influence on relapse of socio-environmental factors. It has clearly been established that variables such as expressed emotion and time spent in face to face contact with a significant relative will increase the risk of relapse and that the protective effects of neuroleptic medication only become evident in settings of high expressed emotion (Vaughn & Leff, 1976; Tarrier, Vaughn, Lader & Leff, 1979). Unless such potent variables are matched, or at least recorded, in drug and placebo groups, the interpretation of the effects of drug on relapse rate might be very difficult. Controlling out all possible variables in a complex but realistic environmental setting may not always be desirable. As Leff (1976) has forcefully pointed out, controlling for all social influences in the study design might deprive the investigator of very useful information about interactions between non-controlled environmental factors and test drug. Careful recording of environmental variables may thus be preferable to trying to allocate them equally between drug and placebo groups (Leff, 1976).

Functional ratings in the chronic illness

An aspect of drug evaluation to which far too little attention has been devoted is the influence of medication on deficits in everyday practical performance in chronic schizophrenia. In the context of the contemporary focus on community care this is obviously important. Here the experimenter is not dealing with the efficacy of the test drug in suppressing florid symptomatology but the facilitation of rehabilitation in the setting of the defect state or 'chronic poverty syndrome' of flattened affect, poverty of speech, slowness, underactivity, social withdrawal and lack of motivation (Wing, 1978). In addition to affecting general social performance, the chronic poverty syndrome may seriously affect work output and therefore bear on the all important issue of employment prospects. Very few studies have attempted to address this question, but the report by Harper & Chacon (1976) shows how this can be done in a straightforward and sensible way. The effects of phenothiazine medication were assessed on work performance in the form of nut and bolt assembly and carton assembly. Dexterity, concentration, skill and productive effort were all rated as separate items of performance. The value of assessing such practical performance items was demonstrated by the fact that, in this study, whereas active drugs had no superiority over placebo in ameliorating clinical indices of the defect state, a clear drug effect was evident on work performance (Harper & Chacon, 1976).

Even in terms of structured clinical scales, the investigator interested in assessing the effects of a new drug on ward behaviour in long-stay patients will be hard pressed to find many satisfactory instruments. In a recent review of twenty-nine English language scales, Hall (1980) found only four which satisfied the criteria of validity, reliability, availability of normative data and statement of a recommended observation period. Of these four, that of Wing (1961) had the further recommendations of brevity and speed of application.

Platelet aggregation as a therapeutic index

If an objective biological variable could be identified which changed consistently in association with clinically effective drug treatment in schizophrenic illness then several important possibilities would present themselves. At the practical level, such a biological indicator might obviate the need for measuring plasma concentrations of the anti-schizophrenic drug—the biological effect would signify the attainment of potentially therapeutic tissue levels of drug. At the theoretical level, the biological variable might afford a fresh insight into the pharmacodynamic principle of the drug.

Just such intriguing possibilities seemed to be emerging with the report by Boullin, Woods, Grimes, Grahame-Smith, Wiles, Gelder & Kolakowska (1975) that chronic chlorpromazine treatment was associated with a curious effect on 5-hydroxytryptamine (5-HT)-induced blood platelet aggregation. When added *in vitro*, chlorpromazine had been known to inhibit 5-HT-induced platelet aggregation (Mills & Roberts, 1967). However, Boullin, Woods *et al.* (1975) reported that in platelet-rich plasma prepared from the blood of nine patients receiving chlorpromazine (150–900 mg/day) for periods in excess of 3 years, the 5-HT response was significantly enhanced rather than inhibited. Furthermore, this enhancement disappeared 3 weeks after drug withdrawal and re-appeared 3 weeks after re-institution of chlorpromazine treatment. A companion report (Boullin, Grahame-Smith, Grimes & Woods, 1975) described further experiments in which platelets harvested from chlorpromazine-treated patients were resuspended in control plasma and these showed that the enhanced aggregation response persisted. The conclusion was that chronic chlorpromazine treatment changed, in some enduring way, the membrane characteristics of the platelet. The significance of these preliminary reports on small numbers of patients was strengthened by the findings that the enhanced aggregation response was also found in patients receiving other anti-schizophrenic drugs (α-flupenthixol, fluphenazine and thioridazine) and that the platelet index correlated with clinical state in chronic schizophrenic patients (Orr & Boullin, 1976; Boullin & Orr, 1976). The clinical state of eighteen chronic schizophrenic patients who had received injections of fluphenazine decanoate for longer than 6 months was evaluated on the BPRS, and the presence of extrapyramidal side-effects was also recorded. It was found that only ten out of eighteen patients showed the enhanced platelet aggregation phenomenon and that in these responders there was significantly more psychopathology but fewer extrapyramidal side-effects (Orr & Boullin, 1976). The authors suggested at that time that platelet response might be a marker for a subgroup of schizophrenic patients who require chronic medication. Boullin, Orr & Peters (1978) further reported that the time-course of development of the abnormal platelet response in some recently admitted patients correlated with the time course of clinical change in response to chlorpromazine. A replication study, however, showed that platelet responders were much less prevalent than had been reported in earlier studies (Boullin et al., 1978). Most recently, an extensive study has been undertaken, involving 139 patients receiving not only phenothiazines but also butyrophenones and thioxanthenes (Orr, Knox, Allen, Gelder & Grahame-Smith, 1981). Inconsistency in platelet response was disappointingly wide; none of a group of fifteen patients on trifluoperazine showed the platelet effect, only eight out of forty patients receiving chronic chlorpromazine therapy now showed it and, most worrying of all, three out of twenty-four drug-naive controls showed the platelet effect (Orr et al., 1981). This time there was no relationship between platelet index and clinical response in recently-admitted patients and the platelet aggregation phenomenon varied over time within patients. In an attempt to understand these puzzling inconsistencies, some artefactual explanation was sought by investigating several technical variables in the platelet assay (Knox, Orr, Allen, Gelder & Grahame-Smith, 1981). It was found that platelet dilution had a powerful effect on 5-HT-induced aggregation. Abnormally enhanced responses could be normalised simply by diluting platelet-rich plasma from neuroleptic treated patients by 30% with platelet-free plasma from the same patients. Thus minor variations in centrifugation speeds, which determine platelet yield, might have contributed to previous inconsistencies by producing false-negative results (Knox et al., 1981). However, even when this variable is attended to, the abnormal response appears unlikely to be found in the majority of chlorpromazine-treated patients, and it is clearly not a phenomenon typical of all anti-schizophrenic drugs.

Thus the early promise of this phenomenon as an objective marker for therapeutic response and as a biological index of anti-psychotic activity has not been borne out. As the authors have put it: 'while an interesting and intriguing pharmacological phenomenon in itself, it is unlikely to be of value as an empirical guide to treatment' (Orr, et al. 1981).

Assessing extra-pyramidal complications

Extrapyramidal dysfunction is a price paid by many patients for the clinical treatment of their psychosis. This was realised soon after the introduction of chlorpromazine (Delay & Deniker, 1952) and the general association of extrapyramidal side-effects with anti-schizophrenic activity has held true for most anti-schizophrenic drugs developed since then. Where apparent exceptions have occurred, the explanation lay in the possession of atropinic as well as anti-dopaminergic properties by the same drug (Miller & Hiley, 1974; Snyder, Greenberg & Yamamura, 1974; Yamamura, Marian & Snyder, 1976). While it is now generally agreed that overt extrapyramidal side-effects are not a 'conditio sine qua non' for therapeutic effectiveness (Marsden et al., 1981), any novel antipsychotic agent which substantially inhibits central dopaminergic transmission will carry the risk of such disorders, acute and chronic. It has thus become a convention that the assessment of extrapyramidal function is a facet of any clinical evaluation of a new antipsychotic agent. Methods of assessment have been fully reviewed in an earlier article in this series (Marsden & Schachter, 1981).

1. Acute toxicity

(a) *Acute dyskinesias* The acute dystonic reactions are dramatic and easily reversible. Their recognition should present little diagnostic problem to the trained observer (Marsden et al., 1981), and recording their presence probably requires no formal rating instrument.

(b) *Akathisia* This essentially subjective disorder has never been rigorously defined nor are there any proper rating instruments available with which to quantify its intensity. Nonetheless, it is a common accompaniment of anti-psychotic medication and one that can be misinterpreted as an exacerbation of psychotic agitation. Investigators should thus be alive to this possibility when investigating the clinical profile of any new drug.

(c) *Bradykinesia* This is an especially common side-effect (Ayd, 1961) and, like akathisia, may present problems of diagnosis and misinterpretation. Rifkin, Quitkin & Klein (1975) have described it as 'a behavioural state of diminished spontaneity characterised by few gestures, unspontaneous speech, and, particularly, apathy and difficulty with initiating usual activities'. It may be the only sign of pseudo-Parkinsonism to occur (Ayd, 1961) and since the total clinical picture may include disturbances of affect and motivation it may be mistaken for a schizophrenic defect state (Marsden et al., 1981).

'Akinetic depression' is a term coined by Van Putten & May (1978) to capture the negative subjective accompaniment to Parkinsonian poverty of movement. Assessment of this complication of neuroleptic drug treatment is imprecise. The purely motor impoverishment can be rated on the 'gait' item of the Simpson & Angus (1970) scale, on the clinical assessment of facial expression and of gait in the scale of Mindham, Gaind, Anstee & Rimmer (1972), or on items assessing daily activities and speed of action in the scale of Godwin-Austen, Tomlinson, Frears & Kok (1969). Van Putten & May (1978) suggest that constriction of handwriting may be a useful correlate of the subjective state which might be labelled 'depression', and they also report an association between drowsiness and drug-induced akinesia. More interpretative ratings of accompanying defects in motivation may be made with simple nurse-related scales such as NOSIE ('shows interest in activities around him') or the scale of Ellsworth and Clayton (1959) (along the 'active, restless *v* listless, apathetic' axis) but the definition of such items is very vague. The apparent lack of detailed rating scales of demonstrated reliability and validity is a serious gap in this complex area. The phenomenological similarity between drug-induced bradykinesia and the schizophrenic defect state raises the possibility of serious misinterpretation. It is vital to distinguish a drug-induced Parkinsonian syndrome, which may be amenable to anticholinergic medication, from a natural feature of the psychotic illness. A brief diagnostic trial with an anticholinergic anti-Parkinson agent probably represents the only straightforward means available by which to make such a distinction, but this approach is very crude.

(d) *Pseudo-Parkinsonism* Most attention is usually devoted to the full-blown drug-induced facsimile of classical Parkinson's disease in which the cardinal features of rigidity, tremor and bradykinesia co-exist with a variety of subsidiary features such as disordered gait and hypersalivation. Many scales have been developed for assessing the signs of true Parkinsonism but those of the drug-induced syndrome are often milder and more subtle, necessitating specially designed rating instruments (Mindham, 1976). The scale developed by Simpson & Angus (1970) was designed specifically for this purpose and has been shown to be probably valid and reasonably reliable. Ten signs and symptoms are each rated on a 5-point (0-5) scale and a clear glossary of definitions is provided (Simpson & Angus, 1970). However, in the writer's experience, items such as 'arm dropping', 'leg pendulousness' and 'shoulder shaking' are difficult to rate in practice, especially in the face of variable co-operation by the patient. Others have tried to tackle the problem of assessment by including in their scales certain objective

performance tests such as a timed walk, inflation of sphygmomanometer cuff, manipulating beads and tapping a stylus (Mindham, Gaind, Anstee & Rimmer, 1972; Simpson, Amuso, Blair & Farkas, 1964; Horne, 1973; Onuaguluchi, 1964; Mindham, 1976). Various tests of handwriting have been claimed to be particularly sensitive to extrapyramidal disorder (Angus & Simpson, 1970) and have the virtue of ease of administration. However, performance tests reflect a complex mixture of various neurological impairments, being influenced by tremor, rigidity, difficulty in initiating movement, and so on. Unfortunately, they have been shown to correlate rather poorly with clinical signs and to be, in fact, generally less sensitive to change (Marsden *et al.*, 1981).

A recent and technically sophisticated refinement seeks to quantify objectively the earliest signs of drug-induced Parkinsonism. This involves the measurement of finger tremor using a piezoelectric accelerometer with computerised power spectral analysis (Collins, Lee & Tyrer, 1979)). The authors have demonstrated that clinical signs of extrapyramidal impairment correlate closely with a reduction in the frequency of finger tremor from the physiological range (10 Hz) to the Parkinsonian range (5–6 Hz). Of particular interest is the finding that the frequency shift precedes the emergence of clinically detectable signs and so may represent a sensitive predictor of extrapyramidal disorder in the course of drug-treatment (Collins *et al.*, 1979). However, validity remains an open question and it is hardly a technique which recommends itself by its simplicity.

While the clinical scale of Chouinard, Annable, Ross-Chouinard & Kropsky (1979) is possibly the most sensitive for detecting minimal signs of Parkinsonism, and hence the most generally suitable scale for drug studies (Marsden *et al.*, 1981), it has to be acknowledged that at the present time the structured methods available for assessing extrapyramidal disorder are not well developed (Mindham, 1976).

2. Chronic toxicity

Here the problem facing the clinical investigator with a new drug is the practical one of time-scale. Anti-schizophrenic medication tends to be given chronically and patients may be exposed to such medication for a large fraction of their lives. Chronic tardive dyskinesia provides a good example of late-onset toxicity, a side-effect which was not evident in the early clinical trials of neuroleptic drugs.

Chronic oro-facial dyskinesia was first described five years after the introduction of chlorpromazine for the treatment of psychotic illnesses (Schoenecker, 1957). Few experimenters would contemplate this sort of time-scale in any clinical drug evaluation programme. The recognition of tardive dyskinesia as an iatrogenic disorder was delayed for many reasons, not least due to a reluctance by the medical fraternity to accept that useful anti-psychotic agents might be neurologically dangerous drugs. However, even given the delay in public recognition of this particular side-effect, impartial and close scrutiny might not have been expected to uncover evidence of serious and potentially irreversible neuronal toxicity within a period of less than 2 years of chronic medication. Animal models of chronic drug-induced oro-facial dyskinesia now exist (Marsden *et al.*, 1981) but it is doubtful if the motor abnormalities observed in animals after 6 to 12 month periods of neuroleptic medication would ever have been taken seriously had not the clinical casualties occurred first.

Clinicians are now more sensitive to the chroinic neurological complications of anti-schizophrenic chemotherapy and thus, hopefully, the dangers of any new anti-schizophrenic agent in this respect will be appreciated quicker. It is mandatory that a close watch is kept on the neurological status of all patients exposed chronically to any new drug—for periods of at least 2 years. A period of drug withdrawal may be required before tardive dyskinesia becomes evident, and this liability must be assessed in an organised long-term surveillance which might therefore include brief drug-holidays.

The diagnosis and rating of late-onset dyskinesia is not always easy (Marsden *et al.*, 1981); Mackay & Sheppard, 1979) but obvious cases present little difficulty. The scale of Kidger, Barnes, Trauer & Taylor (1980) is simple and reliable and ideally suited to rating from video-taped material. Regular assessment of video-tapes from a cohort of patients exposed to any new anti-schizophrenic drug over a 2 year period (including drug holidays) would seem to offer a reasonable strategy for long-term assessment of neurological toxicity.

Tardive dyskinesia is a syndrome with which we are now familiar. As new generations of anti-psychotic agents come to clinical testing it is essential that investigators remain alive to the possibility of new syndromes which may be of late onset. In addition to direct chemical toxicity, the chronic administration of any psychopharmacological agent seems likely to provoke a biological reaction from the brain which may eventually become maladaptive and disabling. Late onset toxicity is often the most serious and thus chronic 'maintenance' medication must always be evaluated with the utmost care.

Future targets

The drug industry has been firmly preoccupied with the dopamine receptor antagonist paradigm for the development of new neuroleptic agents. The reasons are quite understandable—chlorpromazine and its offspring are effective at dispelling psychotic delusions and hallucinations in the majority of acutely ill patients. However, the results of pharmacological development over the past two decades can hardly be described as impressive—new families of neuroleptic agents whose only claims to novelty have been improved potency and some variations in secondary pharmacodynamic profile. This is not surprising since the very screening procedures used to identify possible candidates at the preclinical stage require any new agent to fulfil one essential criterion; that of dopamine receptor antagonist activity. The recent definition of more than one dopamine receptor seemed to provide a timely direction and promise for the development of new anti-dopaminergic drugs; an opportunity perhaps to dissociate anti-psychotic actions and extrapyramidal actions. However, unhappily, this does not now appear to be a likely outcome of dopamine receptor dualism. One sort, the D_2 receptor, seems to mediate both the wanted and unwanted effects in man (Schachter, Bedard, Debono, Jenner, Marsden, Price, Parkes, Keenan, Smith, Rosenthaler, Horowski & Dorrow, 1980; Snyder & Goodman, 1980). It may be that developing 'bigger and better' dopamine receptor antagonists has gone as far as it should. A change in emphasis is required, and the clinical target for this must surely be the schizophrenic defect state. This, more than any other syndrome, shows up the serious limitations of contemporary developments in anti-psychotic medication.

'If you discover a new treatment for schizophrenia make sure you use it on acute schizophrenic patients, for they will surely improve under it'—thus has Kety paraphrased Laennaec's dictum in an allusion to the current preoccupation of psychopharmacology with acute psychosis rather than with classical schizophrenia (Kety, 1980). Most popular diagnostic scales place emphasis on florid positive symptomatology of the Schneiderian sort and thus the clinical population in which new anti-schizophrenic drugs tend to be evaluated is characterised by acute, and environmentally reactive, symptomatology. Most placebo-controlled drug trials in acute schizophrenia report a majority response to medication and also a high level of placebo response (see, for example, Johnstone *et al.*, 1978). The dopamine antagonist performs well here. The situation is very different in chronic schizophrenia where the negative features of the chronic poverty syndrome form the prevailing clinical presentation. Here the response to medication is dismal, the dopamine antagonist largely impotent (Hughes & Little, 1967; Letemendia & Harris, 1967), except in reducing the probability of a florid psychosis. Were the term schizophrenia to be restricted to the fundamental features outlined by

Kraepelin and Bleuler (a chronic disorder of thought and feeling, with insidious onset, characteristic premorbid personality and pernicious deterioration) then most contemporary psychopharmacological research would be irrelevant to that particular illness (Mackay & Crow, 1980). The relative impotence of modern psychopharmacology in classical schizophrenia suggests the target for the future. Frequent reference has been made to the lack of good scales for the diagnosis and rating of the negative syndrome and its behavioural manifestations. Clinicians must concentrate their efforts into clarifying the phenomenological definition in this area and to devising informative rating scales for the chronic patient. The drug companies can justifiably continue to seek neurologically safer antipsychotic drugs which

will continue to help the majority of acutely ill patients, but in addition they must shift their focus from the florid psychoses to the chronic disability. This is already happening on the European Continent where at least one completely novel agent is being evaluated mainly for its efficacy in the defect state (Deniker, 1978).

The defect state is one of the greatest remaining challenges to psychopharmacology and any chemotherapeutic strategy which might emerge with the sort of efficacy which is already evident in drugs used against the florid psychosis would have enormous impact in rehabilitation. To this end, not only will pathophysiological theories need to be revised but the tools of clinical assessment will need to be made more suitable.

References

ATKINSON, A.J. & KUSHNER, W. (1979). Clinical pharmacokinetics. Ann. Rev. Pharmac. Tox., 19, 105–127.

AYD, F. (1961). A survey of drug-induced extrapyramixal reactions. J. Am. med. Ass. 175, 1054–1060.

ANGUS, J.W.S. & SIMPSON, G.M. (1970). Handwriting changes and response to drugs—a controlled study. Acta Psychiat. Scand. Suppl., 212, 28–37.

BLACKWELL, B. (1972). For the first time in man. Clin. Pharmac. Ther., 13, 812–823.

BOULLIN, D.J., GRAHAME-SMITH, D.G., GRIMES, R.P.J. & WOODS, H.F. (1975). Resuspension of platelets: enhanced 5-hydroxytryptamine-induced aggregation in chlorpromazine treated patients due to changes in platelet properties. Br. J. clin. Pharmac., 2, 37–39.

BOULLIN, D.J., KNOX, J.M., PETERS, J. & ORR, M.W. (1978). Platelet aggregation and chlorpromazine therapy. Br. J. clin. Pharmac., 6, 538–540.

BOULLIN, D.J. & ORR, M.W. (1976). Effects of aspirin and prostaglandin E₂ on secondary phase aggregation responses in schizophrenic patients treated with chlorpromazine. Br. J. clin. Pharmac., 3, 929–933.

BOULLIN, D.J., ORR, M.W., & PETERS, J.R. (1978). The platelet as a model for investigating the clinical efficacy of centrally acting drugs; relations between platelet aggregation and clinical condition in schizophrenics treated with chlorpromazine. In Platelets: A multidisciplinary approach, eds Gaetano, S.E. & Garattini, S. New York: Raven Press.

BOULLIN, D.J., WOODS, H.F., GRIMES, R.P.J., GRAHAME-SMITH, D.G., WILES, D., GELDER, M.G. & KOLAKOWSKA, T. (1975). Increased platelet aggregation responses to 5-hydroxytryptamine in patients taking chlorpromazine. Br. J. clin. Pharmac., 2, 29–35.

CHOUINARD, G., ANNABLE, L., ROSS-CHOUINARD, A. & KROPSKY, M.L. (1979). Ethopropazine and benztropine in neuroleptic-induced Parkinsonism. J. clin. Psychiat., 40, 147–152.

COLLINS, P., LEE, I. & TYRER, P. (1979). Finger tremor and extrapyramidal side effects of neuroleptic drugs. Br. J. Psychiat., 134, 488–493.

DELAY, J. & DENIKER, P. (1952). 38 cas de psychoses traitées par la cure prolongée et continué de 4560 RP, Le Congrés de Psychiat. Neurol. de Lange Française (Luxembourg, 1952) in C.R., 503–513, Ed. Masson.

DENIKER, P. (1978). Impact of neuroleptic chemotherapies on schizophrenic psychoses. Am. J. Psychiat., 135, 923–927.

ECDEU ASSESSMENT MANUAL (1976). Early clinical drug evaluation programme assessment manual for psychopharmacology. ed. Giu, W., Maryland: U.S. Department of Health, Education and Welfare.

ELLSWORTH, R.B. & CLAYTON, W.H. (1959). Measurement of improvement in mental illness. J. consult. Psychol., 23, 15–20.

FALLOON, I., WATT, D.C. & SHEPHERD, M. (1978). A comparative controlled trial of pimozide and fluphenazine decanoate in the continuation therapy of schizophrenia. Psychol. Med., 8, 59–70.

FEIGHNER, J.P., ROBINS, E., GUZE, S.B., WOODRUFF, R. A., WINOKUR, G. & MUNOZ, R. (1972). Diagnostic criteria for use in psychiatric research. Arch. gen. Psychiat., 26, 57–63.

GAUTIER, J., JUS, A. & VILLENEUVE, A. (1977). Influence of the antiparkinsonian drugs on the plasma levels of neuroleptics. Biol. Psychiat. 12, 389–399.

GODWIN-AUSTEN, R.B., TOMLINSON, E.B., FREARS, C.C. & KOK, H.W.L. (1969). Effects of L-DOPA in Parkinson's disease. Lancet, ii, 165–168.

GREENBLATT, D.J. (1979). Predicting steady state serum concentrations of drugs. Ann. Rev. Pharmac. Toxi., 19, 347–356.

HALL, J.N. (1980). Ward rating scales for long-stay patients: a review. Psychol. Med., 10, 277–288.

HARPER, P. & CHACON, C. (1976). Work performance versus clinical assessment in the evaluation of phenothiazine treatment. Br. J. clin. Pharmac., 3, (Suppl.) 50–55.

HIRSCH, S.R., GAIND, R., RHODE, P.D., STEVENS, B.C. & WING, J.K. (1973). Outpatient maintenance of chronic schizophrenic patients with long-acting fluphenazine. Double-blind placebo trial. Br. med. J., 1, 633–637.

HOGARTY, G.E. & GOLDBERG, S.C. (1973). Collaborative Study Group: Drugs and sociotherapy in the aftercare of schizophrenic patients; one year relapse rates. *Arch. gen. Psychiat.*, **28**, 54–64.

HOGARTY, G.E., GOLDBERG, S.C., SCHOOLER, N.R. & ULRICH, R.F. (1974). The Collaborative Group: Drugs and sociotherapy in the aftercare of schizophrenic patients II; two-year relapse rates. *Arch. gen. Psychiat.*, **31**, 603–608.

HOLLISTER, L.E. (1962). Studies of delayed-action medication. 1. Meprobamate administered as compressed tablets and as two delayed-action capsules. *New Engl. J. Med.*, **266**, 281–283.

HOLLISTER, L.E. (1972). Prediction of therapeutic uses of psychotherapeutic drugs from experiences with normal volunteers. *Clin. Pharmac. Ther.*, **13**, 803–808.

HOLLISTER, L.E., KANTER, S.L. & WRIGHT, A. (1968). Comparison of intramuscular and oral administration of chlorpromazine and thioridazine. *Arch. int. Pharmacodyn.*, **144**, 571–578.

HONIGFELDT, G. & KLETT, C. (1965). The Nurses' Observation Scale for In-patient Evaluation (NOSIE): A new scale for measuring improvement in chronic schizophrenia. *J. clin. Psychol.*, **21**, 65–71.

HORNE, D.J. de L. (1973). Sensorimotor control in Parkinsonism. *J. Neurol. Neurosurg. Psychiat.*, **36**, 742–746.

HUGHES, J.S. & LITTLE, J.C. (1976). An appraisal of the continuing practice of prescribing tranquillizing drugs for long-stay psychiatric patients. *Br. J. Psychiat.*, **113**, 867–873.

JOHNSTONE, E.C., CROW, T.J., FRITH, C.D., CARNEY, M. W. P. & PRICE, J. S. (1978). Mechanism of antipsychotic effect in acute schizophrenia. *Lancet*, **i**, 848–851.

JOHNSTONE, E.C., BOURNE, R.C., COTES, P.M., CROW, T.J., FERRIER, I.N., OWEN, F. & ROBINSON, J.D. (1980). Blood levels of flupenthixol in patients with acute and chronic schizophrenia. In *Drug Concentrations in Neuropsychiatry*, Ciba Foundation Symposium 74 (New series), pp. 99–111 Oxford: Excerpta Medica.

KETY, S.S. (1980). The syndrome of schizophrenia: Unresolved questions and opportunities for research. *Br. J. Psychiat.*, **136**, 421–436.

KIDGER, T., BARNES, T.R.E., TRAUER, T. & TAYLOR, P.J. (1980). Sub-syndromes of tardive dyskinesia. *Psychol. Med.*, **10**, 513–520.

KNOX, J.M., ORR, M.W., ALLEN, R., GELDER, M.G. & GRAHAME-SMITH, D.G. (1981). The reliability of 5-hydroxytryptamine-induced platelet aggregation responses in schizophrenic patients treated with neuroleptic drugs. *Br. J. clin. Pharmac.*, **11**, 261–263.

KRAWIECKA, M., GOLDBERG, D. & VAUGHAN, M. (1977). A standardised psychiatric assessment scale for rating chronic psychotic patients. *Acta Psychiat. Scand.*, **55**, 299–308.

LEFF, J. (1976). Assessment of drugs in schizophrenia. *Br. J. clin. Pharmac.*, **3**, (Suppl.) 75–78S.

LEFF, J.P. & WING, J.K. (1971). Trial of maintenance therapy in schizophrenia. *Br. med. J.*, **3**, 599–604.

LENTZ, R.J., PAUL, G.L. & CALHOUN, J.F. (1971). Reliability and validity of three measures of functioning with 'hard core' chronic mental patients. *J. abn. Psychol.*, **78**, 69–76.

LETEMENDIA, F.J.J. & HARRIS, A.D. (1967). Chlorpromazine and the untreated chronic schizo-phrenic: a long-term trial. *Br. J. Psychiat.*, **113**, 940–958.

LYERLY, S.B. (1973). *Handbook of Psychiatric Rating Scales*, Edition 2. Bethesda, Maryland, U.S.A.: National Institutes of Mental Health.

McGLASHAN, T. (1973). In *The Documentation of Clinical Psychotropic Drug Trials*, ed. McGlashan, T. Rockville, Maryland: National Institute of Mental Health.

MACKAY, A.V.P. & CROW, T.J. (1980). Positive and negative schizophrenic symptoms and the role of dopamine. *Br. J. Psychiat.*, **137**, 379–386.

MACKAY, A.V.P. & SHEPPARD, G.P. (1979). Pharmacotherapeutic trials in tardive dyskinesia. *Br. J. Psychiat.*, **135**, 489–499.

McNAIR, D.M. (1973). *Self-evaluation of anti-depressants*. Report prepared for the American College of Neuro-psychopharmacology, Subcommittee of the Task Force on Antidepressants.

MARSDEN, C.D., MINDHAM, R.H.S. & MACKAY, A.V.P. (1981). Extrapyramidal movement disorders produced by antipsychotic drugs. In *The pharmacology and treatment of schizophrenia*, eds. Bradley, P.B. & Hirsh, S.R. London: Oxford University Press. (in press.)

MARSDEN, C.D. & SCHACHTER, M. (1981). Assessment of extrapyramidal disorders. *Br. J. clin. Pharmac.*, **11**, 129–152.

MILLER, R.J. & HILEY, R. (1974). Antimuscarinic properties of neuroleptics and drug-induced Parkinsonism. *Nature*, **248**, 596–579.

MILLS, D.C.B. & ROBERTS, G.C.K. (1967). Membrane active drugs and the aggregation of human blood platelets. *Nature*, **213**, 35–38.

MINDHAM, R.H.S. (1976). Assessment of drug-induced extrapyramidal reactions and of drugs given for their control. *Br. J. clin. Pharmac.*, **3**, (Suppl). 395–400S.

MINDHAM, R.H.S., GAIND, R., ANSTEE, B.H. & RIMMER, L. (1972).Comparison of amantidine, orphenadrine, and placebo in the control of phenothiazine-induced Parkinsonism. *Psychol. Med.*, **2**, 406–413.

NAKRA, B.R.S., BOND, A.J. & LADER, M.H. (1975). Comparative psychotropic effects of metolopramide and prochlorperazine in normal subjects. *J. clin. Pharmac.*, **15**, 499–454.

ONUAGULUCHI, G. (1964). *Parkinsonism*. London: Butterworth.

ORR, M.W. & BOULLIN, D.J. (1976). The relationship between changes in 5-HT induced platelet aggregation and clinical state in patients treated with fluphenazine. *Br. J. clin. Pharmac.*, **3**, 925–928.

ORR, M.W., KNOX, J.M., ALLEN, R., GELDER, M.G. & GRAHAME-SMITH, D.G. (1981). The effects of neuroleptic drugs on 5-hydroxytryptamine-induced platet aggregation in schizophrenic patients. *Br. J. clin. Pharmac.*, **11**, 255–259.

OVERALL, J.E. (1976). The brief psychiatric rating scale in psychopharmacologic research. In *ECDEU Assessment Manual*, ed. Guy, W. pp. 166–169. Maryland: U.S. Department of Health, Education and Welfare.

OVERALL, J.E. & GORHAM, D.R. (1962). The brief psychiatric rating scale. *Psychol. Rep.*, **10**, 799–812.

QUITKIN, F., RIFKIN, A., KANE, J., RAMOS-LORENZI, J.R. & KLEIN, D.F. (1978). Long-acting oral versus injectable antipsychotic drugs in schizophrenics. *Arch. gen. Psychiat.*, **35**, 889–892.

RIFKIN, A., QUITKIN, F. & KLEIN, D.F. (1975). Akinesia. *Arch. gen. Psychiat.*, **32**, 672–674.

RIVERA-CALIMLÍM, L., NASRALLAH, H. & STRAUSS, J. (1976). Clinical response and plasma levels: effect of dose, dosage schedules and drug interactions on plasma chlorpromazine levels. *Am. J. Psychiat.*, **133**, 646–652.

ROBINSON, S.E., BERNEY, S., MISHRA, R. & SULSER, F. (1979). The relative role of dopamine and norepinephrine receptor blockade in the action of antipsychotic drugs: metoclopramide, thiethylperazine and molindone as pharmacological tools. *Psychopharmac.*, **64**, 141–147.

SAINSBURY, P. & KREITMAN, N. (1975). *Methods of psychiatric research*, Second Edition. London: Oxford University Press.

SCHACHTER, M., BEDARD, P., DEBONO, A.G. JENNER, P., MARSDEN, C.D., PRICE, P., PARKES, J.D., KEENAN, J., SMITH, B., ROSENTHALER, J., HOROWSKI, R. & DORROW, R. (1980). The role of D-1 and D-2 receptors. *Nature*, **286**, 157–159.

SCHNEIDER, K. (1959). *Clinical Psychopathology*, English translation Hamilton, M.W. & Anderson, E.W., pp. 89–114. New York: Grune & Stratton.

SCHONECKER, M. (1957). Ein eigenümliches Syndrome in oralen Bereich bei Megaphenaplikation. *Nerventartz*, **28**, 35.

SIMPSON, G.M. & ANGUS, J.W.S. (1970). A rating scale for extrapyramidal side-effects. *Acta Psychiat. Scand.*, *Suppl.*, **212**, 11–19.

SIMPSON, G.M., AMUSO, D., BLAIR, J.H. & FARKAS, T. (1964). Phenothiazine-produced extrapyramidal system disturbance. *Arch. gen. Psychiat.*, **10**, 127–136.

SIMPSON, G.M., COOPER, T.B., BARK, N., SUD, I. & LEE, J.H. (1980). Effect of antiparkinsonian medication on plasma levels of chlorpromazine. *Arch. gen. Psychiat.*, **37**, 205–208.

SNYDER, S.H. & GOODMAN, R.R. (1980). Multiple neurotransmitter receptors. *J. Neurochem.*, **35**, 5–15.

SNYDER, S.H., GREENBERG, D. & YAMAMURA, H.I. (1974). Antischizophrenic drugs and brain cholinergic receptors. *Arch. gen. Psychiat.*, **31**, 58–61.

SPITZER, R.L. & ENDICOTT, J. (1975). Psychiatric rating scales. In *Comprehensive Textbook of Psychiatry*, eds Freedman, A.M., Kaplan, H.I. & Sadock, B.J. **2**, 2nd Edition, pp. 2015–2031. Baltimore: The Williams & Wilkins Co.

SPITZER, R., ENDICOTT, J. & ROBINS, E. (1975). Research Diagnostic Criteria. Instrument No, 58, New York: New York State Psychiatric Institute.

STRAUSS, J.S. & GIFT, T.E. (1977). Choosing an approach for diagnosing schizophrenia. *Arch. gen. Psychiat.*, **34**, 1248–1253.

TARRIER, N., VAUGHN, C., LADER, M.H. & LEFF, J.P. (1979). Bodily reactions to people and events in schizophrenics. *Arch. gen. Psychiat.*, **36**, 311–315.

TUCKER, G.T. (1980). Principles of pharmacokinetics. In *Drug concentrations in neuropsychiatry*, Ciba Foundation Symposium 74 (new series), pp. 13–26. Oxford: Excerpta Medica.

TYRER, P.J. (1976). Screening procedures in volunteers and patients. *Br. J. clin. Pharmac.*, Suppl., **3**, 35–40S.

VAN PUTTEN, T. & MAY, P.R.A. (1978). 'Akinetic depression' in schizophrenia. *Arch. gen. Psychiat.*, **35**, 1101–1107.

VAUGHN, C.E. & LEFF, J.P. (1976). The influence of family and social factors on the course of psychiatric illness. *Br. J. Psychiat.*, **129**, 125–137.

WING, J.K. (1961). A simple and reliable subclassification of chronic schizophrenia. *J. ment. Sci.*, **107**, 862–875.

WING, J.K. (1978). The social context of schizophrenia. *Am. J. Psychiat.*, **135**, 1333–1339.

WING, J.K., COOPER, J.E. & SARTORIUS, N. (1974). *The measurement and classification of psychiatric symptoms*. London: Cambridge University Press.

WODE-HELGODT, B., BORG, S., FIJRO, B. & SEDVALL, G. (1978). Clinical effects and drug concentrations in plasma and cerebrospinal fluid in psychotic patients treated with fixed doses of chlorpromazine. *Acta Psychiat. Scand.*. **58**, 149–173.

YAMAMURA, H.I., MARIAN, A.A. & SNYDER, S.H. (1976). Muscarinic cholinergic receptor binding: influence of pimozide and chlorpromazine metabolites. *Life Sci.*, **18**, 685–692.

THE CLINICAL ASSESSMENT OF ANALGESIC DRUGS

D.W. LITTLEJOHNS & D.W. VERE

Department of Pharmacology and Therapeutics,
The London Hospital Medical College,
London E1 2AD

To strike a proper balance between the efficacy and the adverse effects of an analgesic, it is obviously necessary but notoriously difficult to weigh those two factors individually. Any study of analgesic efficacy in man requires a measure of the subjective variable pain, or pain relief. The difficulty of forming even a satisfactory definition of pain (Fordyce, 1978) should warn of the conceptual problems that can lead to measures lacking the intended validity. Early studies in healthy volunteers are often needed, and require some means of inducing pain as well, if analgesic efficacy is to be demonstrated. The ethical problems involved in these, and in the essential studies of analgesic effect in clinical pain, are perhaps more dramatic than complex. Biometric problems can trap the unwary, even when relevant measures have been employed. So it is fortunate that at least the prediction, detection and evaluation of the adverse effects of analgesics, and their pharmacokinetics, are beset with only a few difficulties peculiar to this group of drugs.

What do you mean by 'pain'?

Methods of pain measurement began to be developed in a form suitable for the assessment of analgesics about 30 years ago, and the work of that decade is still a useful introduction to the subject (Hewer, Keele, Keele & Nathan, 1949; Hardy, Wolff & Goodell, 1953; Beecher, 1957; Lasagna, 1960). More recent reviews incorporate more work comparing one method with another (Huskisson, 1974b), or provide a higher level of psychometric sophistication (Wolff, 1978).

How pain is measured depends on how it is regarded. A scheme is presented in Figure 1 which employs a terminology adapted from Loeser (1980). It can be regarded as compatible with, but as being a simplified version of, the map of pain experience offered by Melzack & Dennis (1978), which was derived from somewhat speculative correlations between neurophysiological mechanisms of pain sensation and psychological observations on the dimensions of pain experience. The fine detail of neurophysiology (Nathan, 1977; Melzack & Dennis, 1978), valuable to mode of action studies (e.g. Yaksh & Rudy, 1978), cannot be resolved by the coarse methods of investigation available in man. On the other hand, further simplification would obscure differences between the information provided by different modes of measurement, whereas the specificity of the measure, for instance, is always of particular concern when dealing with subjective variables. It is of interest that the plan employed here resembles that used similarly by Hindmarch (1980) in this series to

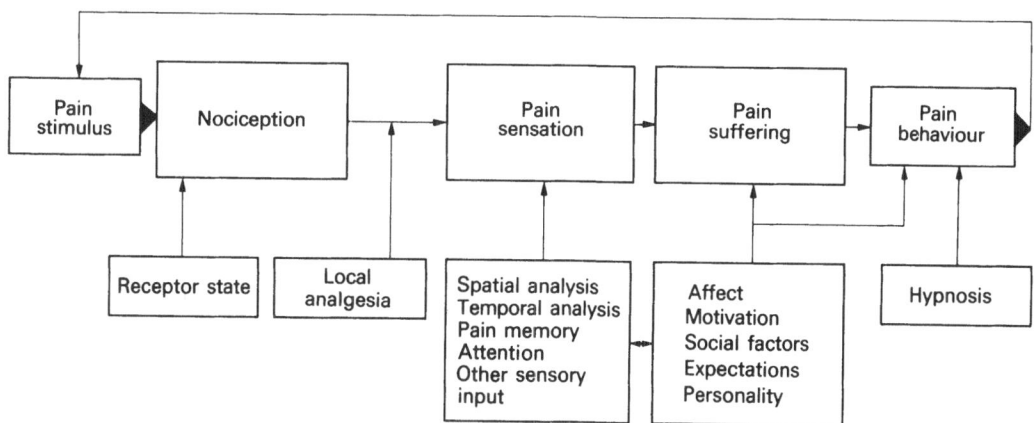

Figure 1   Relationships between the events in pain perception.

order the relationships between tests of psychomotor function, though the two were independently conceived and are not expressed alike.

Though it is seldom obvious that an exact choice has been consciously made, it is possible to choose to measure the stimulus, or nociception, or pain sensation, or pain suffering, or pain behaviour, as seems most appropriate. The use of more than one measure can help in the interpretation of results, especially if those measures have a different specificity within the above range. Those targets, gathered under the generic term 'pain', require to be defined more closely.

(i) The *pain stimulus* is accessible to measurement only when employing induced pain; then, it can often be measured with some precision. For analgesic studies it must be combined with a measure of response, and, though it is attractive to demonstrate analgesic efficacy as a blunting of the stimulus-response relationship, it is not straightforward to design such studies to be sensitive to drug effects.

(ii) *Nociception* is the sequence of processes in the periphery by which noxious stimuli are detected by receptors and converted into impulses carried by small-fibre ($A\delta$ and C) afferent nerves. These processes have so far proved largely inaccessible to measurement in man, though sensory nerve recording, while difficult, has for some time been possible (Valbo & Hagbarth, 1968).

(iii) *Pain sensation* is nociceptive input, further modulated by another series of processes, but this time in the spinal cord and brain, and emerging as a sensory experience. The quest to measure it has made it at times seem the Holy Grail of pain research. While some advocates of Signal Detection Theory have felt they were close (Chapman, 1977), others less committed have expressed fundamental doubts (Rollman, 1977). Another view is that cognitive, evaluative processes can precede and influence sensory perception (Melzack & Dennis, 1978); it would follow that attempts to separate completely the sensory and judgmental aspects of pain is more like the search for the end of the rainbow. Nevertheless, any method of measurement that diminishes the judgmental and affective ('attitudinal') elements would have obvious value in the assessment of analgesics.

(iv) *Pain suffering* is close to the pragmatic clinical concept of pain as being a subjective experience, defined by the patient rather than the doctor. It comprises not only pain sensation, but also the associated distress, the essential unpleasantness of pain, and the affective response—typically anxiety, anger and/or depression. The measures of pain most widely used reflect chiefly pain suffering. To what extent they represent pain sensation is unknowable, but probably varies among both individuals and methods. Distress from any cause other than pain is apt to intrude into all measures of pain suffering, rendering them less specific than intended.

(v) *Pain behaviour* has less frequently been measured. Like stimulus recording, it is susceptible to very precise and objective measurement but is remote from what matters to the patient or subject. Spontaneous verbal responses have been much studied, although particularly affected by social, cultural and environmental factors (Craig, 1978). It is possible to measure the purely physiological responses to pain; there is reason to suppose that they are linked to pain suffering rather than to pain sensation.

Table 1 Differences between acute and chronic pain

	Acute pain	Chronic pain
Conduction pathways	Rapid	Slow
Tissue injury	Clearly causal	Minor or absent
Autonomic response	Present	Absent
Biological value	High	Low
Mood	Anxiety	Depression, anxiety
Social effects	Slight	Marked
Effective treatment	Analgesics	Variable, sometimes none

The *duration* of pain influences analgesic effects. There are substantial differences between acute and chronic pain (Table 1), though the pains due to advancing malignancy may persist for many months and still have predominantly the characteristics of acute pain. Moreover, it is useful to subdivide acute pain into *first (phasic) pain* (carried by $A\delta$ fibres) and *second (tonic) pain* carried by C fibres. Nitrous oxide relieves both, but morphine chiefly the second (Melzack & Dennis, 1978), and most clinical pain is in this second category (Mumford & Bowsher, 1976).

The *intensity* of pain may also affect the results of analgesic assessment. The low pain levels most acceptable in experimentally-induced pain are one factor in making clinical pain more susceptible to analgesics than experimental pain, and the pain tolerance level more sensitive to analgesics (Smith, Lowenstein, Hubbard & Beecher, 1968; Wolff, 1977) than pain threshold. Even the placebo effects of medication are more marked at high pain intensities (Levine, Gordon, Bornstein & Fields, 1979).

If the generic term 'pain' thus requires a more specific definition, so does the generic term 'analgesic'. For instance, should an antidepressive drug that diminishes chronic pain by alleviating the depression associated with it be regarded as having analgesic properties? It is clear that relief of pain suffering makes a drug clinically useful; relief of pain sensation implies a mechanism of benefit. A drug that influenced only pain behaviour, without relieving pain suffering, might be useful, but perhaps it should not be regarded as an analgesic; there is some evidence that the relief of pain by hypnosis falls into this category (Hilgard, 1978).

Pain stimulus

The physical measurement of the pain stimulus seldom causes problems, but the stimulus is inevitably somewhat remote from the processed and modulated phenomena of pain suffering which concern the patient. Indeed, experimentally-induced pain is likely to be registered more as pain sensation, compared to the more threatening, and often more severe, pain due to disease, and it is often of the 'first pain' type. These reasons presumably underlie the difficulty of demonstrating the effects of even well-known analgesics under experimental conditions. Within these limitations, the criteria for an appropriate stimulus have been discussed for many years (Hardy *et al.*, 1953; Beecher, 1959; Wolff, 1978). It is widely agreed that any stimulus should have these properties:

(i)   it should be convenient to apply
(ii) it should be recognised as painful, whatever other sensations it produces, and the pain should be diminished by known analgesics.
(iii) the measurable content of the stimulus should be closely associated with the changes causing pain.
(iv) its intensity should be measurable physically with greater precision than sensory discrimination can achieve.
(v)   its intensity should range from providing threshold to maximum tolerable pain.
(vi) it should provide a reproducible measure of pain threshold under standard conditions.
(vii) repetitions even above the threshold level should not affect subsequent determinations, which implies the avoidance of tissue damage.

Of these criteria (v) and (vii) are particularly difficult to meet, but four methods of pain induction come close enough to the ideal to be widely used.

Electrical stimulation

The sensation produced is more discomfort than pain, and the associated sensations are unlike those to any other stimulus. Healthy tooth pulp is widely used, but fingers, hand, forearm and deep stimulation to the gluteus maximus have all been used. The stimulator should be given a constant current, since contact resistance varies and the stimulus is related more to current than voltage. The subject must be electrically isolated for safety. Responses are highly repeatable (Wolff, 1978) but the validity of the sensation is open to question.

Radiant heat

The original paper describing this method is well known (Hardy, Wolff & Goodell, 1940) and most instruments have continued to use the principle of controlled heat and light focussed from a projector bulb onto any non-hairy, blackened skin surface. The flexor surface of the forearm, the forehead or the back are suitable sites. Heart intensity is measured as mcal s^{-1} cm^{-2}, and is controlled by a variable resistance. The subject can indicate the time to pain threshold and to maximum pain tolerance by pressing buttons, the button for tolerance terminating the stimulus by closing a shutter. Above about 400 mcal s^{-1} for 3 s tissue damage is likely, being shown by subsequent erythema (Hardy, Wolff & Goodell, 1947). Responses are acceptably repeatable.

Pressure algometer

A spring-loaded plunger of standard size and shape is pressed at a constant rate of increase in force onto the skin against a bony surface e.g. forehead, knuckle, medial malleolus (Keele, 1954). The stimulus measured is the force (as the distance the spring is depressed) that has to be applied for pain threshold and tolerance. The method provides acceptably repeatable results for both variables (Merskey & Spear, 1964).

Cold water pain

The skin temperature of one hand is standardised by putting it into water at a given temperature (e.g. 37°C) for a few minutes; then it is plunged into a stirred bath of ice fragments in water. The subject indicates the onset of pain and the end of tolerance; these times are the measurements. The method is, of course, also used for studies of cardiovascular responses, and especially the hypertensive response to pain. The stimulus is standard but not physically quantified. It cannot be rapidly repeated, but the pain appears to resemble that due to disease, and it is a sensitive test of analgesic activity.

Other methods

A variety of other methods has been employed, but none has been so generally successful. The slow onset of pain at four different intensity levels after standard arm exercise while the arterial supply is occluded has been used to demonstrate the effects of analgesics (Smith, Egbert, Marcowitz, Mosteller & Beecher, 1966; Smith *et al.*, 1968) but few investigators have used it and it has not been proved to be repeatable. The same is true of inflating a sphygmomanometer cuff with internal projections (Poser, 1962). The application of chemicals to a blister produced by cantharidin (Armstrong, Dry, Keele & Monkham, 1953) is more a technique for studying peripheral mechanisms of nociception, but could be used to test analgesics. It can also be used to test local anaesthetics (Mongar, 1955).

Pain sensation

Two approaches to the measurement of pain sensation are possible. One is to measure both pain suffering itself and those factors (see Figure 1) which modify pain sensation to result in pain suffering, and subtract their influence; the other is to measure pain sensation directly. The former method would involve non-pain measurements almost as controversial as those of pain itself, with no way of predicting accurately in the individual case how powerfully these entities influence pain suffering. However, it is advantageous to make at least some measurements of relevant personality and affective factors when measuring pain suffering; marked differences in them might illuminate the pain measurements. For example, lessened anxiety can reduce pain suffering more than aspirin does (von Graffenried, Adler, Abt, Nuesch & Spiegel, 1978).

The only method that might seem to offer a measure of pain sensation is Signal Detection Theory (SDT). It originated in the statistics of hypothesis testing, and was developed by radar engineers interested in the detection of a weak signal against background noise. Lucid descriptions of an admittedly complex subject by Swets (1973) introduced the concepts to sensory psychology, and a helpful introduction to its use in pain studies has been written by Clark (1974). It is sometimes known as sensory decision theory.

The basic assumptions of SDT are that:

(i) the sensory experience to a standard stimulus is not fixed but variable, with a median value and some dispersion, and so can be represented best by a distribution curve (Figure 2).

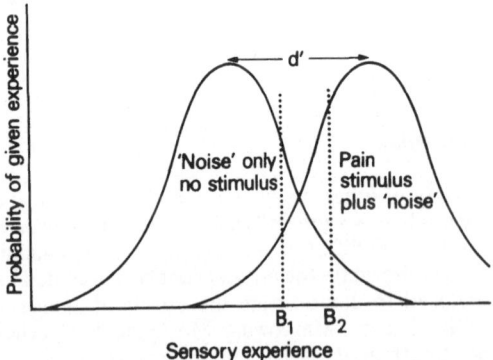

Figure 2 The variable sensory experience in the absence of a stimulus is regarded as 'noise'. The discriminability (d') between a repeated mild pain stimulus and this noise depends on how large the difference in pain sensation is. For a near-threshold stimulus, overlap of experience means that reports of 'pain' and 'no pain' do not perfectly match 'stimulus' or 'no stimulus'. Different settings of response bias (B_1 and B_2) alter the proportion of false negative and false positive reports.

(ii) increasing stimuli give distribution curves with a displaced median, but all share the same dispersion; the discriminability of two stimuli then depends on the difference in the two medians (d' in Figure 2).

(iii) there is at any time a particular value of sensory experience which corresponds to a person's report of a threshold (e.g. between 'no pain' and 'pain', or between 'tolerable pain' and 'intolerable pain'). This is referred to as response bias (B_1 and B_2 in Figure 2), or criterion, and it is influenced by cultural factors, mental attitude, expectancy of pain etc. For instance, in Figure 2 any value of B will involve some 'false positive' and/or 'false negative' reports of pain, but B_2 represents greater stoicism than B_1—fewer false positives, at the cost of more false negatives.

The method of SDT is to present pairs of stimuli repeatedly, record the reported responses, and analyse to give values for discriminability and response bias. It is attractive because it seems that all the attitudinal influences are gathered together as 'response bias'. The calculations may assume normal distributions, or use non-parametric methods, and a variety of procedures is possible (Swets, 1973; Chapman, 1978).

On the whole, it does seem that analgesics change discriminability whereas psychological modifiers and psychotropic drugs change response bias (Wolff, 1978). But nitrous oxide changes both measures (Chapman, Murphy & Butler, 1973), as do morphine and diazepam, though diazepam has more effect on response bias and morphine more on discriminability (Yang, Clark, Ngai, Berkowitz & Spector, 1979). Though these methods are obviously useful, the criticisms of the validity of additional assumptions that it is easy to make from SDT Theory are a necessary warning (Rollman, 1977). For instance, to measure discriminability is to measure something related to pain sensation, but it does not measure pain sensation itself. It would be an error to define analgesics as substances that reduced the discriminability of pain stimuli. It is easy to commit this error, because as most stimuli increase, so does the difference between just-discriminable stimuli, as measured in linear physical units; logarithmic units such as decibels are the result of the logarithmic Weber-Fechner Law. But the calculations are upset by adaptation (the sensory equivalent to tachyphylaxis) as shown by Rollman (1979), and a drug might blunt the discriminatory ability of the CNS without altering sensation.

Pain suffering

When measured as a response to a pain stimulus, two points on the intensity scale are fairly clearly fixed—the pain threshold and pain tolerance. The former contains the greater amount of information about pain sensation, but the latter is more valuable in analgesic studies. The measurement of clinical pain is more problematical, but by no means impossible.

Pain threshold

This is usually determined by the method of limits, though other methods are possible. Starting with very weak stimuli, stimulus strength is gradually increased in successive trials until pain is reported; then a stronger stimulus is applied, followed by a descending series, noting when pain is no longer felt. The threshold of the ascending and the descending series is averaged. The reliability of the result depends on the subject, the method of inducing pain (Lynn & Perl, 1977), the interval between measurements, and the number of pairs of trials—e.g. five pairs of trials are sufficient for work with radiant heat, and the first value is best disregarded as it shows the greatest variance about the same mean.

Pain threshold measurements impose least discomfort on the experimental subject, and thresholds have been extensively studied, with divergent results (Beecher, 1959; Woodforde & Merskey, 1972). Keele (1968) found the pain of myocardial infarction related to pain threshold, but Huskisson & Hart (1972) using the same method found it accounted for only about 5% of the variance in analgesic consumption in patients with rheumatoid arthritis, and this may have been due to pain threshold correlating with disease severity. Thus it does not seem to be a major determinant of clinical pain, and though it can be used to detect the effects of analgesics, it is not particularly sensitive to them (Smith *et al.*, 1968; Wolff, Kantor, Jarvick & Laska, 1969; Wolff, 1977).

Pain tolerance

Pain tolerance is the point at which the subject feels obliged to end the pain stimulus. It is more easily modulated by psychological factors than is pain threshold, and so it has a rather higher variance, but is more sensitive to analgesic effects and is therefore an important measure in the study of analgesics, despite the risk of tissue damage and the discomfort to the subject. Obviously, to use it is ethical only if the subject can terminate the stimulus.

Wolff (1977) has used an intermediate point on the scale, the *drug request point*—e.g. the pain level at which the subject would normally take an over-the-counter analgesic if the pain occurred spontaneously. This measure is also sensitive to analgesic effects, but the sensitivity may depend on how close it lies to pain tolerance.

Ordinal pain scales

The pain produced by radiant heat applied to the forehead or forearm can be divided into a series of 21 'just noticeable differences' (JNDs) ranging between threshold pain and the maximum pain possible with this technique (Hardy *et al.*, 1947). Since such precise measurement was possible only under ideal conditions, two JNDs were considered to be the practical pain unit, called a 'dol'. However, these observations have not been validated for other pain stimuli, and the 10-point scale of pain has not been widely used.

In measurements of clinical pain, a 5-category ordinal scale is well understood and easily used (Keele, 1948), though it is effectively a 4-point scale because the highest value is seldom used. We have found the words 'no pain/slight pain/moderate pain/severe pain/excruciating pain' are seldom misunderstood. It is not difficult to apply such scales to the assessment of analgesics, an observer asking the patient to rate the pain at regular intervals (Hewer *et al.*, 1949; Beecher, 1957; Wallenstein, Heidrich, Kaiko & Houde, 1980; Dundee, 1980). It may be useful to represent the scale as a series of lights (Nayman, 1979). Scales any more finely divided are difficult to provide with suitable words to each category, but Downie, Leatham, Rhind, Wright, Branco & Anderson (1978a) employed a 'numerical rating scale' of adjacent boxes labelled from 1 to 10 and showed advantages from using this. The novel numerical scale may have attracted more interest and explanation from the experimenters, but would be of interest if the results can be repeated by others. A similar technique is to use a numerical scale with zero as 'no pain', 10 as pain tolerance, but open to higher scores, with no top limit (Hilgard, 1978).

Visual analogue scale (VAS)

Visual analogue scales were introduced into medical use for the measurement of feelings (Aitken, 1969; Aitken & Zealley, 1970). High reliability and validity had already been shown in other contexts, and Aitken added other experiments on validity, using loaded breathing; not all have agreed about validity (Downie, Leatham, Rhind, Pickup & Wright, 1978b). Aitken pointed out the advantages of greater sensitivity of such scales compared to verbal category scales, and a more recent opinion (Nicholson, 1978) is that VAS methods are valuable, though it is not safe to rely on them when used alone. Validity for pain is impossible to estimate, but there is good agreement between ordinal pain scales and visual analogue scales both for spontaneous pain changes and those due to analgesics, but the VAS is more sensitive (Downie *et al.*, 1978a; Ohnhaus & Adler, 1975; Joyce, Zutshi, Hrubes & Mason, 1975; Woodforde & Merskey, 1972; Scott & Huskisson, 1976). A 100 mm scale with the ends marked, for example, 'No pain/Pain as bad as it could be' is now widely used, and is usually measured to the nearest millimetre (Huskisson, 1974b). Some authors have found it difficult to use, but we and many others have had few difficulties even with patients of low intelligence. A standard introduction is useful—e.g. 'This is a way of showing me how bad your pain is, without having to use words. A mark here (indicates 'No pain' end) means you are completely free from pain. Marks along the line (moves pointer along it) would mean gradually worse pain, until at this end (indicates other end) is the most extreme pain imaginable. Please, would you put a stroke through the line at the place that shows what your pain is like now.' Subsequent use requires no instruction.

The visual analogue scale has been much studied. Words set beside the scale merely attract a high density of responses close to them (Scott & Huskisson, 1976), and a 50 mm line is less discriminatory than 100 mm (Revill, Robinson, Rosen & Hogg, 1976); either change reduces the sensitivity of the measure. There is no appreciable difference between a scale set vertically and one set horizontally (Downie *et al.*, 1978a). It is usual to prevent the subject being able to see previous pain ratings, which users may prefer, but this precaution is unnecessary or perhaps deleterious (Joyce *et al.*, 1975). Memory for a random mark is good even 24 hours later, but consistency in rating a previous pain is better still, and is unaffected by pethidine 150 mg intramuscularly (Revill *et al.*, 1976).

Verbal responses

Spontaneous verbal responses are better classified as pain behaviour, but in measuring pain it is usual for structured responses to be elicited for that purpose alone. The only method widely used is the McGill Pain Questionnaire (Melzack, 1975), which takes some time to administer, and is unsuitable for frequent use in single-dose analgesic studies; it was designed for the evaluation of clinical pain, and is concerned with many factors other than pain intensity. The subject is asked to mark any of 102 adjectives which have been found to be reliable in their meaning independent of age, culture etc. in somewhat limited validation studies (Melzack & Torgerson, 1971). As many are marked as seems appropriate to the subject.

The number of words marked provides one index of response, and a pain rating index calculated from numerical values given to each word provides another. A 5-point ordinal pain scale is also included. Unfortunately, the words employed were originally chosen by the investigators rather than being selected from those used by patients, and some (e.g. 'lancinating') are not in common use. It has been suggested that the analysis of the questionnaire results could be more appropriately performed using somewhat different factors, derived experimentally rather than rationally (Crockett, Prkachin & Craig, 1977). Verbal reports contain considerable information about the affective and sensory aspects of pain; intensity is by no means as predominant a factor as might

be supposed (Bailey & Davidson, 1976). Although the McGill Questionnaire is thus open to improvement, chosen adjectives for pain do seem to be surprisingly reliable indicators of sensory intensity (Gracely, McGrath & Dubrier, 1978a), and are changed as would be expected by diazepam (Gracely, McGrath & Dubrier, 1978b). As a measure of dental pain it was effective, though the subscales contained rather too much common information (van Buren & Kleinknecht, 1979), and head pain was accurately recalled when using it on occasions up to 5 days apart (Hunter, Philips & Rachman, 1979). The McGill Questionnaire would probably be a useful assessment measure in an analgesic trial carried out over a day or longer.

Stimulus matching

It is possible for the subject to match clinical pain with a second pain due to another, variable stimulus (Kast, 1962), or alternatively to express pain as a proportion or multiple of a standard pain stimulus. The latter method avoids the danger of causing physical injury by a stimulus of an intensity as high as that of clinical pain, but it is not easy to match two pain stimuli that differ in other sensory qualities, and most methods of inducing experimental pain involve equipment too cumbersome to bring to the bedside. Pain intensity can also be expressed in terms of the magnitude of another sensory modality (e.g. brightness, loudness), but the value of this is limited (Woodforde & Merskey, 1972). Armstrong, Dry, Keele & Monkham (1953) used the force of squeezing a sphygmomanometer cuff, and adapted this to graphical recording. The visual analogue scale uses linear distance likewise, and has already been discussed.

Pain behaviour

Pain behaviour can conveniently be regarded as activities consequent on pain, not necessarily under voluntary control, but of a sort not especially introduced for the purposes of measurement. The objec-

Table 2 Physiological responses used as measures of pain

Physiological response	Sample reference
Cortical evoked response	Sitaram *et al.* (1977)
	Buchsbaum *et al.* (1977)
Skin conductance	Craig & Neidermayer (1974)
Plasma cortisol	Lascelles *et al.* (1974)
Urine catecholamines	Huskisson (1974a)
Serum non-esterified fatty acid	Knitza *et al.* (1979)
Serum β-lipoproteins	Keele & Stern (1973)
Acid-base balance	Evans (1972)
Vital capacity	Parkhouse & Holmes (1973)

tivity of an external observer may indeed reduce the impact of emotional factors (Houde, Wallerstein & Rodgers, 1960) or prevent some patients exaggerating their pain (Parkhouse & Holmes, 1963) but there is no valid way in which an observer can consistently conclude from pain behaviour what the pain sensation may be; the most valid measures of a subjective sensation are subjective responses. In practice, the chief effect is to increase variance, but if observation of analgesic effects by an observer is carried out on a large enough scale, analgesic effects can be detected (Jick, Slone, Shapiro, Lewis & Siskind, 1971).

Physiological responses have the advantage of precise and objective measurement, and the disadvantages of uncertain validity. Some examples are given in Table 2. Many are related to the activity of the autonomic nervous system. These are poor measures of first pain, being extinguished by repetition of the stimulus when the pain is not (Wolff, 1978). They might be more valid in clinical pain, but it is commonly observed that the most easily-measured autonomic responses are increasingly diminished as pain persists longer. Cortical evoked responses are an attractive measure, but magnitude and latency may well reflect arousal, the most likely explanation for the effect of physostigmine (Sitaram, Buchsbaum & Gillin, 1977).

Biometric problems

In any biometric work it is necessary to consider:
(i) what is measured—its biological identity (validity)
(ii) the measures and the measurers—to minimise bias
(iii) the mathematical properties of the measures, including aspects related to (i)
(iv) sensitivity and repeatability.

Pain measurement is particularly difficult in each respect; despite this striking progress has been made in the field. Pain measurements can now yield monotonic results (i.e. measures move in a uniform direction in relation to one another, and to stimulus intensity, when that is known), the variances of measurements can be strikingly small, and the predictive power of research for clinical practice can be substantial (Wallenstein *et al.*, 1980). Nevertheless, close attention to detail is needed to ensure useful results.
(i) In relation to *what is measured*, there must be careful consideration of:
(a) the intensity levels of the studied pain
(b) the clinical type of pain (Beaver & McMillan, 1980)
(c) the relationship of analgesic blood levels to the onset, peak and duration of drug effect, and
(d) the place of the observed data within the range of possible drug effects (Beaver & McMillan, 1980).

Any experiment in which these features are ill-matched is likely to fail. For example, a measurement of analgesic effects in one type of pain may not predict them for another, variable-dose tests crowded into one end of the range of biological response will fail to shown sensitivity to differences in pain stimuli, tests made with single doses of a cumulative drug will show a surprising lack of effect, and so on. Recurring pain behaves differently from non-recurring (Dundee, 1980) and expectations may depend upon the time of day at which measurements are made (Glynn & Lloyd, 1976). Obviously, variance of the results is minimised by measuring the effect of an analgesic on a similar pain stimulus in each subject. This is most easily achieved when pain is experimentally-induced, but the value of such methods is limited (see above and Figure 3), and so studies of clinical pain are more than just ways of generating paper for regulatory authorities. A number of clinical situations have been investigated in some detail, notably post-partum pain (Bloomfield, Barden & Mitchell, 1976; Sunshine, 1980), dental pain (Cooper & Beaver, 1976; Levine *et al.*, 1979) and cross-over studies in cancer pain (Twycross, 1975). Instances in which pain is likely to be more variable, but which represent important uses of analgesics, are headache (von Graffenried & Nuesch, 1980), rheumatoid and osteoarthritis (Deodhar, Dick, Hodgkinson & Buchanan, 1973) and post-operative pain (Nayman, 1979; Gómez-Jiménez, Franco-Patino, Chargoy-Vera & Olivares-Sosa, 1980).

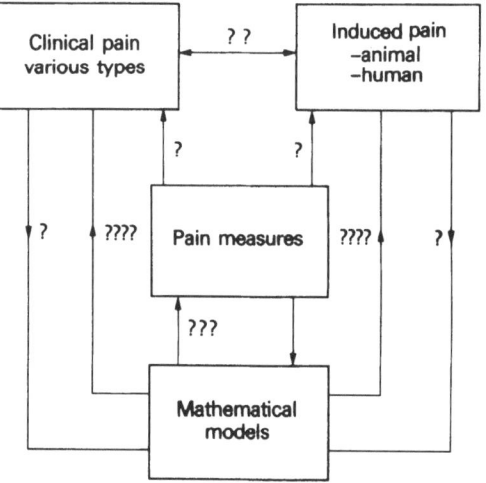

Figure 3 Relationships between components of pain measurement. The arrows represent inferences, and the more question marks associated with each, the more are they open to doubt.

(ii) The *measures* used are awkward for several reasons, not least because the same measure may at times yield data nearly normally-distributed and suitable for parametric analysis, but at other times yield data having a highly skewed distribution (Twycross, 1975). The *measurers* are involved partly because pain is an emotive matter, likely to lead to bias in reporting, but mostly for the reason that in varying degrees pain measurements are made through at least two minds, those of the person in pain and the observer, which can lead to bias compounded by a sort of folie à deux. It is often rightly stressed that double-blind conditions are essential in analgesic trials to avoid this, but the effectiveness of the blindfold should be tested. In Figure 3 the complexity of the measurement problems is stressed by separating out the components of pain measurement, and by indicating by the number of question marks on the arrows between them which inferences are most susceptible to logical errors.

(iii) The *mathematical properties* involved are the problems set by non-normal distributions, by the use of mathematical models, and by the occurrence of time-dependent variation. There is no problem when ordinal data, or VAS scales are analysed using appropriate non-parametric statistical tests, which make no assumptions about the distribution of the measurements, albeit at the sacrifice of some statistical power. For instance, the VAS using a 'No pain/Worst pain imaginable' scale is unipolar, and it is not surprising if the measurements are sometimes crowded towards the 'No pain' end. If pilot trials suggest that only one end of the scale is much used, it may be better to devise another scale on which they are more evenly spread. Certainly, if a distribution is skewed or bimodal (see Figure 4), it would be misleading to

attempt any simple parametric analysis of the data. Bimodal responses may be found because there was ambiguity. Patients then include two kinds of response upon the same scale (e.g. pain and suffering). It may be possible to separate these responses later, but usually it is best to repeat the observations, having changed the scales so as to avoid ambiguity. If the data are simply skewed (there are now tests for skewness and kurtosis in the statistical packages available for many programmable calculators) a transformation (also now an easy thing to do) may be required to render the data suited to parametric analysis. Although Aitken (1969) mentioned an arc-sine transform for VAS data, the choice of transform is quite arbitrary, and the methods were discussed at length by Oldham (1968). The arc-sine transform is described and tabled in the Geigy Tables (Diem & Lentner, 1970). Many workers ignore it as conferring no discriminative advantage upon these methods. In summary, the ways around the problems of non-normality of data distributions are to look for non-normality, and, should it be present, design another scale, or use a distribution-free test statistic, or a normalising transform, as seems appropriate to the problem.

It has been said already that the practice of putting words or marks along the course of a VAS has several measurement effects which are mostly disadvantageous. It is not always realised that these marks also change the nature of the data. Their effect is to convert interval into ordinal data (so losing information) and to change their distribution from a continuous to a stepped form (i.e. moving towards a rating scale). An impressive result of this is that parametric tests are no longer applicable; only non-parametric methods should be used; once more there is then a small sacrifice of power. This may be worthwhile if it improves comprehension. Dundee (1980) gives a figure with several alternative forms of VAS. These may be satisfactory alternative measures, but it must be realised that their results should probably be analysed in different ways.

Model fitting and model forcing

Often experimental data are well fitted by a model; the model used most frequently is a straight line, but a logarithmic or other curve is sometimes better. The logic of using models often seems ill-understood. It is essential to realise that there are two kinds of model, an arbitrary one which just happens to fit the data well (an empirical model), and one with an implied chemical, physiological or pharmacological meaning (a bio-theoretic model). An example would be a log dose-response curve, where a straight line may be found to give a good fit over the central 60% of the curve *either* because it happens to be almost straight, *or* because such a line would be expected from mass-

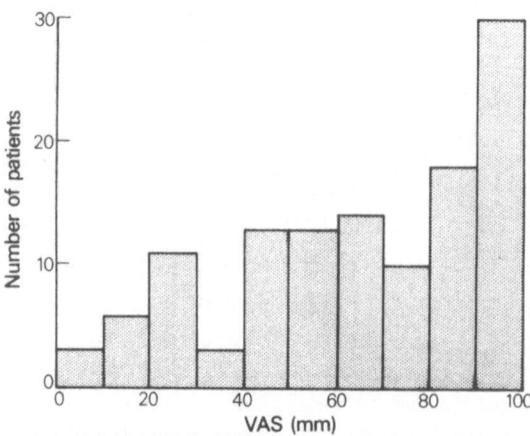

Figure 4 Distribution of marks made by 123 hospital inpatients with pain on a visual analogue scale for pain intensity.

action receptor kinetics, or both. It happens that the monotonic relationship between visual analogue and ordinal pain scales is curved; curved lines give a significantly better fit than straight lines, and a power function:

$$y = ax^n$$

where y is the VAS, x is the numerical pain rating score and a and n are constants, gives a better fit than a logarithmic curve:

$$y = f (\log x) \text{ (Wallenstein } et al., 1980)}$$

However, it is important not to infer from what is known or pain in other situations—that it behaves as a power function of stimulus intensity (Tursky, 1975; Gracely *et al.*, 1978a)—to what its behaviour *should* be in numerical or VAS measures of clinical pain. The model may fit well for purely arbitrary mathematical reasons (e.g. a sigmoid log dose-response curve can be fitted equally well by a mass-action law formula, by a hyperbolic tangent, by a probit, or by a cubic curve). Indeed, there might be reasons to expect the curve which relates VAS to rating scores to be sigmoid because the scales are tied at both ends, and there is even a suggestion that this could be so in Figure 7 of Wallenstein *et al.* (1980). What is worse, a sigmoid fitted to such data would be sure to yield a better fit than the power curve; a curve with two bends can always accommodate varied data better than a curve with only one. However, this does not suggest that a sigmoid should be used as a better bio-theoretic model. It is therefore not possible to agree with Wallenstein *et al.* (1980) that 'categorical reports of pain and magnitude estimates of pain are best described in terms of power curve relationship'; it seems wise to suspend judgment on the point until much more is known. The logical point is exposed with full rigour in Gödels Theorem, but is illustrated in less formal ways by many examples of clinical 'reasoning' (Hofstadter, 1979). It is quite safe to use a model simply because it happens to fit the data, and to stop the chain of inference there.

Another major difficulty is *time-dependent variation* or self-modification of recorded pain. The features of a single episode of pain may depend on other pain which precede it and adaptation to a pain stimulus is a well-known psychological observation. Methods exist to study self-dependent variation; they are a particular form of Bayes' logic. When the probability of a given event depends only on that of the event which precedes it immediately, the sequence of events is called a Markov chain (Lindley, 1965). But if within that sequence of events each is independent, the appropriate mathematical model for counting numbers of attacks is that used to describe the likelihood of radioactive decay (Vincent, 1973). These two probabilistic approaches provide mathematical models against which to test biological event patterns to test whether or not they are indistin-

guishable from the independent or Markovian models. We are unaware of any clinical attempts to do this, but the relevance to topics such as pain is obvious. Thus, Sunshine (1980) discusses whether patients should be asked to rate their pain in abstract, or in relation to the severity of the last pain they experienced. The problem also arises in cross-over trials, if inadequate 'wash-out' periods are used, since the second course of treatment is then influenced by the first (Hills & Armitage, 1979).

Cross-over designs are indeed prevalent in pain assessment because, in such a subjective field, it is hoped that each subject is best used at his own control. Sophisticated methods, such as the twin crossover design (Finney, 1964) adapted to pain measurement (Wallenstein & Houde, 1975) can be very useful provided that the power of the analysis of variance (ANOVA) test is computed, and provided tests for sequential effects are made (Laska & Sunshine, 1973). It is not always realised that when the same subjects appear in more than one cell of the ANOVA design, the ordinary computation must be modified to cope with the loss of independence amongst the data. (The situation is a development from the simpler 'related' and 'unrelated' forms of the *t*-test familiar to clinical investigators). A description is given in any standard work on ANOVA, e.g. Dixon & Massey (1969). Moreover, a significant ANOVA test reveals merely an inhomogeneity amongst the means somewhere in that block of data. The site of the inhomogeneity must then be sought amongst all pairs of data sets using *t*-tests; it may not be found to reside amongst the single treatment contrasts at all. Indeed, this seems to have been the basis for the difference between claims of analgesic effects of codeine between Bloomfield *et al.* (1976) and Sunshine (1980). Problems readily arise if biostatistical 'packages' are applied routinely to data without careful attention to their properties, or if statistical advice is obtained without giving a full explanation of the biological problem to the statistician.

(iv) The *sensitivity and reliability* of pain measures can be tested very well provided that positive and negative controls (i.e. a known analgesic and a placebo) are both incorporated in each test, and moreover several doses are used to obtain a graded response. This 'belt and braces' approach is unnecessary to show only that a drug has analgesic efficacy, but is advisable to determine relative potencies (Sunshine, 1980). As we have remarked, it still does not suffice for a drug which cumulates appreciably (Prescott, 1980a).

Often, measures of drug effects are modified to provide derived indices. An example is the S.P.I.D. (Sum of Pain Intensity Differences) (Sunshine, 1980). Such indices may have obvious clinical value in interpreting pain alteration as it applies to the patient, but any index will have different statistical properties from those of the measures from which it is derived. For example, the S.P.I.D. is in fact a cusum, and might better be called that, since the term is standard and the statistics of its use well studied (Van Dobben de Bruyn, 1968). If we have:

$$I = \text{initial pain score}$$
$$H_i = \text{hourly pain scores}$$

$$\text{then S.P.I.D.} = \sum_{o}^{t} |H_i - I|$$

The 'variable percentage S.P.I.D.' is also used, which is:

$$\frac{\text{S.P.I.D. found}}{\text{S.P.I.D. max}} \times 100$$

Sunshine (1980) states that analysis of variance was done upon such scores. However, problems readily arise when scores from different individuals are combined (Oldham, 1968); ANOVA is applicable only when data are drawn from subjects randomly chosen from populations having roughly equal variances (Dixon & Massey, 1969); and interactions between data groups radically alter the ways in which ANOVA can be applied.

Now it is important to note the effects of taking indices upon these measures. If someone's initial score is close to the maximum, his pain has more room to improve than someone whose initial score was well below the maximum. The point is illustrated in Figure 5. Who had more relief of pain? What is the appropriate statistical test for such data?

Such problems become extremely difficult to analyse when the variance of the results depends on initial value (one form of heteroscedasticity). Often it is impossible to tell from published methods how indices have been derived, or what their statistical properties might be. It is therefore essential to publish individual and unmodified data in addition to the indices, advice which will be resented by journal editors but which is essential to assess the scientific merit of original work (Oldham, 1968).

Ethics of analgesic studies

This was recently discussed by Dundee (1980). It is essential that the subject should be fully informed. This does not prejudice double-blind technique, for it is necessary to conceal only the timing, not the fact, of placebo use. There must be a voluntary escape mechanism by which a subject can either discontinue an induced pain stimulus, or take 'rescue' medication, as soon as spontaneous pain becomes intolerable, even though this causes difficulty in analysing the results (Lasagna, 1980). Even with this provision, it is still important to design experiments to avoid

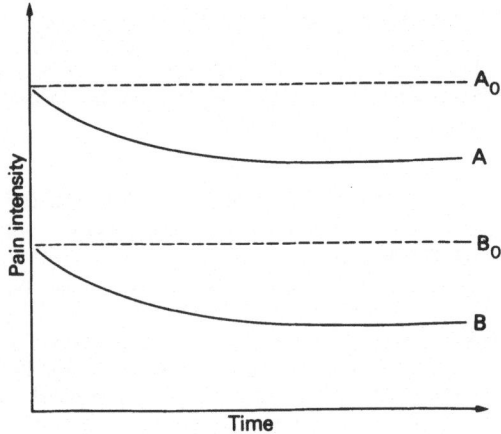

Figure 5 Imaginary pain scores in two subjects, A and B, differing in the initial intensities (A_0 and B_0) of their pains. A obtains 25% pain relief, B obtains 50%, but both have the same SPID index.

injury during analgesic treatment. For example, even if a radiant heat stimulus to blackened skin can be turned off by the subject he may not do so before he has been burned if he has taken a strong analgesic.

Individuals may volunteer for pathological reasons; it is difficult to protect someone who volunteers for masochistic reasons or from false heroism. It helps to know personally the group from whom volunteers are chosen and to elicit consent singly and in private, perhaps through a neutral person. People vary greatly in the 'gains' which give them satisfaction and provide their inner drives. These comments have special relevance to tests of narcotic analgesics. Particularly dangerous methods include routine approaches, where everyone who has undergone a certain operation is asked to volunteer, without regard to their personal differences. Substantial financial rewards can elicit a conditioned acceptance response from many people, but pharmaceutical companies commonly find themselves unable to test a promising new analgesic unless they offer high rewards. It seems equally unwise to ignore the motives that might attract experimenters into this field. So much depends on how the experiment is done, and not just on what is done, that Ethics Committees would be wise to expect particularly detailed protocols before giving such work their approval, and to consider who will make the actual tests as well as the person who submitted the protocol.

Adverse effects

Such adverse effects as are predictable by the investigator of a new analgesic will, of course, be indicated by its preclinical pharmacology and by the pattern of adverse effects of any familiar compounds related to it in chemical structure or mode of action. Some can be investigated in early human pharmacology, but others must await larger-scale investigation. It is easy to measure the histamine-releasing potency of opioids in man by intradermal injection of them in solution, measuring the size of the weal and/or flare, and using classical bioassay methods of calculation (Paton, 1957; Fowle, Hughes & Knight, 1971). The measurement of respiratory depression is not easy (Jennett, 1968; Saunders, 1980), but the use of respiratory minute volume or blood gas estimations is an important safeguard in initial tolerance studies. Useful observations of haemostasis, including platelet aggregation, can also be made on small numbers of subjects (e.g. Mielke, Kahn, Muschek, Tighe, Ng & Minn, 1980). Nausea and vomiting may also be noted early on, and can be measured with ordinal scale and VAS methods in normal volunteers, similarly and at the same time as pain; a central emetic effort may be missed if the subjects are not free to move about, as movement exaggerates this effect of opioids. In later trials, the number of subjects experiencing nausea and/or vomiting may be merely counted, probably a more valid measure, since individual susceptibility varies greatly, and a small sample of subjects may easily be misleading.

Compounds that inhibit cyclo-oxygenase may reasonably be expected to have some gastro-intestinal toxicity and to induce asthma in susceptible subjects. It is helpful and possible to study both before marketing. The controversy concerning gastrointestinal toxicity has recently been succinctly reviewed (Duggan, 1980), and comparison of occult gastrointestinal blood loss due to the new drug with that from standard compounds possessing and lacking an effect on platelets may represent the best index of such an adverse effect that can be obtained until the results of post-marketing surveillance are available (Johnson, 1980). Asthma induced by mild analgesics is not rare nor impossible to test in suitable subjects (Szczeklik, 1980).

Animal pharmacology now goes some way to predicting the abuse liability of opioid analgesics, and studies in previously opioid-dependent subjects can provide further information (Jasinski, 1979). Nephrotoxicity of mild analgesics is due to a less predictable form of dependence, and in some countries is a fairly common disorder (Nanra, 1980), chiefly due to formulations of analgesics in combination. Animal models can help to predict the likelihood of analgesics being nephrotoxic (Axelsen, 1980), but little information can be gained from studies in normal subjects or patients. The hepatotoxicity of paracetamol sets a similar problem of a relevant animal model but no human data can be obtained for such a threshold phenomenon, save by drug abuse (Prescott, 1980b); with the type of hepatotoxicity due to salicylates we lack even the animal model.

After marketing, there is an important difference between the numbers needed to detect an unwanted effect and the far larger number required to assess its incidence, though the two are closely related (Wardell, 1977). Detection requires a significant signal-to-noise ratio; it depends critically on the variance, the 'noise' level (false adverse reaction reports, perhaps due to biological ambiguities) and any bias in reporting (Finney, 1971). Neither data from circumscribed clinical experiments, nor clinical trials of the size usual in Britain, furnish sufficient data to detect or measure drug adverse reactions occuring less often than about one in a hundred users, but such measurements can be made very successfully in major trials of the size which national research councils can produce. Those interested in methods of detecting adverse reactions in larger populations will find a discussion of appropriate statistical techniques in papers by Mantel & Haenzsel (1959), Pike & Morrow (1970), Miettinen (1974) & Wardell (1977).

Pharmacokinetics

As with other classes of drugs, pharmacokinetic investigation can greatly illuminate efficacy studies, though it is particularly important that any body fluid samples are obtained painlessly, if pain is also being measured. Studies with salicylates are reviewed by Levy (1980), and with paracetamol by Prescott (1980a). Opioid analgesics have been less extensively studied, but some data are available (Berkowitz, 1976), interpretation of the results being hampered by the limited relevance of plasma drug levels for drugs that act within, and may be sequestered by, the central nervous system.

References

AITKEN, R.C.B. (1969). Measurement of feelings using visual analogue scales. *Proc. Roy. Soc. Med.*, **62**, 989–993.

AITKEN, R.C.B. & ZEALLEY, A.K. (1970). Measurement of moods. *Br. J. hosp. Med.*, **4**, 215–224.

ARMSTRONG, D., DRY, R.M.D., KEELE, C.A. & MONKHAM, J.W. (1953). Observations on chemical excitants of cutaneous pain in man. *J. Physiol.*, **120**, 326–351.

AXELSEN, R. (1980). Nephrotoxicity of mild analgesics in the Gunn strain of rat. *Br. J. clin. Pharmac.*, **10**, 309S–312S.

BAILEY, C.A. & DAVIDSON, P.O. (1976). The language of pain: Intensity. *Pain*, **2**, 319–324.

BEAVER, W.T. & McMILLAN, D. (1980). Methodological considerations in the evaluation of analgesic combinations: Acetoaminophen (paracetamol) and hydrocodone in postpartum pain. *Br. J. clin. Pharmac.*, **10**, 215S–223S.

BEECHER, H.K. (1957). The measurement of pain. Prototype for the quantitative study of subjective responses. *Pharmac. Rev.*, **9**, 59–209.

BEECHER, H.K. (1959). *Measurement of Subjective Responses.* New York: Oxford University Press.

BERKOWITZ, B.A. (1976). The relationship of pharmacokinetics to pharmacological activity: Morphine, methadone and naloxone. *Clin. Pharmacokin.*, **1**, 219–230.

BLOOMFIELD, S., BARDEN, T. & MITCHELL, J. (1976). Aspirin and codeine in two post-partum pain models. *Clin. Pharmac. Ther.*, **20**, 499–503.

BUCHSBAUM, M.S., DAVIS, G.C. & BUNNEY, W.E. (1977). Naloxone alters pain perception and somatosensory evoked potentials in normal subjects. *Nature*, **270**, 620–622.

CHAPMAN, C.R. (1977). Sensory decision theory methods in pain research: a reply to Rollman. *Pain*, **3**, 295–305.

CHAPMAN, C.R. (1978). Pain: the perception of noxious events. In *The Psychology of Pain*, ed. Sternbach, R.A., pp. 169–202. New York: Raven Press.

CHAPMAN, C.R., MURPHY, T.M. & BUTLER, S.H. (1973). Analgesic strength of 33 per cent nitrous oxide: A signal detection theory evaluation. *Science*, **179**, 1246–1248.

CLARK, W.C. (1974). Pain sensitivity and the report of pain: An introduction to sensory decision theory. *Anesthesiology*, **40**, 272–287.

COOPER, S.A. & BEAVER, W.T. (1976). A model to evaluate mild analgesics in oral surgery outpatients. *Clin. Pharmac. Ther.*, **20**, 241–250.

CRAIG, K.D. (1978). Social modeling influences on pain. In *The Psychology of Pain*, ed Sternbach, R.A., pp. 73–109. New York: Raven Press.

CRAIG, K.D. & NEIDERMAYER, H. (1974). Autonomic correlation of pain thresholds influenced by social modelling. *J. Pers. Soc. Psychol.*, **29**, 246–252.

CROCKETT, D.J., PRKACHIN, K.M. & CRAIG, K.D. (1977). Factors of the language of pain in patient and volunteer groups. *Pain*, **4**, 175–182.

DEODHAR, S.R., DICK, W.C., HODGKINSON, R. & BUCHANAN, W.W. (1973). Measurement of clinical response to anti-inflammatory drug therapy in rheumatoid arthritis. *Quart. J. Med.*, **166**, 387–401.

DIEM, K. & LENTNER, C. (Ed) (1970). *Documenta Geigy: Scientific tables.* 7th Edition, p. 69. Basle: J.R. Geigy.

DIXON, W.J. & MASSEY, F.J.J. (1969). *Introduction to Statistical Analysis,* 3rd Edition. New York: McGraw-Hill.

DOWNIE, W.N., LEATHAM, P.A., RHIND, V.M., WRIGHT, V., BRANCO, J.A. & ANDERSON, J.A. (1978a). Studies with pain rating scales. *Ann. Rheum. Dis.*, **37**, 378–381.

DOWNIE, W.W., LEATHAM, P.A., RHIND, V.M., PICKUP, M.E. & WRIGHT, V. (1978b). The visual analogue scale in the assessment of grip strength. *Ann. Rheum. Dis.*, **37**, 382–384.

DUGGAN, J.M. (1980). Gastrointestinal toxicity of minor analgesics. *Br. J. clin. Pharmac.*, **10**, 407S–410S.

DUNDEE, J.W. (1980). Clinical evaluation of mild analgesics. *Br. J. clin. Pharmac.*, **10**, 329S–334S.

EVANS, R.J. (1972). Acid-base changes in patients with intractable pain and malignancy. *Can. J. Surg.*, **15**, 37–42.

FINNEY, D.J. (1964). *Statistical Methods in Biological Assay,* 2nd Edition, pp. 266–272. New York: Hafner.

FINNEY, D.J. (1971). Statistical logic in the monitoring of reactions to therapeutic drugs. *Methods of Information in Medicine* (Stuttgart), **10**, 237–245.

FORDYCE, W.E. (1978). Learning processes in pain. In *The Psychology of Pain*, ed. Sternbach, R.A., pp. 49–72. New York: Raven Press.

FOWLE, A.S.E., HUGHES, D.T.D. & KNIGHT, G.J. (1971). The evaluation of histamine antagonists in man. *Eur. J. clin. Pharmac.*, **3**, 215–220.

GLYNN, C.J. & LLOYD, J.W. (1976). The diurnal variation in perception of pain. *Proc. Roy. Soc. Med.*, **69**, 369–372.

GOMEZ-JIMENEZ, J., FRANCO-PATINO, R., CHARGOY-VERA, J. & OLIVARES-SOSA, R. (1980). Clinical efficacy of mild analgesics in pain following gynaecological or dental surgery: Report on multicentre studies. *Br. J. clin. Pharmac.*, **10**, 355S–358S.

GRACELY, R.H., McGRATH, P. & DUBNER, R. (1978a). Ratio scales of sensory and affective verbal pain descriptors. *Pain*, **5**, 5–18.

GRACELEY, R.H., McGRATH, P. & DUBNER, R. (1978b). Validity and sensitivity of ratio scales of sensory and affective verbal pain descriptors: manipulation of affect by diazepam. *Pain*, **5**, 19–29.

HARDY, J.D., WOLFF, H.G. & GOODELL, H. (1940). Studies on pain: A new method for measuring pain threshold: Observations on spatial summation of pain. *J. clin. Invest.*, **19**, 649–657.

HARDY, J.D., WOLFF, H.G. & GOODELL, H. (1947). Studies on pain: discrimination of differences in intensity of a pain stimulus as a basis of a scale of pain intensity. *J. clin. Invest.*, **26**, 1152–1158.

HARDY, J.D., WOLFF, H.G. & GOODELL, H. (1953). *Pain Sensations and Reactions.* Baltimore: Williams and Wilkins.

HEWER, A.J.H., KEELE, C.A., KEELE, K.D. & NATHAN, P.W. (1949). A clinical method of assessing analgesics. *Lancet*, **ii**, 431–435.

HILGARD, E.R. (1978). Hypnosis and pain. In *The Psychology of Pain*, ed. Sternbach, R.A., pp. 219–240. New York: Raven Press.

HILLS, M. & ARMITAGE, P. (1979). The two-period crossover clinical trial. *Br. J. clin. Pharmac.*, **8**, 7–20.

HINDMARCH, I. (1980). Psychomotor function and psychoactive drugs. *Br. J. clin. Pharmac.*, **10**, 189–209.

HOFSTADTER, D.R. (1979). *Gödel, Escher, Bach.* Hassocks, Sussex: Harvester Press.

HOUDE, R.W., WALLENSTEIN, S.L. & RODGERS, A. (1960). Clinical pharmacology of analgesics: 1. A method of assaying analgesic effect. *Clin. Pharmac. Ther.*, 1, 163–174.

HUNTER, M., PHILIPS, C. & RACHMAN, S. (1979). Memory for pain. *Pain*, 6, 35–46.

HUSKISSON, E.C. (1974a). Catecholamine excretion and pain. *Br. J. clin. Pharmac.*, 1, 80–82.

HUSKISSON, E.C. (1974b). Measurement of pain. *Lancet*, ii, 1127–1131.

HUSKISSON, E.C. & HART, F.D. (1972). Pain threshold and arthritis. *Br. med. J.*, 4, 193–195.

JASINSKI, D.R. (1979). Human pharmacology of narcotic analgesics. *Br. J. clin. Pharmac.*, 7, 287S–290S.

JENNETT, S. (1968). Assessment of respiratory effects of analgesic drugs. *Br. J. Anaesth.*, 40, 746–756.

JICK, H., SLONE, D., SHAPIRO, S., LEWIS, G.P. & SISKIND, V. (1971). A new method for assessing the clinical effects of oral analgesic drugs. *Clin. Pharmac. Ther.*, 12, 456–463.

JOHNSON, P.C. (1980). A comparison of the effects of zomepirac and aspirin on fecal blood loss. *J. clin. Pharmac.*, 20, 401–405.

JOYCE, C.R.B., ZUTSHI, D.W., HRUBES, V. & MASON, R.M. (1975). Comparison of fixed interval and visual analogue scales for rating chronic pain. *Eur. J. clin. Pharmac.*, 8, 415–420.

KAST, E.C. (1962). The measurement of pain: A new approach to an old problem. *J. New Drugs*, 2, 344–351.

KEELE, K.D. (1948). The Pain Chart. *Lancet*, ii, 6–8.

KEELE, K.D. (1954). Pain-sensitivity tests: The pressure algometer. *Lancet*, i, 636–639.

KEELE, K.D. (1968). Pain complaint threshold in relation to pain of cardiac infarction. *Br. med. J.*, 1, 670–673.

KEELE, K.D. & STERN, P.R.S. (1973). Serum lipid changes in relation to pain. *J. Roy. Coll. Physcns.*, (Lond.), 7, 367–372.

KNITZA, R., CLASEN, R. & FISCHER, F. (1979). Pain-induced alterations in the individual non-esterified fatty acids in serum. *Pain*, 6, 91–97.

LASAGNA, L. (1960). The clinical measurement of pain. *Ann. N.Y. Acad. Sci.*, 86, 28–37.

LASAGNA, L. (1980). Analgesic methodology: A brief history and commentary. *J. clin. Pharmac.*, 20, 373–376.

LASCELLES, P.T., EVANS, P.R., MERSKEY, H. & SABUR, M.A. (1974). Plasma cortisol in psychiatric and neurological patients with pain. *Brain*, 87, 533–538.

LASKA, E. & SUNSHINE, A. (1973). Anticipation of analgesia—a placebo effect. *Headache*, 13, 1–11.

LEVINE, J.D., GORDON, N.C., BORNSTEIN, J.C. & FIELDS, H.L. (1979). Role of pain in placebo analgesia. *Proc. Nat. Acad. Sci.*, 76, 3528–3531.

LEVY, G. (1980). Clinical pharmacokinetics of salicylates: A re-assessment. *Br. J. clin. Pharmac.*, 10, 285S–290S.

LINDLEY, D.V. (1965). *Introduction to probability and statistics. Part 1. Probability*, pp. 25 & 215–235. Cambridge: Cambridge University Press.

LOESER, J.D. (1980). Perspectives on pain. In *Clinical Pharmacology & Therapeutics. Proceedings of the First World Conference*, ed. Turner, P., pp. 313–316. London: Macmillan.

LYNN, B. & PERL, E.R. (1977). A comparison of four tests for assessing the pain sensitivity of different subjects and test areas. *Pain*, 3, 353–365.

MANTEL, N. & HAENSZEL, W. (1959). Statistical aspects of the analysis of data from retrospective studies on disease. *J. National Cancer Institute*, 22, 719–727.

MELZACK, R. (1975). The McGill Pain Questionnaire: Major properties and scoring methods. *Pain*, 1, 277–299.

MELZACK, R. & DENNIS, S.G. (1978). Neurophysiological foundations of pain. In *The Psychology of Pain*, ed. Sternbach, R.A., pp. 49–72. New York: Raven Press.

MELZACK, R. & TORGERSON, W.S. (1971). On the language of pain. *Anesthesiology*, 34, 50–59.

MERSKEY, H. & SPEAR, F.G. (1964). The reliability of the pressure algometer. *Br. J. Soc. clin. Psychol.*, 3, 130–136.

MIELKE, C.H., KAHN, S.B., MUSCHEK, L.D., TIGHE, J.J., NG, K.T. & MINN, F.L. (1980). Effects of zomepirac on hemostasis in healthy adults and on platelet function *in vitro*. *J. clin. Pharmac.*, 20, 409–417.

MIETTINEN, O.S. (1974). Simple interval-estimation of risk ratio. *Am. J. Epidemiol.*, 100, 515–516.

MONGAR, J.L. (1955). A study of two methods for testing local anaesthetics in man. *Br. J. Pharmac.*, 10, 240–246.

MUMFORD, J.M. & BOWSHER, D. (1976). Pain and protopathic sensibility. A review with particular reference to the teeth. *Pain*, 2, 223–243.

NANRA, R.S. (1980). Clinical and pathological aspects of analgesic nephropathy. *Br. J. clin. Pharmac.*, 10, 349S–368S.

NATHAN, P.W. (1977). Pain. *Br. med. Bull.*, 33, 149–156.

NAYMAN, J. (1979). Measurement and control of postoperative pain. *Ann. Roy. Coll. Surg. Engl.*, 61, 419–426.

NICHOLSON, A.N. (1978). Visual analogue scales and drug effects in man. *Br. J. clin. Pharmac.*, 6, 3–4.

OHNHAUS, E.E. & ADLER, R. (1975). Methodological problems in the measurement of pain: a comparison between the verbal rating scale and the visual analogue scale. *Pain*, 1, 379–384.

OLDHAM, J.D. (1968). *Measurement in Medicine*. London: English University Press.

PARKHOUSE, J. & HOLMES, C.M. (1963). Assessing postoperative pain relief. *Proc. Roy. Soc. Med.*, 56, 579–583.

PATON, W.D.M. (1957). Histamine release by compounds of simple chemical structure. *Pharmac. Rev.*, 9, 269–328.

PIKE, M.C. & MORROW, R.H. (1970). Statistical analysis of patient-control studies in epidemiology: factor under investigation an all-or-none variable. *Br. J. Prev. Soc. Med.*, 24, 42–44.

POSER, E.G. (1962). A simple and reliable apparatus for the measurement of pain. *Am. J. Psychol.*, 75, 304–305.

PRESCOTT, L.F. (1980a). Kinetics and metabolism of paracetamol and phenacetin. *Br. J. clin. Pharmac.*, 10, 291S–298S.

PRESCOTT, L.F. (1980b). Hepatotoxicity of mild analgesics. *Br. J. clin. Pharmac.*, 10, 373S–379S.

REVILL, S.I., ROBINSON, J O., ROSEN, M. & HOGG, M.I.J. (1976). The reliability of a linear analogue for evaluating pain. *Anaesthesia*, 31, 1191–1198.

ROLLMAN, G.B. (1977). Signal detection theory measurement of pain: A review and critique. *Pain*, 3, 187–211.

ROLLMAN, G.B. (1979). Signal detection theory pain measures: empirical validation studies and adaptation-

138

level effects. *Pain*, **6**, 9–21.

SAUNDERS, K.B. (1980). Methods in the assessment of the control of breathing. *Br. J. clin. Pharmac.*, **9**, 3–9.

SCOTT, J. & HUSKISSON, E.C. (1976). Graphic representation of pain. *Pain*, **2**, 175–184.

SITARAM, N., BUCHSBAUM, M.S. & GILLIN, C. (1977). Physostigmine analgesia and somatosensory evoked responses in man. *Eur. J. Pharmac.*, **42**, 285–290.

SMITH, G.M., EGBERT, L.D., MARCOWITZ, R.A., MOSTELLER, F. & BEECHER, H.K. (1966). An experimental pain method sensitive to morphine in man: The submaximal effort tourniquet technique. *J. Pharmac. exp. Ther.*, **154**, 324–332.

SMITH, G.M., LOWENSTEIN, E., HUBBARD, J.H. & BEECHER, H.K. (1968). Experimental pain produced by the submaximal tourniquet technique: Further evidence of validity. *J. Pharmac. exp. Ther.*, **163**, 468–474.

SUNSHINE, A. (1980). Clinical evaluation of mild analgesics in post partum pain. *Br. J. clin. Pharmac.*, **10**, 335S–337S.

SWETS, J.A. (1973). The relative operating characteristic in psychology. *Science*, **182**, 990–1000.

SZCZEKLIK, A. (1980). Analgesics, allergy and asthma. *Br. J. clin. Pharmac.*, **10**, 401S–405S.

TURSKY, B. (1975). The development of a pain perception profile: A psychophysical approach. In *Pain: New Perspectives in Therapy and Research*, eds Weisenberg, M. & Tursky, B., pp. 171–194. New York: Plenum Press.

TWYCROSS, R.G. (1975). *The evaluation of narcotic analgesics in patients with terminal cancer*. Paul Martini Award Essay.

VALBO, A.B. & HAGBARTH, K.-E. (1968). Activity from skin mechanoreceptors in awake human subjects. *J. exp. Neurol.*, **21**, 270–289.

VAN BUREN, J. & KLEINKNECHT, R.A. (1979). An evaluation of the McGill Pain Questionnaire for use in dental pain assessment. *Pain*, **6**, 23–33.

VAN DOBBEN de BRUYN, C.S. (1968). *Cumulative Sum Tests: Theory and Practice*. London: Griffin.

VINCENT, C.H. (1973). *Random Pulse Trains, their measurement and statistical properties* I.E.E. Monograph Series, No 13. London: Peter Peregrinus.

VON GRAFFENRIED, B., ADLER, R., ABT, K., NUESCH, E. & SPIEGEL, R. (1978). The influence of anxiety and pain sensitivity on experimental pain in man. *Pain*, **4**, 253–263.

VON GRAFFENRIED, B. & NUESCH, (1980). Nonmigrainous headache for the evaluation of oral analgesics. *Br. J. clin. Pharmac.*, **10**, 225S–231S.

WALLENSTEIN, S.L., HEIDRICH, G., KAIKO, R. & HOUDE, R.W. (1980). Clinical evaluation of mild analgesics: The measurement of clinical pain. *Br. J. clin. Pharmac.*, **10**, 319S–327S.

WALLENSTEIN, S.L. & HOUDE, R.W. (1975). The clinical evaluation of analgesic effectiveness. In *Methods in Narcotics Research*, eds. Ehrenpreis, S. & Neidle, A., pp. 127–145. New York: Marcel Dekker.

WARDELL, W.A. (1977). Post-marketing surveillance: case-study approach. In *Drug Monitoring*, ed. Gross, F.H. & Inman, W.H.W. London: Academic Press.

WOLFF, B.B. (1977). Analgesic drug and dose discriminations by experimental human pain response parameters. *Clin. Pharmac. Ther.*, **21**, 123–132.

WOLFF, B.B. (1978). Behavioural measurement of human pain. In *The Psychology of Pain*, ed. Sternbach, R.A., pp. 129–168. New York: Raven Press.

WOLFF, B.B., KANTOR, T.G., JARVIK, M.E. & LASKA, E. (1969). Response of experimental pain to analgesic drugs: III. Codeine, aspirin, secobarbital, and placebo. *Clin. Pharmac. Ther.*, **10**, 217–228.

WOODFORDE, J.M. & MERSKEY, H. (1972). Some relationships between subjective measures of pain. *J. psychosom. Res.*, **16**, 173–178.

YAKSH, T.L. & RUDY, T.A. (1978). Narcotic analgesics: CNS sites and mechanisms of action as revealed by intracerebral injection techiques. *Pain*, **4**, 299–359.

YANG, J.C., CLARK, W.C., NGAI, S.H., BERKOWITZ, B.A. & SPECTOR, S. (1979). Analgesic action and pharmacokinetics of morphine and diazepam in man. *Anesthesiology*, **51**, 495–502.

METHODS OF ASSESSMENT OF ANTIEPILEPTIC DRUGS

NORMAN MILLIGAN

Clinical Pharmacology Unit, Institute of Neurology,
Queen Square, London WC1

ALAN RICHENS

Department of Clinical Pharmacology and Materia Medica,
Welsh National School of Medicine, Heath Park, Cardiff CF4 4XN

Epilepsy is a symptom with protean manifestations and as such it is a difficult disease in which to carry out a therapeutic trial. The methods available to research workers for the assessment of new antiepileptic drugs are hampered by the fact that epilepsy is a fluctuant condition. Although it is a chronic disorder open to study using cross-over trials and within-patient comparisons, accurate assessments cannot be easily made at any one point in time. Research workers are therefore automatically placed at a time factor disadvantage and this is especially so for those searching for quick methods of evaluating new compounds. The need for a quick and reliable method of assessing a new antiepileptic drug has long been appreciated. This article will discuss the methods currently available and we will begin by considering the most commonly used method of assessment with particular reference to some of the problems involved in conducting a controlled clinical trial in epilepsy.

Assessment by seizure counting

The traditional method of assessing response to an antiepileptic drug is by demonstrating an improvement in fit frequency. Ideally this requires a double-blind, placebo-controlled cross-over study and takes several months to complete. The proper design of clinical trials involves clearly defining the objectives of the study, attention to randomisation, removal of bias from data collection, thought of statistical analysis to be used and the fulfilment of strict criteria for patient entry to and also withdrawal from the clinical trial. The fundamental principles inherent to the design of clinical trials are detailed elsewhere (Cereghino & Penry, 1972; ILAE Commission on Antiepileptic Drugs, 1973; Bulpitt, 1975; Richens, 1975).

Patient selection

Clinical trials in epilepsy are best done on in-patients where both patient and drug supervision are more reliable. In practice, such trials of long duration are only possible in institutions for residential patients. Ideally one should look at groups of patients with a single seizure type, e.g. tonic-clonic or complex partial seizures. Unfortunately this is not always possible as many patients have more than one type of fit. It is, of course, mandatory to examine individual seizure types as some fits may improve more than others. This will help in the design of future studies and may identify those groups of epileptic patients most likely to benefit from the new drug. As the method of assessment will be fit frequency it is essential that each patient's fits be clearly defined. A change in seizure severity can sometimes be as important as a change in seizure frequency. The use of demerit points in which each fit is scored according to its type and severity provides a method of comparing several treatments in a highly controlled manner (White, Plott & Norton, 1966). Gastaut's international classification is probably the most satisfactory for the purposes of defining the type of fit

Table 1 Classification of the epilepsies, modified from Marsden (1975)

---

1. *Generalized seizures*
   A. Tonic-clonic seizures (grand mal)
   B. Absence seizures (petit mal)
   C. Myoclonic and akinetic seizures.

2. *Partial seizures (focal fits)*
   A. With simple symptoms
      (i) Motor seizures
      (ii) Sensory seizures
         (a) Somatosensory
         (b) Visual
         (c) Auditory
         (d) Olfactory and gustatory
         (e) Visceral and autonomic
   B. With complex symptoms
      (complex partial seizures)
         (a) Automatisms
         (b) Psychic experiences (psychomotor, psychosensory)
         (c) Emotional and mood changes
   C. With impaired consciousness.

3 *Partial seizures secondarily generalized*
   Indicated by:
   A. Aura preceding tonic-clonic fit.
   B. Focal EEG discharge preceding generalized discharge.
   C. Focal events during or prefacing a tonic-clonic fit.
   D. Focal aftermath to tonic-clonic fit.

(Gastaut, 1969). A simplified version of this is shown in Table 1.

During phase 2 clinical trials the subjects will usually have more severe and poorly controlled epilepsy. This is a harsh test for a new drug but any definite improvement in such patients is all the more encouraging (Richens & Ahmad, 1975). It is usual at this stage to administer the new drug as an add-on to pre-existing medication as physicians are reluctant to withdraw therapy for fear of making matters worse. The likelihood of adverse effects and drug inter-actions is increased by such measures. Unsatisfactory though they are, these trials form the foundation for the preliminary evaluation of new antiepileptic drugs in man. Once the new compound has shown useful results in these patients it can then be used on a wider scale in phase 3 clinical trials. Evaluation studies at this stage will include the less severe cases whose fits have not been satisfactorily controlled by established drugs and those with newly diagnosed and previously untreated epilepsy. Whether those patients already taking antiepileptic drugs should receive the new compound as sole therapy is not easy to answer although this may be possible if there is doubt about the effectiveness of established medication. It may also be justifiable to include patients with well con-trolled epilepsy if the new drug is likely to produce fewer adverse effects for the same degree of control. The use of the new compound as sole treatment in newly diagnosed cases presents fewer ethical objec-tions for here there are no problems from drug with-drawal. The assessment of a new antiepileptic drug in newly diagnosed patients has been little explored. Approximately 80% of such patients respond to monotherapy using conventional medication (Shor-von, Chadwick, Galbraith & Reynolds 1978). There is here a pool of relative responders and it is surprising that no trials of new compounds have been published using this model. Indeed, there is a paucity of con-trolled trials of the established antiepileptic drugs in newly diagnosed patients. This is an extraordinary omission and reflects the generally poor quality of trials of drugs used in epilepsy.

Subjects who have had only a single fit could also be included in clinical trials at this stage (see below) though there are practical problems as not all patients will go on to have subsequent fits. However, in a clinic of sufficiently large size this should not be a major difficulty provided the number of such patients is small. In practice, the opportunity of studying patients presenting after a single fit is difficult and is influenced by factors not easily controlled, e.g. speed and accuracy of diagnosis, speed of referral and hospital out-patient waiting lists. Moreover, referral policy in general practice is such that patients are often not referred until they have had two or more fits and by the time they reach the out-patient clinic many are already receiving medication.

Choice of control treatment

In the clinical trial of a new antiepileptic drug there are two choices of control treatment, an identical placebo or an established antiepileptic drug. Com-paring a new compound against an established drug will indicate whether it is more active, less active or equivalent in effectiveness to the established drug. This presupposes that the efficacy of the control treat-ment has been proved beyond doubt but this may not necessarily be the case. There is still much con-troversy about the relative merits of the established antiepileptic drugs in the treatment of complex partial seizures. The effect of new drugs on complex partial seizures has previously been compared against phenobarbitone and primidone at a time when the efficacy of the control treatment had not been fully evaluated in a controlled trial in this seizure type (Richens, 1976). If both new and established drugs are found to be equally effective (without comparison against placebo) the interpretation that neither drug is effective is as plausible as that both drugs are producing benefit. Comparison of a new drug against placebo at some stage is essential and if necessary this should be done as a separate study.

The use of placebo, however, can pose ethical problems. A placebo given as a control as an add-on to pre-existing medication is entirely justified but difficulties arise when considering the use of a placebo as sole therapy in patients presenting for the first time. One method might be to use placebo following the first fit and change to active treatment after the occurrence of the second fit. There are no ethical objections here as patients are not considered epileptic until after their second fit at which point the trial ends as continued treatment with placebo becomes unethical. The method of assessment might be the time interval between the institution of placebo treatment and the occurrence of the next fit compared with the time interval between fits on active treatment. It is likely that the duration and number of patients included in this type of study will both need to be large if accurate statistical conclu-sions are to be drawn. The justification for using a placebo as a control treatment (sole therapy) in chronic or newly diagnosed epileptic patients, i.e. those having two or more fits, is more difficult although this may be possible where subjects have relatively non-harmful seizures, e.g. absences and complex partial seizures without secondary generali-sation. Patients with tonic-clonic seizures should probably receive an established antiepileptic drug as a control.

Serum level monitoring and drug dosage

It is essential that serum levels of both established antiepileptic drugs and the new compound be monitored throughout the study as any change in fit control may occur due to drug interactions. This is especially important where subjects are already taking antiepileptic drugs in combination. In the case of sulthiame, it was a much appreciated clinical observation that this drug exerted its most beneficial effect when given in combination with other anti-epileptic drugs. Much of the evidence for its anti-epileptic effect came from uncontrolled add-on studies with no pharmacokinetic data (Green & Kupferberg 1972). The inhibition of phenytoin meta-bolism by sulthiame was only discovered subse-quently (Houghton & Richens 1974 a, b). Further-more, unless serum levels are monitored any toxic effects due to drug interaction may be erroneously attributed to the new compound (Jeavons & Clark, 1974; Richens & Ahmad, 1975).

The dose to be used in a clinical trial is usually based on data from pilot studies done on an open basis. Clinical trials involving a fixed dosage schedule do not take into account patient variables such as differing rates of absorption, metabolism and elimination. However, this type of study would be useful when comparing a new drug against placebo where the aim is to determine if the new compound has antiepileptic properties. Furthermore it is diffi-cult to build in a dosage adjustment scheme when a placebo is included. In comparisons of new and estab-lished drugs it is better to allow dosage adjustment to suit each patient. The rules to be adopted in changing doses and the minimum interval between increments in dosage will be based on the pharmacokinetic properties of the new drug. These are necessary to allow a steady state serum level to be achieved and assessment of fit frequency should be made only after this point. The duration of each treatment period should be long enough to allow adequate assessment of fit frequency and to look for tolerance if this is suspected.

Once a steady state level in the serum has been reached following initial administration of the drug continued stability at that level is not assured. For example, a steady state level of carbamazepine has been shown to drift downwards to a lower level during chronic administration in normal volunteers due to enzyme induction (Levy, Pitlick, Troupin, Green & Neal, 1975). This partially explains why adverse reactions at the initiation of treatment tend to improve over ensuing weeks. Patients may also have a good therapeutic response initially only to find an increase in seizures subsequently which parallels the decrease in serum levels. Tolerance to the effect of antiepileptic drugs given on a long term basis may also lead to a decline in fit control (Browne & Penry, 1973). In addition, the half-life of new compounds when administered to patients receiving other anti-epileptic drugs may be significantly shorter (and occasionally longer) than when the drug is admin-istered to drug-free volunteers (Cereghino, Van Meter, Brock, Penry, Smith & White, 1973; Patel, Levy & Cutler, 1980).

Although several antiepileptic drugs are most effective when serum concentrations are maintained within the therapeutic range it does not necessarily follow that such rules will apply to all newly developed compounds. The therapeutic range of a new compound may not be known for certain during its preliminary evaluation and in later studies such estimates may not be directly related to its anti-epileptic effect. In practice, maintenance of serum levels within the therapeutic range can be difficult to achieve especially if the drug has a short half-life when marked fluctuations in serum concentration can be expected. In the case of sodium valproate, a drug with a relatively short half-life, there is evidence to suggest that the antiepileptic effect is not closely re-lated to its concentration in the serum (Jeavons, Clark & Maheshwari, 1977; Rowan, Binnie, de Beer-Pawlikowski, Goedhart, Gutter, Van Parijs, Meinardi & Meijer 1978) although some authors express a different view (Grant & Barot 1976; Gram, Flachs, Würtz-Jorgensen, Parnas & Andersen, 1979). Using photosensitivity as a model Rowan, Binnie, Warefield, Meinardi & Meijer (1979) have shown that an acute oral administration of sodium valproate has both a delayed and prolonged effect which can persist long after the drug is detectable in the serum. Indeed, some physicians recommend single daily doses of sodium valproate (Covanis & Jeavons, 1980). This does not appear to affect seizure control adversely and may improve patient com-pliance.

Trial design

The measures of efficacy to be examined should be clearly defined at the trial design stage. The duration of the trial will depend on factors such as frequency of seizures in the sample studied and degree of superiority of one drug over another. New com-pounds which are only marginally better than their counterparts will require trials of long duration to demonstrate a significant difference between treat-ments especially if newly diagnosed patients with re-latively infrequent fits are included. Similarly, calcu-lations of sample size should take these factors into account and numbers should be sufficient to allow for unavoidable drop-outs and non-responsiveness. Tables are available for estimating the size of samples required to achieve results at different levels of significance. It may seem banal to mention basic principles of trial design but clinical trials which are too short and contain too few numbers are extremely common (Ambroz, Chalmers, Smith, Schroeder, Frieman & Shareck, 1978). The importance of these considerations is discussed elsewhere (Altman, 1980).

In a traditional placebo controlled add-on study it

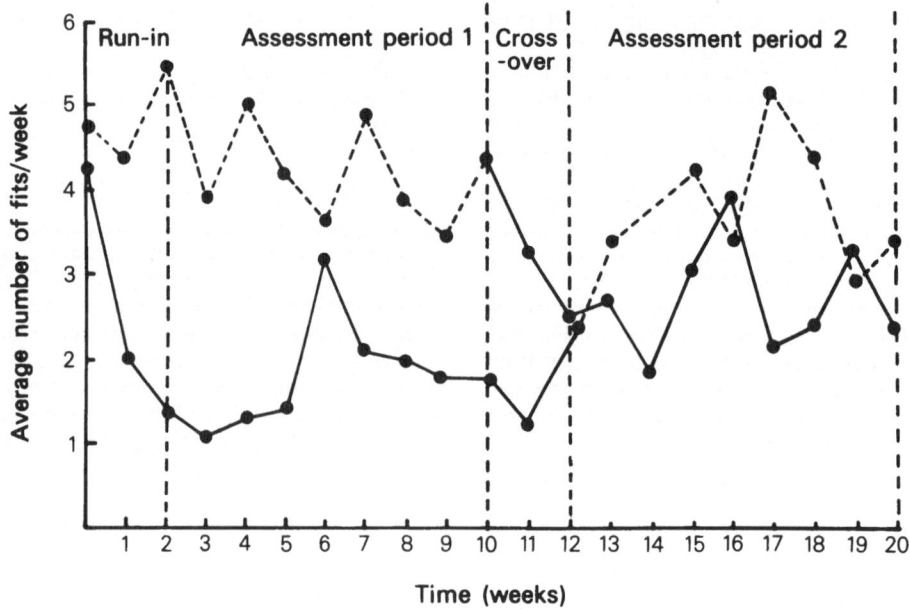

Figure 1 Double-blind cross-over trial of sodium valproate (●—●) with placebo (●--●) in 20 institutionalised patients with uncontrolled epilepsy. Following the run-in and cross-over periods which allowed gradual introduction or change of the treatment, a fixed dose of 1200 mg of sodium valproate was compared with a matching placebo. The mean frequency of tonic-clonic fits is illustrated. Analysis of variance indicated a significant difference between treatments ($P < 0.001$). (Reproduced from Richens (1976) with permission).

is usual to use a cross-over design to allow within-patient comparisons to be made. A cross-over period is desirable also so that one drug can be tailed off while gradually introducing another. This reduces the risk of precipitating status epilepticus which might otherwise occur on abrupt withdrawal of an anti-epileptic drug. It may be necessary to adjust the duration of the cross-over period to the magnitude of the risk involved. The trial should also have a run-in period so that dosage increments can be made gradually, thereby lessening the appearance of adverse effects. It may be wise to precede the actual trial with a run-in placebo period and if the patient successfully completes this period he could then enter the study (Bulpitt, 1975). Any carry-over effect of active drug into placebo period will be minimised by proper trial design. However, unexpected problems can arise especially if hitherto unknown properties of the new compound are at play. The delayed and prolonged effect of sodium valproate on photosensitivity has already been mentioned. Figure 1 illustrates the results of a double-blind placebo-controlled cross-over study showing the effects of sodium valproate on fit frequency in chronic institutionalised epileptic subjects. There is a significant improvement of fit frequency in patients taking sodium valproate. Had the authors been looking at photosensitivity and not fit frequency a cross-over or wash-out period of two weeks may have been insufficient to eliminate totally

a carry-over effect and the results may then have been more difficult to interpret. Such difficulties are hardly foreseeable at the early stage of assessment of a new drug and depend on the model being examined.

Between-subjects trials offer an alternative to the traditional cross-over study. Such a trial would be useful in the comparison of a relatively new compound against an established drug, both given as sole therapy. The duration of this type of trial would depend on factors previously mentioned but it is likely to be substantially longer than the more usual cross-over trial (Shorvon *et al.*, 1978). This is a disadvantage. It also precludes the use of a placebo as control treatment. As only between-patient comparisons are possible, careful matching of patients is a *sine-qua-non* for this type of trial. The use of this design deserves consideration at some stage but it will clearly depend on the question to be answered.

When ethical considerations are of major concern and it is necessary that a trial be concluded quickly the main objective is to show that drug A is better than drug B. Sequential analysis offers a technique where results can be available rapidly and analysed at once. Following the analysis of each patient's results the decision is made whether to stop the trial or continue. Birket-Smith, Lund, Mikkelsen, Vestermark, Zander-Olsen & Hulm (1973) used this method under single-blind conditions to demonstrate the effectiveness of clonazepam in complex partial seizures. The technique can be adapted to suit a within subjects, cross-over design using fit frequency but in other situations only between-patient comparisons are possible. This method is ideally suited for the assessment of drugs used in status epilepticus where subjects can be admitted to the trial serially. Sequential trials, however, are of little additional value when patients have to be followed for long periods and the fluctuant nature of epilepsy may impose limitations on the usefulness of this technique. Careful model selection is clearly important if sequential analysis is to be used.

Counting clinical seizures is satisfactory for dramatic events such as tonic-clonic or partial motor fits but in other situations this may not be so appropriate, e.g. nocturnal convulsions. Attempts to count clinical absences in patients with absence seizures are notoriously difficult and inaccurate as many attacks are so brief they pass unnoticed even by experienced observers. Research workers have therefore had to search for more objective methods of assessing response to medication and inevitably they turned towards the electroencephalogram.

Assessments based on changes in the EEG

Random EEG recordings

The EEG is primarily used as a diagnostic tool but many attempts have been made to correlate paroxysmal epileptiform activity in the EEG with seizure frequency. In 1935 Gibbs, Davis & Lennox introduced the theory of ictal and inter-ictal ('larval') activity and although there is still debate about the precise significance of inter-ictal paroxysmal activity the concept has persisted. The fluctuant nature of both spontaneous seizures and electroencephalographic inter-ictal activity make it difficult if not impossible to draw any conclusions from random EEG recordings. Clinical and paroxysmal EEG abnormalities occur at any time within a 24 h period but random 20 min EEG recordings sample only a small fraction of the paroxysmal activity that may occur during an entire day. Assessments of therapeutic response based on random EEGs are therefore likely to be inaccurate (Binnie, 1980).

Assessment of response to antiepileptic drugs based on random EEG recordings is compounded also by the effect of drugs on the EEG. Some drugs (carbamazepine) are reputed to cause a deterioration in the EEG whilst at the same time improving fit control. Such comments however, need to be seen in perspective. Early statements that the EEG was 'worse' during therapy with carbamazepine were based on the simplistic assumption that slow waves are somehow worse than spikes or sharp waves. Subsequent studies have given more specific information.

Cereghino, Brock, Van Meter, Penry, Smith & White (1974) demonstrated that there was no reduction in paroxysmal abnormalities during therapy with carbamazepine despite an improvement in seizure frequency. This observation was confirmed by Rodin, Rim & Rennick (1974) who, in contrast, also demonstrated a fall in spike counts in subjects treated with phenytoin which seemed to parallel increasing serum levels. More recent investigations have confirmed earlier impressions. In a double-blind cross-over study Wilkus, Dodrill & Troupin (1978) compared the effects of phenytoin and carbamazepine on the EEG. Each treatment period lasted four months. There was a significant increase in both generalised slow wave activity and generalised epileptic discharges in patients taking carbamazepine. This occurred without a corresponding increase in seizure incidence. Focal epileptic abnormalities were not significantly altered however. The discrepancy between the EEG and seizure control in patients taking carbamazepine serves to underline the point that single and even repeated random 20 min EEG recordings are poor indicators in the assessment of a clinical response to antiepileptic drugs.

Inter-ictal spike frequency

There is general agreement that disappearance of inter-ictal spikes from the EEG should parallel an improvement in fit control although the evidence for this is often controversial (Bancoud, Ribet & Chagot, 1975; Carrie, 1976). Rowan, Pippenger, McGregor & French (1975) observed an increase in paroxysmal epileptiform activity in relation to various stages of sleep with suppression during REM periods. There was a marked increase in activity shortly after waking which responded to an increase in antiepileptic drug, the largest dosage being given at bedtime. The subsequent clinical and EEG improvement paralleled an increase in serum concentration throughout the night and in the morning. It is reasonable therefore to assume that disappearance of spikes is of clinical significance provided the EEG is sufficiently prolonged. Quantitation of spike frequency over several hours of EEG recording requires a system of automated analysis if its use is to become widespread. Many methods of computerised spike frequency analysis have been devised but all run into problems in differentiating true cerebral spikes from muscle activity and other artefacts. More recently Gotman has developed an automatic recognition system based on rectification of the EEG signal into half-waves and the measurement of the duration, amplitude and sharpness relative to the background. These measures are then combined to determine whether a wave is a possible spike or sharp wave. Preliminary evaluation indicates that the reliability of this method is variable but the problems are not insurmountable (Gotman,

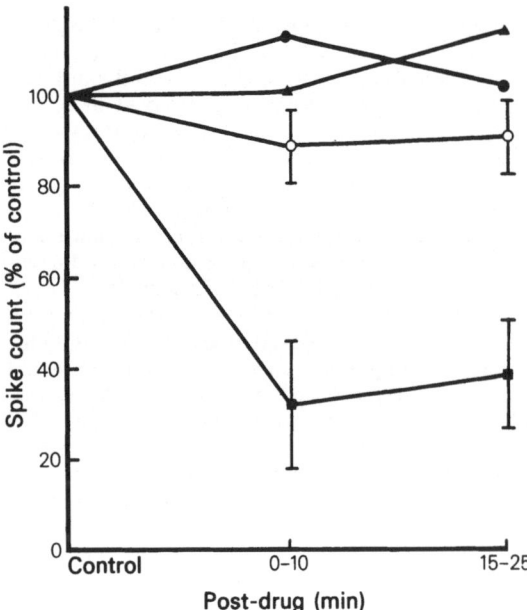

Figure 2 Results of a double-blind trial in six epileptic patients who exhibited frequent interictal spikes in their EEGs. Intravenous injections of (+)-propranolol (50 mg, ▲) (the non-β-adrenoceptor blocking isomer of propranolol) and mexiletine (100 mg,●) were compared with diazepam (5 mg, ■) and saline (O). Assessment was by spike counting in 10 min of control EEG, and two 10-min periods following intravenous administration of the drugs. Observations after diazepam— significantly different from those after saline ($P < 0.05$). (Reproduced from Ahmad et al. (1977) by kind permission of the editor).

Ives & Gloor, 1979). Such a method, if reliable, would help in the study of relationships between inter-ictal spike activity and seizures, stages of sleep and level of medication. Further evaluation studies are clearly necessary and are awaited with interest.

An alternative approach to automatic spike recognition is to count the spikes by eye. Obviously this is very laborious and time consuming but the method can be adapted to suit the needs of the investigator. Ahmad, Perucca & Richens (1977) demonstrated a significant reduction in inter-ictal spike frequency following intravenous diazepam (Figure 2). This technique provides a useful and quick method for the preliminary assessment of an antiepileptic drug. The main limitations are that it can only be used in patients who have frequent inter-ictal spikes in their EEG and with drugs that penetrate rapidly into the brain. Preliminary results from more prolonged studies evaluating the effect of rectal administration of diazepam on inter-ictal spikes over a 3 h period suggests that there are marked spontaneous fluctua-

tions in spike counts (Milligan & Richens, unpublished results). The instability of inter-ictal spike frequency complicates the assessment of drugs over prolonged periods especially those that do not have a dramatic effect. The large variance of spike frequency may make statistical analysis impossible if small numbers are studied. Drugs which have a delayed onset of action or are effective after conversion to active metabolites may therefore not be suitable for assessment using this method.

It may be possible, however, to use this technique for drugs which do not penetrate quite so rapidly into the brain as diazepam or which need to be given slowly. For example, phenytoin should be given intravenously only by slow infusion, preferably under ECG control. Assessment of inter-ictal spike frequency would need to take into account the distribution time of phenytoin which is longer than that of diazepam. In the assessment of a new drug care needs to be taken to ensure that the distribution time is not excessive otherwise a situation may be reached which is little better than random recording.

Paroxysmal spike-wave activity

Although the relationship between inter-ictal spikes and clinical epilepsy is open to question the same cannot be said of paroxysmal spike-wave (S-W) activity in absence seizures. There is abundant evidence to indicate that the frequency of absences closely parallels the amount of paroxysmal S-W activity in the EEG. In no other field of epilepsy does the relationship between EEG epileptiform activity and clinical epilepsy exist with such clarity. The EEG is potentially the most reliable tool for assessing response to medication in patients with absence seizures. This topic will therefore be considered in some detail.

An absence seizure can be defined as a brief impairment of consciousness during which the subject will interrupt his activities and then carry on as if nothing had happened (simple absence) or he may exhibit semi-purposeful movements (complex absence). During an absence seizure the EEG exhibits generalised S-W activity, classically at 3 per second. The difficulties of clinical assessment have already been mentioned. However, neuropsychological assessments made during paroxysmal epileptiform activity are often abnormal, generalised discharges producing greater abnormality than focal discharges (Wilkus & Dodrill, 1976). The generalised S-W activity during an absence seizure is virtually always accompanied by a measurable impairment of mental ability (Goode, Penry & Dreifuss 1970; Porter, Penry & Dreifuss, 1973). Browne, Penry, Porter & Dreifuss (1974) found that auditory reaction times were impaired in 57% of cases at the onset of a S-W paroxysm. This increased to 80% after a delay of

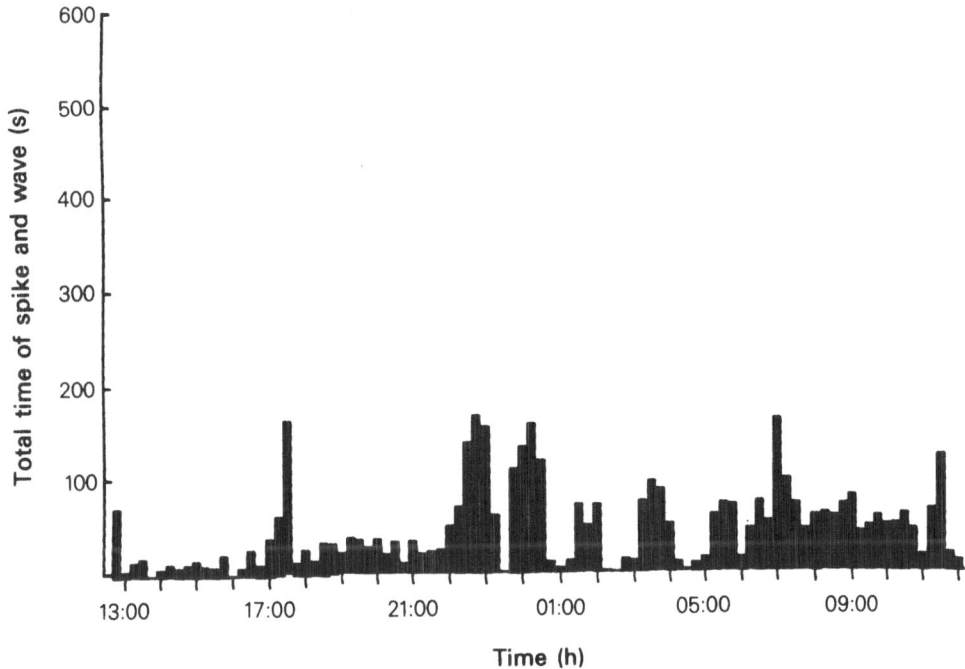

Figure 3 Computer print out showing distribution of spike-wave activity over a 24 h period beginning at 12.45 h in an epileptic patient who showed frequent paroxysms of atypical spike-wave activity in his EEG. Each bar represents the number of seconds of spike-wave activity in 15 min. Note the periodicity of spike-wave discharges during sleep (22.00–06.00 h). Each cycle lasts approximately 1.25 h. Total spike-wave = 4262 s in 24 h.

0.5 seconds into a paroxysm. Interestingly, the degree of maximal impairment of reaction time was the same in paroxysms of both long and short duration. Thus paroxysmal S-W discharges represent true ictal activity, quantification of which enables a more objective assessment of seizure occurrence to be achieved. Long periods of EEG registration are again necessary if the inaccuracies of random recordings are to be avoided. This can be achieved using radio or cable telemetry (Porter, Wolf & Penry, 1971). Serial recordings can then be done to demonstrate a reduction in S-W activity in response to medication (Penry, Porter & Dreifuss 1971). Therapy should aim at controlling all S-W discharges and not just the longer paroxysms as even shorter duration bursts can impair consciousness. Cable telemetry is to be preferred as this provides 'cleaner' recordings. The disadvantages of both systems are their expense and that the subject has to be confined within a restricted area during recordings.

More recently it has become possible to monitor the EEG in freely moving subjects (Ives & Woods, 1975). This removes the restrictions imposed by telemetry and enables recordings to be done in the home environment. A system of automatic analysis is again required if the large quantities of EEG data are to be analysed rapidly. A technique for monitoring S-W activity using ambulatory taped EEG recordings and computerised analysis has been developed at the National Hospital for Nervous Diseases, Queen Square (Quy, Willison, Fitch & Gilliatt, 1980). The EEG is recorded using head mounted pre-amplifiers and a four channel cassette recorder (Oxford Medical Systems Medilog Recorder). The EEG recordings are replayed at sixty times real time with S-W activity being quantified by an analogue detection system. Arbitrary thresholds are pre-set for both spike and wave components independently so that the occurrence of a paroxysmal discharge will result in simultaneous opening of both spike and wave gates and detection by the computer. Spike and wave detector thresholds are set according to the individual morphology of the paroxysmal discharge relative to the background and to the amount and type of artefact. Once the detector thresholds have been determined a single 24 h tape can be analysed in 20 min. Bar charts of the amount of S-W activity over 24 h are automatically plotted by microcomputer and dot matrix printer. The result is a histogram showing the amount of S-W activity in 15 min epochs over 24 h (Figure 3). This provides both a numerical and graphical representation of S-W activity over a 24 h period. The site for electrode placement is determined from the resting EEG. Complete technical details are reported elsewhere (Quy, Fitch & Willison, 1980).

Preliminary experience indicates that the reliability of this system is variable and depends on the 'cleanness' of the recordings. The limitations of this technique are therefore similar to those encountered in automated inter-ictal spike detection *viz.* differentiation of true paroxysmal epileptiform activity from artefact. In addition, this system is useful only for those patients whose EEGs show well defined and frequent paroxysms of S-W activity on a relatively normal background. Movement artefact can be reduced using head mounted preamplifiers (Quy, 1978) but other types of artefact, particularly chewing artefact, can be more of a problem. The high amplitude electromyographic artefact from chewing can only be reduced by siting the electrodes away from the temporalis muscles. Whether or not this is feasible depends on how clearly defined the S-W paroxysms are at other sites. An alternative solution is not to use the ambulatory monitoring equipment during meals. Instead at meal times the patient can be positioned in front of a video play back unit linked to an EEG recording system. This will reduce considerably inaccuracies from chewing artefact but it will also require more expensive and sophisticated equipment and in some ways this detracts from the basic principles of ambulatory monitoring.

Reduction of S-W activity following appropriate therapy is the best indicator of a therapeutic response in patients with absence seizures. However, changes in total S-W activity over isolated 24 h periods can be misleading. Recordings done over several consecutive days in chronic institutionalised epileptic subjects with uncontrolled epilepsy indicate marked spontaneous fluctuations of S-W activity over 24 h periods (Milligan & Richens, unpublished results). Unless the drug administered is highly effective in reducing S-W paroxysms, any partial beneficial effect could well be masked by the variability of S-W activity in these subjects. As in the case of random 20 min EEG recordings, single 24 h recordings may not be sufficient to demonstrate a definitive improvement with medication. The problem of variability of S-W discharges complicates considerably the assessment of patients especially those that are relative non-responders and underlines the difficulty of drawing conclusions from studies using chronic institutionalised epileptic subjects.

It must be admitted, however, that the variability study referred to was conducted in a non-standardised environment. Ideally, drug studies in absence seizures should be conducted in a standard environment but these are difficult to design especially over long periods. Standardised structured activities are equally difficult to design and what is interesting to one patient may be boring to another. Confining subjects within a restricted area where they are allowed to do various activities (watching television, playing cards etc.) at different times and in differing sequence falls far short of the ideal standard environment. Certainly structured activities and behavioural changes do influence S-W paroxysms (Luborsky, Docherty, Todd, Knapp, Mirsky & Gottschalk, 1975; Sato, Penry & Dreifuss, 1976), but patients' interest and time spent in such activities vary from day to day as do television programmes. Whether S-W activity recorded under these conditions is representative of or significantly different from recordings done in the natural environment is unclear although any unstructured situation, characterised by boredom and lack of direction, tends to have a facilitatory effect on paroxysmal discharges.

One further problem in data analysis concerns the activity recorded during sleep. Most patients will have more epileptiform activity during the night than during the day. This consists largely of high amplitude, short duration spike and wave discharges which bear little morphological resemblance to diurnal paroxysmal activity. Such discharges are closely related to slow wave sleep with relative suppression during REM periods. Figure 3 clearly shows that nocturnal epileptic activity exhibits a cyclical pattern throughout the night. True ictal activity does not demonstrate such periodicity. Nocturnal discharges should therefore be regarded as inter-ictal. Furthermore, patients do not have absence seizures whilst asleep. It is for these reasons that the authors believe that activity recorded during sleep ought to be excluded from calculations of total S-W activity when using this system in assessing a clinical response to medication. This can easily be done by reference to the numerical computer print out which lists the number of seconds of S-W activity in each 15 minute epoch. Subtraction of nocturnal epileptic activity from the total gives the amount of diurnal S-W activity. It may not be possible to determine the exact onset of sleep from the computer print out in which case recordings or calculations should be made over a fixed number of hours of wakefulness.

Nocturnal epileptiform activity may not be entirely without value, however, in assessing response to medication. A proportion of patients with absence seizures have excessive and often prolonged fits on waking. Although the relationship of absence seizures to arousal is well recognised, the pathophysiology is quite unknown. Of the subjects who have absences on waking some show a characteristic pattern distribution of nocturnal epileptic activity with cyclical augmentation, attenuation and augmentation of S-W discharges throughout the night in relation to slow wave sleep. If the final augmentation of S-W discharges occurs just before arousal it is often continued into wakefulness and manifests itself clinically (Kellerway, Frost & Crawley, 1980).

Alteration of the time modulation of nocturnal epileptic discharges may protect those patients prone to frequent seizures on waking. It seems logical to suggest that timing of medication may be important here and perhaps the patients at risk ought to receive the bulk, if not all, of their tablets at bedtime. Although the actual amount of nocturnal epileptiform activity may not be significantly reduced by such regimes (Rowan et al., 1978) it is perhaps the alteration in pattern distribution which is more important than the total number of seconds. Clinicians often prescribe medication to slot in with the fit distribution in certain individual patients. A clinical improvement is very gratifying although the reasons for this may be far from clear. Study of the time modulation of S-W discharges and its alteration by drugs may provide an explanation.

A further advantage of the ambulatory monitoring equipment is that it allows detailed study of individual patients. Using a simple trial design, a single subject prone to frequent and prolonged absences has been studied during fits. He is electively connected to the monitoring equipment whilst well and he wears it continually, though not operating, until an absence 'series' occurs. The tape recorder can then be started and treatment given, in this case either diazepam or a placebo administered rectally. An automatic recognition system is not required as for such a short study the tape can be played out on paper and the S-W paroxysms counted by eye. This increases the accuracy of the results. Preliminary observations indicate that diazepam administered rectally is highly effective in terminating an absence series as judged by disappearance of S-W activity (Milligan & Richens, unpublished results). The disadvantages of this technique are that the equipment is inoperative during the waiting period and that serial absence seizures are extremely uncommon in the general epileptic population.

Photosensitivity

Photosensitivity is defined as an abnormal electro-encephalographic or clinical response to light. The relationships between photosensitivity and epilepsy have been investigated since the 1940s and stroboscopic stimulation is now widely used in routine EEG practice to uncover potential epileptiform abnormalities. Photosensitive patients are typically young females often with a family history of photosensitivity or epilepsy. In general, the relatively young age of patients with photosensitivity may act as an obstacle to the assessement of new drugs, particularly those still under preliminary evaluation. The discovery of the Senegalese baboon *Papio papio* has provided research workers with an animal model on which to study photosensitivity. A wide variety of agents have been administered to *Papio papio* to explore the neuropharmacological mechanisms of photosensitivity. These include neurotransmitters, neurotransmitter blocking agents, neurotransmitter agonists and antagonists (Newmark & Penry, 1979). Several of these agents have been found to have a profound effect on photosensitivity although a specific biochemical abnormality has not been demonstrated. Many antiepileptic drugs have also been tested in *Papio papio* and thorough reviews are available (Killam, Matsuzaki & Killam, 1973; Meldrum, Anlezark, Balzamo, Horton & Trimble, 1975). Most antiepileptic drugs block or reduce the clinical response to photic stimulation in over 75% of animals. Phenytoin, however, is effective only in chronic doses. Most studies include mild myoclonus as a clinical measure in addition to generalised tonic-clonic convulsions. This is in contrast to the human model where responses are based essentially on specific changes in the EEG. Direct comparisons between animal and human studies are therefore difficult as different phenomena are being compared. Several authors have also noted variability in the photosensitivity of *Papio papio* which can further complicate interpretation of results. Daily, weekly and other cyclical fluctuations may appear despite standardised testing conditions (Killam, Killam & Naquet, 1967; Wada, Terao & Booker, 1972). The differing responses and variability of photosensitivity together with their expense and somewhat irascible nature makes *Papio papio* less suitable for study than the human model.

In clinical practice photosensitivity is assessed by demonstrating a photoconvulsive response (PCR) to intermittent photic stimulation (IPS). Studies show that abnormal photic responses occur in patients with a wide variety of seizure disorders. The most frequently accompanying seizure disorders in adults are of the generalised type, either generalised tonic-clonic or absence seizures. Among children the PCR is associated with a much wider variety of seizures and no seizure type predominates (Newmark & Penry, 1979). In contrast to animal studies, most antiepileptic drugs have little effect on abnormalities induced by IPS. Ethosuximide reduces the response in approximately 50% of cases. Sodium valproate is more effective, though it is often necessary to give a relatively large dose to abolish the PCR completely. In a comprehensive study, Harding, Herrick & Jeavons (1978) demonstrated complete control or significant improvement (greater than 78% reduction) of photosensitivity in 78% of subjects taking sodium valproate.

Markedly photosensitive patients are usually sensitive to light within clearly defined limits of flash frequency (sensitivity limits). The lower sensitivity limit (i.e. the lowest flash frequency which consistently evokes a PCR) is more reliable and reproducible as photic stimulators tend to produce subharmonic modulations at higher frequencies (Jeavons & Hard-

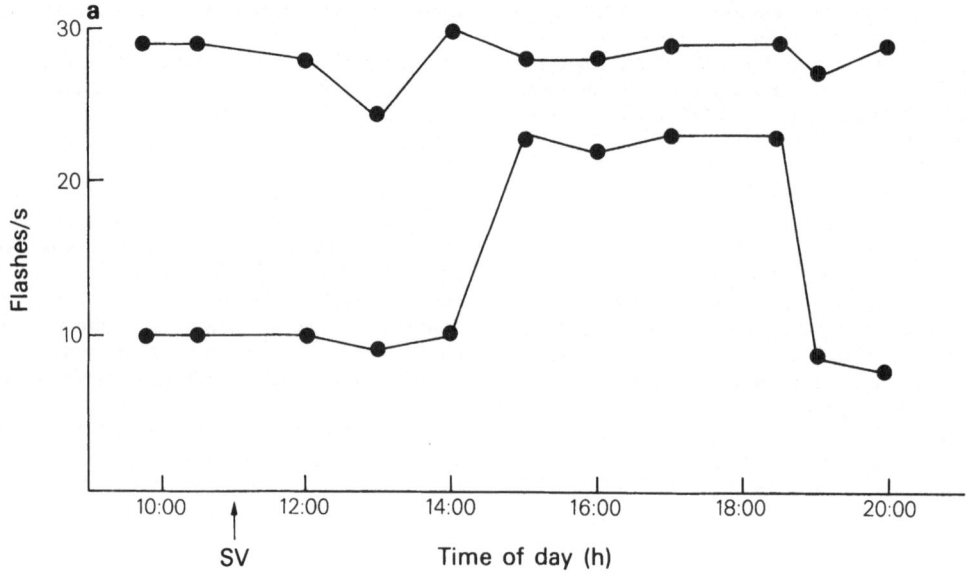

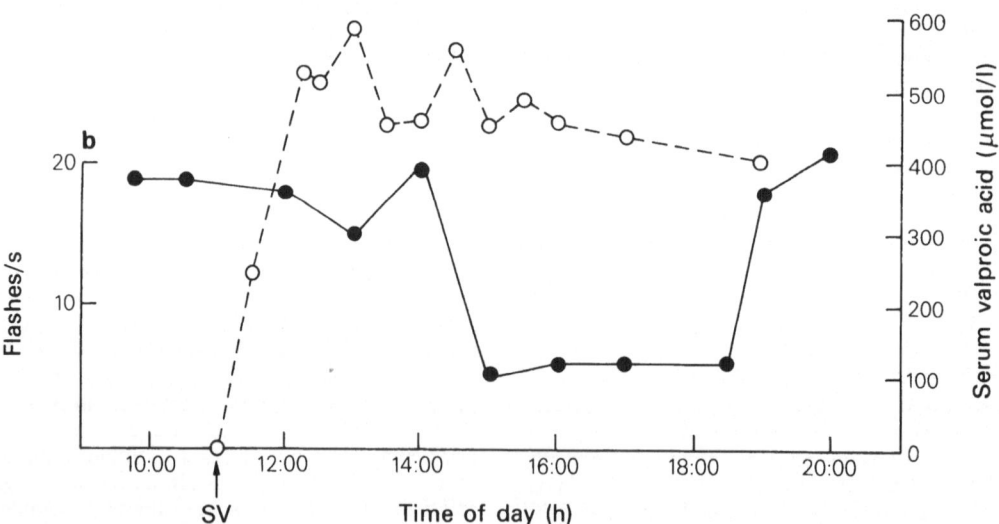

Figure 4 (a) Effect of a single oral dose of 600 mg of sodium valproate on the upper and lower limits of photosensitivity (sensitivity limits). The drug, sodium valproate (SV), was administered at 11.00 h. A photoconvulsive response was seen between the threshold limits (indicated in flashes/s). There is elevation of the lower sensitivity limit following sodium valproate administration, and the sensitivity range (i.e. the difference between the upper and lower sensitivity limits) is narrowed.

(b) Sensitivity range depicted as a single curve (●—●) with serum levels of valproic acid (O···O). Depression of the sensitivity range persists for 4.5 h but does not occur until 3 h after administration of the drug and 1 h after peak serum concentration is reached.

ing, 1975). Imperfect equipment can thus produce a falsely high upper sensitivity limit of 60 flashes/s when the actual value is 30 flashes/s. The sensitivity range, obtained by subtracting the lower from the upper sensitivity limit, can be used as a measure of photosensitivity, high values indicating more marked sensitivity than low values. Figure 4 shows the effect of a single dose of sodium valproate on the PCR of a patient with marked sensitivity to IPS. There is depression of the sensitivity range which does not begin until 3 h after administration of sodium valproate and 1 h after the peak serum concentration (Figure 4b). The effect persists for 4.5 h and in this case is due to elevation of the lower sensitivity limit (Figure 4a). Depression of the sensitivity range may be more prolonged and occasionally persists after the drug is no longer detectable in the serum. These changes are most evident in valproate naive patients but they do not disappear entirely in those on chronic therapy (Rowan *et al.*, 1979). Furthermore, improvement in the upper sensitivity limit can be maintained for 3 months after withdrawal of chronic medication (Harding *et al.*, 1978).

In studies of this kind it is vital to have a clear understanding of what constitutes a PCR. Generalised spike or polyspike and wave discharges are regarded by most as significantly abnormal responses. Bursts of bilateral high amplitude slow waves without spikes have also been considered abnormal by some (Reilley & Peters, 1973) but these are not universally accepted. Other responses to IPS such as occipital spikes and exaggerated visual evoked potentials should not be misinterpreted for a PCR. Some subjects show a diurnal variation in their sensitivity to IPS with a spontaneous reduction of the sensitivity range in the latter half of the day. It is therefore wise to precede the drug day with a control day if false positive results are to be avoided (Rowan *et al.*, 1979).

The results of photic stimulation strongly depend on the method of testing. Important variables include light intensity, flash frequency, flash duration, colour and size of visual pattern. The importance of these variables and the numerous methods of photic stimulation are reviewed elsewhere (Jeavons & Harding, 1975). Much of the published literature on photosensitivity fails to mention these variables in their methodology. Unless methodological detail is reported in published work, direct comparisons between studies will be difficult. Furthermore, the wide discrepancies between studies often reflects differing definitions of the PCR. Attention to these basic principles is of paramount importance if maximum value is to be derived from the study of photosensitivity. Whether depression of the sensitivity range by sodium valproate can act as an index of therapeutic response in differing seizure types is at present unknown although in general absences show a favourable response to this drug. The technique

provides a quick method of assessing one aspect of the potential antiepileptic effect of a new drug. As the PCR is altered during sleep, being reduced during REM periods and often abolished completely during slow wave sleep (Yamamoto, Furaya, Wakamatsu & Hishikawa, 1971), this method may not be suitable for drugs with marked sedating properties.

The visual evoked response

Study of the visual evoked response (VER) aids considerably the assessment of patients with neuro-ophthalmological disorders. Many conditions affecting the visual pathways will alter the VER and this has been of particular value in demonstrating subclinical demyelinating lesions in early cases of multiple sclerosis. The latency and amplitude of individual response peaks are commonly used parameters. Analysis of the VER in clinical practice is well documented (Halliday & Mushin, 1980) but little work has been done in man on the effect of drugs on the VER.

Analysis of the VER in epilepsy has been controversial and many of the discrepancies are due to differences in technique, terminology and patient populations. The VER in epileptic patients is more variable than normals and most authors report short latencies and increased amplitude of several components. Both normal and seizure populations show marked interindividual variability of the VER, though this is more evident in seizure groups. Patients who have paroxysmal discharges in their resting EEG tend to have a more variable VER than patients who do not. There is no correlation, however, between alterations in the VER and other changes in the EEG; nor is there any typical abnormality for any one group of patients (Lücking, Creutzfeldt & Heinemann, 1970).

A possible exception are patients with photic induced seizures. This group of epileptic patients frequently have increased amplitude and/or reduced latency of several wave forms. Lee, Messenheimer, Wilkinson, Brickley & Johnson (1980) examined specifically change in the VER of photosensitive patients before and after medication and compared the differences to a normal control group. The most striking differences were changes in the morphology of the VER. Normal subjects have a very low amplitude wave immediately following the end of the stimulus. This is in contrast to untreated photosensitive patients whose responses during the immediate post stimulus period remain of high amplitude often with large slow waves. Following treatment with sodium valproate the initial peaks return to normal in configuration and latency and the late responses after the end of the stimulus are much less pronounced. The latencies to various peaks, however, are not significantly different from patients on no medication.

Such studies, interesting though they are, have little relevance to the clinical effect of an antiepileptic drug. There is no information to indicate whether alteration of the VER is indicative of an improvement in seizure control. As the VER shows marked inter-individual variation and is relatively non-specific in most epileptic groups, its usefulness as an indicator of therapeutic response would seem very limited.

Conclusions

In summary, the methods available for the assessment of antiepileptic drugs are either clinical or electroencephalographic. Each has distinct advantages and disadvantages. However, there is at present no quick and wholly reliable method for the assessment of antiepileptic drugs in man. The protracted double-blind cross-over study using fit frequency is still the foundation for the evaluation of new compounds. Other models are open to major criticisms as they are often not directly related to clinical epilepsy.

Paroxysmal S-W activity in absence seizures is an exception. The foremost problem here is accuracy of rapid data analysis and the solution to this lies in the field of the scientist as it is he who will devise improved automatic recognition systems.

Photosensitivity and its influence by drugs is a relatively new area for exploration. A study of sodium valproate in patients selected on the basis of depression of their sensitivity range would be both exciting and potentially very informative. Whilst this may further identify those groups of patients likely to benefit from this drug it may also provide a useful yardstick against which new compounds could be measured.

Changes in the VER following medication indicate a cerebral effect of a drug but in view of the lack of correlation between the VER and clinical epilepsy the value of these data is unknown. As further work is likely to continue, standardisation of both terminology and methods would do much to clarify this rapidly expanding field.

References

AHMAD. S., PERUCCA, E. & RICHENS. A. (1977). The effect of frusemide, mexiletine, (+) propranolol and three benzodiazepine drugs on interictal spike discharges in the electroencephalogram of epileptic patients. *Br. J. clin. Pharmac.*, **4**, 683–688.

ALTMAN, D.G. (1980). Statistics and ethics in medical research. *Br. med. J.*, **281**, 1336–1338.

AMBROZ, A., CHALMERS, T.C., SMITH, H., SCHROEDER, B., FRIEMAN, J.A. & SHARECK, E.P. (1978). Deficiencies of randomised controlled trials. *Clin. Res.*, **26**, 280 A.

BANCOUD, J., RIBET, M.F. & CHAGOT, D. (1975). Comparison between discharges of subclinical spikes and clinical epileptic attacks in patients with epilepsy. *Electroencephalogr. clin. Neurophysiol.*, Soc. Proc. 39, 554.

BINNIE, C.D. (1980). The use of the EEG in the diagnosis of the epilepsies. *J. Electrophysiol. Technol.*, **6**, 59–74.

BIRKET-SMITH, E., LUND, M., MIKKELSEN, B., VESTER-MARK. S., ZANDER-OLSEN. P. & HULM. P. (1973). A controlled trial of Ro 5-4023 (clonazepam) in the treatment of psychomotor epilepsy. *Acta neurol. Scand.*, **49**, Suppl. 53, 18–25.

BROWNE, T.R. & PENRY, J.K. (1973). Benzodiazepines in the treatment of epilepsy: A review. *Epilepsia*, **14**, 277–310.

BROWNE, T.R., PENRY, J.K., PORTER, R.J. & DREIFUSS, F.E. (1974). Responsiveness before, during and after spike-wave paroxysms. *Neurology (Minneap.)*, **7**, 659–665.

BULPITT, C.J. (1975). The design of clinical trials. *Br. J. Hosp. Med.*, **13**, 611–620.

CARRIE, J.R.G. (1976). Computer assisted EEG sharp—transient detection and quantification during overnight recordings in an epileptic patient. In *Quantitative Analytic Studies in Epilepsy*, eds Kellerway, P. & Petersen, I. New York: Raven Press.

CEREGHINO, J.J., BROCK, J., VAN METER, J., PENRY, J.K., SMITH, L. & WHITE, B. (1974). Carbamazepine for epilepsy. A controlled prospective evaluation. *Neurology (Minneap.)*, **24**, 401–410.

CEREGHINO, J.J. & PENRY, J.K. (1972). General principles: testing of anticonvulsants in man. In *Antiepileptic Drugs*, eds Woodbury, D.M., Penry, J.K. & Schmidt, R.P., pp. 63–73. New York: Raven Press.

CEREGHINO, J.J., VAN METER, J., BROCK, J.T., PENRY, J.K., SMITH, L. & WHITE, B.G. (1973). Preliminary observations of serum carbamazepine concentration in epileptic patients. *Neurology (Minneap.)*, **23**, 357–366.

COVANIS, A. & JEAVONS, P.M. (1980). Once-daily sodium valproate in the treatment of epilepsy. *Dev. Med. Child Neurol.*, **22**, 202–204.

GASTAUT, H. (1969). Classification of the epilepsies. Proposal for an international classification. *Epilepsia*, **10**, Suppl. 514–521.

GIBBS, F.A., DAVIS, H. & LENNOX, W.G. (1935). The electroencephalogram in epilepsy and in conditions of impaired consciousness. *Arch. Neurol. Psychiatr.*, **34**, 1133–1148.

GOODE, D.J., PENRY, J.K. & DREIFUSS, F.E. (1970). Effects on paroxysmal spike-wave activity on continuous visual-motor performance. *Epilepsia*, **11**, 241–254.

GOTMAN, J., IVES, J.R. & GLOOR, P. (1979). Automatic recognition of inter-ictal epileptic activity in prolonged EEG recordings. *Electroencephalogr. clin. Neurophysiol.*, **46**, 510–520.

GRAM, L., FLACHS, H., WÜRTZ-JORGENSEN, A., PARNAS, J. & ANDERSEN, B. (1979). Sodium valproate, serum level and clinical effect in epilepsy: a controlled study. *Epilepsia*, **20**, 303–312.

GRANT, R.H.E. & BAROT, N.H. (1976). The use of sodium valproate in severely handicapped patients with epilepsy. In *Clinical and Pharmacological Aspects of Sodium Valproate (Epilim) in the Treatment of Epilepsy*, ed. Legg, N.J. pp. 14–22. Tunbridge Wells: MCS Consultants.

GREEN, J.R. & KUPFERBERG, H.J. (1972). Sulthiame. In *Antiepileptic Drugs*, eds Woodbury, D.M., Penry, J.K. & Schmidt, R.P., pp. 477–485. New York: Raven Press.

HALLIDAY, A.M. & MUSHIN, J. (1980). The visual evoked potential in neuro-ophthalmology. *International Ophthalmology Clinics*, **20**, 155–183. Massachusetts: Little, Brown and Company.

HARDING, G.F.A., HERRICK, C.E. & JEAVONS, P.M. (1978). A controlled study of the effect of sodium valproate on photosensitive epilepsy and its prognosis. *Epilepsia*, **19**, 555–565.

HOUGHTON, G.W. & RICHENS, A. (1974a). Inhibition of phenytoin metabolism by sulthiame in epileptic patients. *Br. J. clin. Pharmac.*, **1**, 59–66.

HOUGHTON, G.W. & RICHENS, A. (1974b). Phenytoin intoxication induced by sulthiame in epileptic patients. *J. Neurol. Neurosurg. Psychiat.*, **37**, 275–281.

ILAE COMMISSION ON ANTIEPILEPTIC DRUGS (1973). Principles for clinical testing of antiepileptic drugs. *Epilepsia*, **14**, 451–458.

IVES, J.R. & WOODS, J.F. (1975). 4-channel 24 hour cassette recorder for long term monitoring of ambulatory patients. *Electroencephalogr. clin. Neurophysiol.* **39**, 88–92.

JEAVONS, P.M. & CLARK, J.E. (1974). Sodium valproate in treatment of epilepsy. *Br. med. J.*, **2**, 584–586.

JEAVONS, P.M., CLARK, J.E. & MAHESHWARI, P. (1977). Treatment of generalised epilepsies of childhood and adolescence with sodium valproate (Epilim). *Dev. Med. Child Neurol.*, **19**, 9–25.

JEAVONS, P.M. & HARDING, G.F.A. (1975). *Photosensitive Epilepsy. A Review of the Literature and a study of 460 Patients*. William Heinemann Books.

KELLERWAY, P., FROST, J.D. Jr. & CRAWLEY, J.W. (1980). Time modulation of spike and wave activity in generalised epilepsy. *Ann. Neurol.*, **8**, 491–500.

KILLAM, K.F., KILLAM, E.K. & NAQUET, R. (1967). An animal model of light sensitive epilepsy. *Electroencephalogr. clin. Neurophysiol.*, **22**, 497–513.

KILLAM, E.K., MATSUZAKI, M. & KILLAM, K.F. (1973). Studies of anticonvulsant compounds in the *Papio papio* model of epilepsy. In *Brain Function*, ed. Sebelli, H.C., pp. 161–171. New York: Raven Press.

LEE, S.I., MESSENHEIMER, J.A., WILKINSON, E.C., BRICKLEY, J.J. Jr. & JOHNSON, R.N. (1980). Visual evoked potentials to stimulus trains: normative data and application to photosensitive seizures. *Electroencephalogr. clin. Neurophysiol.*, **48**, 387–394.

LEVY, R., PITLICK, W., TROUPIN, A., GREEN, J. & NEAL, J. (1975). Pharmacokinetics of carbamazepine in normal man. *Clin. Pharmac. Ther.*, **17**, 657–668.

LUBORSKY, L., DOCHERTY, J.P., TODD, T.C., KNAPP, P.H., MIRSKY, A.F. & GOTTSCHALK, L.A. (1975). A context of analysis of psychological states prior to petit mal EEG paroxysms. *J. Nervous Mental Dis.*, **160**, 282–298.

LÜCKING, C.H., CREUTZFELDT, O.D. & HEINEMANN, U. (1970). Visual evoked potentials of patients with epilepsy and a control group. *Electroencephalogr. clin. Neurophysiol.*, **29**, 557–566.

MARSDEN, C.D. (1975). Neurology. In *A Textbook of Epilepsy*, eds Laidlaw, J. & Richens, A. London and Edinburgh: Churchill Livingstone.

MELDRUM, B.S., ANLEZARK, G., BALZAMO, E., HORTON, R.W. & TRIMBLE, M. (1975). Photically induced epilepsy in *Papio papio* as a model for drug studies. In *Advances in Neurology*, **10**, eds Meldrum, B.S. & Marsden, C.D., pp. 119–132. New York: Raven Press.

NEWMARK, M.E. & PENRY, J.K. (1979). *Photosensitivity and Epilepsy: A Review*. New York: Raven Press.

PATEL, I.H., LEVY, R.H. & CUTLER, R.E. (1980). Phenobarbital—valproic acid interaction. *Clin. Pharmac. Ther.*, **27**, 515.

PENRY, J.K., PORTER, R.J. & DREIFUSS, F.E. (1971). Quantitation of paroxysmal abnormal discharges in the EEGs of patients with absence (petit-mal) seizures for the evaluation of antiepileptic drugs. *Epilepsia*, **12**, 278–279.

PORTER, R.J., PENRY, J.K. & DREIFUSS, F.E. (1973). Responsiveness at the onset of spike-wave bursts. *Electroencephalogr. clin. Neurophysiol.*, **34**, 239–245.

PORTER, R.J., WOLF, A.A. Jr. & PENRY, J.K. (1971). Human electroencephalographic telemetry. A review of systems and their applications and a new receiving system. *Am. J. EEG. Technol.*, **11**, 145–159.

QUY, R.J. (1978). A miniature preamplifier for ambulatory monitoring of the electroencephalogram. *J. Physiol. (Lond.)*, **284**, 23–24.

QUY, R.J., FITCH, P. & WILLISON, R.G. (1980). High speed automatic analysis of EEG spike and wave activity using an analogue detection and microcomputer plotting system. *Electroencephalogr. clin. Neurophysiol.*, **49**, 187–189.

QUY, R.J., WILLISON, R.G., FITCH, P. & GILLIATT, R.W. (1980). Some developments in ambulatory monitoring of the EEG. In *ISAM 1979: Proceedings of the Third International Symposium on Ambulatory Monitoring*, eds Stott, F.D., Raftery, E.B., Sleight, P. & Goulding, L. pp. 393–398. London: Academic Press.

REILLEY, E.L. & PETERS, J.F. (1973). Relationship of some varieties of electroencephalographic photosensitivity to clinical convulsive disorders. *Neurology (Minneap.)*, **23**, 1050–1057.

RICHENS, A. (1975). Clinical pharmacology and medical treatment. In *A Textbook of Epilepsy*, eds Laidlaw, J. & Richens, A. London and Edinburgh: Churchill Livingstone.

RICHENS, A. (1976). *Drug Treatment of Epilepsy*. London: Henry Kimpton.

RICHENS, A. & AHMAD, S. (1975). A controlled trial of sodium valproate in severe major epilepsy. *Br. med. J.*, **4**, 255–256.

RODIN, E., RIM, C. & RENNICK, P. (1974). The effects of

152

carbamazepine on patients with psychomotor epilepsy: Results of a double-blind study. *Epilepsia,* **15**, 547–561.

ROWAN, A.J., BINNIE, C.D., de BEER-PAWLIKOWSKI, N.K.B., GOEDHART, D.M., GUTTER, T.L., VAN PARIJS, J.A.P., MEINARDI, H. & MEIJER, J.W.A. (1978). 24 hour EEG studies with very frequent antiepileptic drug concentration determinations in the study of sodium valproate. In *Advances in Epileptology 1977,* eds Meinardi, H. & Rowan, A.J. Amsterdam and Lisse: Swets and Zeitlinger.

ROWAN, A.J., BINNIE, C.D., WARFIELD, C.A., MEINARDI, H. & MEIJER, J.W.A. (1979). The delayed effect of sodium valproate on the photoconvulsive response in man. *Epilepsia,* **20**, 61–68.

ROWAN, A.J., PIPPENGER, C.E., McGREGOR, P.A. & FRENCH, J. (1975). Seizure activity and anticonvulsant drug concentration. *Arch. Neurol.,* **32**, 281–288.

SATO, S., PENRY, J.K. & DREIFUSS, F.E. (1976). Electroencephalographic monitoring of generalised spike-wave paroxysms in the hospital and at home. In *Quantitative Analytic Studies in Epilepsy,* eds Kellerway, P. & Petersen, I., pp. 237–251. New York: Raven Press.

SHORVON, S.D., CHADWICK, D., GALBRAITH, A.W. & REYNOLDS, E.H. (1978). One drug for epilepsy. *Br. med. J.,* **1**, 474–476.

WADA, J.A., TERAO, A. & BOOKER, H.E. (1972). Longitudinal correlative analysis of epileptic baboon, *Papio papio. Neurology (Minneap.),* **22**, 1272–1285.

WHITE, P.T., PLOTT, D. & NORTON, J. (1966). Relative anticonvulant potency of primidone. A double-blind comparison. *Arch. Neurol. (Chic.),* **14**, 31–35.

WILKUS, R.J. & DODRILL, C.B. (1976). Neuropsychological correlates of the electroencephalogram in epileptics: 1, topographic distribution. *Epilepsia,* **17**, 89–100.

WILKUS, R.J., DODRILL, C.B. & TROUPIN, A.S. (1978). Carbamazepine and the electroencephalogram of epileptics: a double-blind study in comparison to phenytoin. *Epilepsia,* **19**, 283–291.

YAMAMOTO, J., FURAYA, E., WAKAMATSU, H. & HISHIKAWA, Y. (1971). Modification of photosensitivity in epileptics during sleep. *Electroencephalogr. clin. Neurophysiol.,* **31**, 509–513.

CLINICAL ASSESSMENT OF NEUROMUSCULAR TRANSMISSION

J.P. PAYNE

Research Department of Anaesthetics, Royal
College of Surgeons of England, London WC2,
St Peter's Hospitals, London WC2 and the
London Hospital, London E1

R. HUGHES*

Research Department of Anaesthetics, Royal
College of Surgeons of England, London WC2
and St Peter's Hospitals, London WC2

Introduction

The concept of neuromuscular transmission as a separate physiological entity was introduced by Claude Bernard in 1851 when he demonstrated by means of curare that the junction between nerve endings and muscle fibres possessed unique properties. The logic and simplicity of Bernard's experiments have not been surpassed by more modern methods and they still offer a convenient and relatively inexpensive means of screening new drugs with a possible action at the neuromuscular junction. Bernard's studies with curare focused attention on its peripheral actions and its therapeutic possibilities were soon recognised. By 1858 the drug had already been used in the management of tetanus and shortly thereafter albeit with less justification it had been employed in the treatment of a variety of diseases including chorea, epilepsy and hydrophobia.

Curare continued to be used intermittently throughout the remainder of the 19th century and beyond without any proper understanding of its action and without any real evidence of beneficial effect. However where it was used to advantage was in the developing sciences of physiology and pharmacology where the use of such pharmacological techniques as had been described by Bernard had become an essential component in the interpretation of physiological phenomena. None were more adept in the exploitation of these techniques than Henry Dale and his colleagues but it was 1934 before the first definitive evidence was published that established the chemical transmitter acetylcholine as the physiological link between the nerve-endings and the muscle fibres (Dale & Feldberg, 1934; Dale, Feldberg & Vogt, 1936).

Subsequently in a series of well planned experiments Dale and his group succeeded in defining the

*Present address: Pharmacology Department, The Wellcome Research Laboratories, Langley Court, Beckenham, Kent BR3 3BS

pattern of neuromuscular transmission and in so doing laid the foundations for the development of a new pharmacological approach to the management of anaesthesia for thoracic and abdominal surgery.

Mechanism of neuromuscular transmission

Understanding has been helped by the application of modern technology which has enabled the individual constituents of the neuromuscular junction to be identified so that its anatomical structure is now well demarcated. Essentially, when a motor nerve reaches the muscle it supplies, it divides into a series of myelinated axons which in turn break down into branches to supply groups of from 5 to 300 muscle fibres. These branches lose their myelin sheath as they approach the muscle and further sub-divide into fine terminals which end in close approximation to highly localised and specialised areas of the muscle membrane arranged in discrete folds to form the post-synaptic membrane. But even at this stage there is no direct contact between nerve and muscle; they are separated not only by the pre-synaptic membrane which encloses the nerve ending and the post-synaptic muscle membrane but also by a distinct extracellular gap which itself is partitioned by a basement membrane.

The physiological pattern of events at the neuromuscular junction can now be described. The chemical transmitter acetylcholine is formed and stored in the nerve terminal by the action of the enzyme choline acetyltransferase on the simple ammonium quaternary base choline. Storage of acetylcholine occurs as discrete packages or quanta and up to 200,000 such quanta may be accumulated, enough to react to several thousand impulses although only a small fraction of that number is immediately available to respond to individual impulses. The amount of acetylcholine released during repeated nerve stimulation is determined by a series of factors including the quantity present at the time of stimulation, the extent of previous activity and the concentration of calcium ions. The rate at which acetylcholine can continue to be released reflects the balance between the extent to which it can be mobilised from the main stores and the speed at which it is utilised. Once released acetylcholine diffuses across the extracellular gap to occupy the receptor areas on the post-synaptic muscle membrane. The process of occupation stimulates an electrical change and the resting potential of the end-plate becomes less negative. If the electrical change is great enough a critical threshold is reached and an action potential is produced on the surface of the adjacent muscle membrane. This in turn provokes a muscle contraction the strength of which is related to the number of motor units stimulated.

A distinction needs to be made between the mechanism responsible for the end-plate potential and that which brings about the action potential. The end-plate potential is caused by the occupation of the specific receptors by acetylcholine and is not propagated. The action potential is elicited by the increase in membrane permeability provoked by the end-plate potential. The change in membrane permeability results in a rapid movement of sodium into the cell across the cell membrane and a subsequent loss of potassium. Normally a negative potential of around 70 mV is maintained within a resting cell relative to that on the external surface of the membrane by the active exclusion of sodium ions. When this mechanism is disturbed by the action of acetylcholine on the end-plate the shift in ionic balance causes the membrane potential within the cell to fall to zero and then to overshoot so that the interior of the cell becomes positive. This electrical change propagated from cell to cell and described as the depolarisation process produces the muscle contraction. Repolarisation must occur before the muscle can contract again.

Thus neuromuscular transmission will be interrupted if the synthesis of acetylcholine is disturbed, if it fails to be released at the nerve terminals, if that which is released is prevented from occupying the receptors interposed between the nerve endings and the muscle fibres or if the muscle membrane in immediate proximity to the motor end-plate is unable to regain its excitability. In practice block of neuromuscular transmission is achieved with two groups of drugs; the first competes with acetylcholine for access to the motor end-plate and the second produces a persistent depolarisation so that the muscle membrane becomes electrically inexcitable.

Initially the investigation of neuromuscular blocking drugs attracted little interest, despite the enthusiasm of clinicians like Ranyard West (1932) who attempted a quantitative assessment of curare for the treatment of spasticity in neurogenic disease and A.E. Bennett (1941) who used the drug to prevent the traumatic complications of shock therapy in psychiatry. It was not until Griffith and Johnson (1942) used curare as a skeletal muscle relaxant for major abdominal surgery that its place in medicine became established. Its use in surgery was a major step forward; not only did it revolutionise anaesthetic practice by removing the need for deep anaesthesia it also stimulated a new interest in neuromuscular transmission as pharmacologists realised the possibilities of this clinical development.

Quantitative assessment of muscular function

Ranyard West's (1932) assessment of curare was probably the first quantitative evaluation of neuromuscular function in man and was based on a device designed for measuring the force required to extend the leg at the knee joint. The apparatus was designed to be used on a sedentary patient and consisted of two flat boards of suitable dimensions. The first was applied to the anterior aspect of the thigh so that it projected beyond the knee joint at which point the second board was hinged and suspended along the anterior surface of the leg. The degree of extension, which was provided by a spring balance attached to the ankle, was assessed before and after the injection of curare by measuring the force required to produce the extension determined by the angle between the boards.

Such a technique though useful in the assessment of spastic states was scarcely applicable to normal healthy volunteers so that when Paton & Zaimis (1948) introduced decamethonium as a depolarising neuromuscular blocking agent suitable for clinical use the effects of the drug were studied on ventilation and on muscle tone (Organe, Paton & Zaimis, 1949).

A similar approach was adopted by Mushin and his colleagues in the first clinical trial of gallamine (Flaxedil) undertaken in the United Kingdom (Mushin, Wien, Mason & Langston, 1949) but neither group described their techniques in detail. Both these studies attempted to relate muscular power to respiratory effort. Organe and his colleagues compared the effect of the drug on vital capacity with that on hand-grip strength, leg-raising ability and abdominal muscle tone, while Mushin's group compared activity with minute ventilation.

On the basis of preliminary experiments Mushin and his colleagues concluded that in conscious volunteers the contracting power of muscles was best measured by mechanical devices. In the case of the hand muscles a dynamometer was used with a pointer which moved over a scale graduated appropriately. For measuring the ability of the rectus muscles to contract a spring-loaded pad was adjusted in position on the abdomen with the volunteer supine and the knees firmly strapped down. When leg-raising was attempted the recti became taut and the pad was displaced upwards against the spring which in turn moved a pointer over a scale.

These relatively simple techniques have the advantages that they are easy to use, they can be adapted to suit different circumstances and the equipment can be improvised from readily available appliances. For example, Bodman (1952) assessed hand-grip strength by the ability of a volunteer to compress a rubber bulb filled with water and connected to a mercury manometer. Because of the relative incompressibility of water a single compression of the bulb was sufficient to raise the mercury column to produce a reading. The main problem was that intervals of two minutes between compressions were needed to avoid fatigue.

The general disadvantage of such techniques is that they depend on voluntary effort so that the subjects need to be conscious with the corresponding problems associated with such factors as adrenaline release and carbon dioxide retention. In addition the results can only be interpreted as indicating a trend rather than providing fully quantitative data. Nevertheless the use of these techniques did demonstrate the relative resistance of the respiratory muscles to neuromuscular block and made it possible to identify different degrees of muscle sensitivity to the blocking drugs.

Since the respiratory effects are of paramount importance in the assessment of neuromuscular blocking drugs it is not surprising that the measurement of such effects was a prominent feature of the early studies and certainly in anaesthetic practice alterations in pulmonary ventilation were regarded as the most satisfactory index of change in the degree of neuromuscular block (Brennan, 1956). However the distinction needs to be made between techniques suitable for conscious volunteers and those that can be used in anaesthetised patients.

Tests of respiratory function such as the determination of forced expiratory volumes and vital capacity demand the active co-operation of the subject and are therefore suitable only for use with conscious volunteers. In most instances investigators have endeavoured to study a range of variables one of which could be used as the end-point. In one such study, by Johansen, Jorgensen & Molbech (1964) the experiments involved the measurement of four separate functions; head-lift and hand-grip were compared to either maximal inspiratory and expiratory flows or to maximal inspiratory and expiratory pressures. The degree of depression of respiratory muscle power and hand-grip strength was determined when the ability to raise the head was nearly or completely abolished by tubocurarine. In these experiments the strength of head-lift was measured by means of a strap placed around the forehead attached to a strain-gauge dynamometer and registered by an automatic measuring bridge. The hand-grip strength was also determined by a hand dynamometer and recorded in the same way as the head-lift. Maximal inspiratory and expiratory flows were measured on a direct reading gas flowmeter. Maximal inspiratory pressure after maximal expiration and maximal expiratory pressure after maximal inspiration were measured on a simple mercury manometer. The weakness of this approach is that volunteers have to be trained before performing the respiratory function tests if reliable results are to be obtained.

Such techniques are manifestly unsatisfactory in anaesthetised patients and most studies in this field have been restricted to an analysis of the changing respiratory pattern in response to neuromuscular blocking drugs. In one of the earliest studies by Brennan (1956) the reservoir bag of a standard Boyles' anaesthetic machine was inserted through the neck of a sealed aspirating bottle which was connected by widebore tubing to a Benedict-Roth recording spirometer. A continuous record was obtained from which could be derived the respiratory rate and the tidal and minute volumes as required. An alternative method is to substitute the recording spirometer for the rebreathing bag in a closed circle anaesthetic system.

Such methods have the disadvantage that the evidence of neuromuscular block can only be presumptive on the basis of a developing muscle weakness and that a quantitative assessment of the failure of neuromuscular transmission is virtually impossible. It was for these reasons that more precise and more specific methods of measuring interference with neuromuscular transmission were developed. Currently the most widely used method for assessing neuromuscular blockade in man depends on the measurement of the force of skeletal muscle indirectly evoked by the stimulation of the associated motor nerve.

Quantitative assessment of neuromuscular transmission

Single twitch response

The first detailed account of such a method suitable for the accurate assessment of neuromuscular blocking drugs in man was published by Mapleson & Mushin in 1955. The method was based on that described by Bigland & Lippold (1954) for the determination of the tension developed in the small muscles of the thumb supplied by the ulnar nerve when square wave pulses were applied to the nerve at different frequencies. For reasons of convenience in the operating room Mapleson & Mushin preferred to stimulate the median nerve at the wrist and measured the contraction of the small flexor muscles of the thumb when the nerve was stimulated by means of a 'multiwick' electrode placed on the skin over the nerve. Sub-maximal stimuli of 9 ms duration at a frequency of 50 Hz were applied for 1.2 s every 6 s and the resultant contractions were recorded with an ink writer through a mechanically operated system. Poulsen & Hougs (1957) also used sub–maximal tetanic stimuli of the median, tibial and peroneal nerves in their study of the effects of various curarising drugs in conscious volunteers.

A somewhat different approach had been adopted earlier by Thesleff (1952) who measured the twitch response of the ulnar fingers of the hand in anaesthetised patients when supramaximal stimuli were applied to the ulnar nerve at the elbow and this technique was utilised by Payne & Holmdahl (1959) when they demonstrated the development of tachyphylaxis in man after repeated doses of suxamethonium. For this purpose a supramaximal stimulus provided by a square wave pulse of 0.5 ms duration was applied at 10 s intervals through a surface electrode placed over the ulnar nerve in the vicinity of the elbow joint. The voltage required ranged from 70 to 100 volts and it was possible to maintain this type of stimulation for several hours without any obvious ill effects. The contractions were recorded through a metal strip fixed to the two ulnar fingers of the hand and connected through a pivot to a flat steel spring myograph suitably amplified to produce an ink tracing on a rotating drum. Subsequently a more convenient method of measuring the twitch response was described by Katz (1965) who measured the contraction of the adductor pollicis muscle of the thumb following supramaximal stimulation of the ulnar nerve at the elbow or the wrist. Katz studied the electrical and mechanical responses of skeletal muscle to nerve stimulation as well as the integrated abdominal electromyogram and concluded that the mechanical response of the muscle to nerve stimulation was the most accurate, convenient and useful guide to the effects of neuromuscular blocking drugs.

Later work by Gissen & Katz (1969) has demonstrated that the single twitch is a less sensitive index of neuromuscular transmission than is the response to tetanic stimulation in the frequency range 20–200 Hz.

Train of four

In an attempt to overcome the relative insensitivity of single twitch measurements Ali, Utting & Gray (1970) introduced the concept of 'the train of four' for the assessment of neuromuscular block. The method is based on the fact that under conditions of partial neuromuscular blockade it is possible to show that if a steady state of twitch height is obtained at a particular frequency of stimulation a change to a higher frequency lowers the twitch height and a new lower steady state is usually attained after five stimuli at the

faster rate. In practice Ali *et al.* (1970) recommend the use of trains of four stimuli at a frequency of 2 Hz repeated at 10 s intervals.

This reduction in twitch height in response to repetitive nerve stimulation was first used clinically by Roberts & Wilson (1969) who used a train of four stimuli at a frequency of 4 Hz in myasthenic patients to assess the progress of the disease and to determine the effects of treatment.

The main advantage claimed for the 'the train of four' is the fact that a clinical assessment can be carried out at any time without the need to refer to a control period. There can be no doubt that this is a particularly useful attribute in the clinical field when, for example, the diagnosis of residual block may be in doubt or when an assessment of the response to treatment is needed. However in the quantitative evaluation of neuromuscular block it seems unlikely to offer any advantages over the single twitch response and from that aspect it has yet to prove its value.

Tetanic response

The relative lack of sensitivity in the single twitch response has been a source of anxiety to many investigators and led Cookson & Paton in 1969 to comment that 'the mere recording of muscle twitches under clinical conditions is not likely to yield much further dividends. On the other hand careful study of tetanic and post-tetanic responses under different conditions of block would be very helpful.' Despite the uncertainty about the value of the single twitch it continued to be widely used. Some years were to elapse before a direct simultaneous comparison between tetanic and single twitch responses demonstrated that after the administration of neuromuscular blocking drugs the tetanic and single twitch contractions follow a different pattern of behaviour. In some instances the difference is qualitative as well as quantitative. Further in the presence of marginally adequate neuromuscular transmission tetanic fade increases with the frequency of stimulation even though the twitch response is unaffected. Thus the use of high frequency tetanic stimuli may reveal a failure of transmission not apparent with single twitch contractions. Tetanic fade is defined as the failure to sustain the square wave form of the tetanic contraction in response to tetanic stimulation. As recovery from neuromuscular blockade proceeds tetanic fade progressively disappears until the response is fully sustained. This led to the suggestion that if the maximum benefit was to be derived from studies of neuromuscular blocking drugs both tetanic and single twitch responses should be recorded (Sugai, Hughes & Payne, 1973). Since then these authors have carried out a series of such studies undertaken on patients about to undergo elective surgery and from whom informed consent had been obtained. It is now considered that the tetanic response gives a more accurate assessment not only of the depth but also of the time course of neuromuscular blockade than does the single twitch. Moreover the tetanic response is more physiological since breathing and the movement of skeletal muscles are activated by trains of stimuli rather than by single shocks.

Throughout their studies the small adductor muscles of the thumbs supplied through the ulnar nerve have been used and the investigators have now developed a standard technique for the clinical evaluation of neuromuscular drugs. Adduction of the thumbs is measured by strain-gauge transducers mounted in the hands as first described by Tyrrell (1969). The transducers used are Statham force transducers model UC-3 Gold Cell (Universal transducing cell). For measurement of the force of the tetanic contraction of the adductor pollicis muscle a load cell model UL 4-20 has been combined with the transducer to give a linear response for forces up to 9.1 kg sufficient for the purpose. In the case of the single twitch response a load cell UL 4-5 has been used and this combined with the transducer produces a linear response for forces up to 2.3 kg which is adequate for the measurement of the single twitch response.

Basically the transducer is an unbonded strain-gauge which employs Statham's patented zero-length principle. Very little force or displacement is needed to activate the unbonded strain-sensitive filaments, a characteristic which is particularly appropriate for the measurement of the adduction force of the thumb in almost isometric conditions. A handle has been incorporated round the shaft of the transducer container and a suitably shaped thumb rest attached to the load cell connected to the sensitive tip of the tranducer. When tested the frequency response was flat over the range 0–90 Hz. The transducer is placed in the palm of the hand with the fingers grasping the hand-grip and the thumb mounted on the thumb rest in the extended position to provide a pre-load to the adductor pollicis muscle. The unit is held in position by adhesive tape.

Platinum needle electrodes are then inserted subcutaneously close to the ulnar nerve at the wrist about 20 mm apart. The electrodes are autoclaved before use and the skin suitably sterilised before insertion. The nerve is stimulated by means of a Devices stimulator type 3072 with an isolation unit and a digitimer type 3290. The tetanic stimulation is generated in conjunction with a gated pulse generator type 2521 which can produce repetitive stimulation and single pulse stimulation simultaneously and synchronously. One nerve is stimulated tetanically and the other with a single pulse. Usually the tetanic stimulus is applied at 12 s intervals for one second at a frequency of 50 Hz

with individual pulses lasting for 200 μs. A supramaximal stimulus is used and the voltage is normally of the order of 20 to 30 volts. The twitch stimulus also supramaximal is a single square wave pulse of 200 μs duration applied synchronously with the tetanus at 12 s intervals at 30 to 40 volts. A tetanic stimulus of 50 Hz was selected because tetanic fusion of the adductor pollicis muscle occurs with frequencies of 35 Hz and a frequency of 50 Hz is within the physiological range and so provides tetanic responses without causing undue fatigue.

When the ulnar nerve is stimulated at the wrist in the way described the stimulus affects the adductor pollicis, the deep head of the flexor pollicis brevis, all the interossei and the palmaris brevis muscles. However with the fingers firmly fixed on the hand-grip of the transducer most of the muscle activity acts to stabilise the hand and the movement of thumb adduction can be regarded as an isometric contraction of the adductor pollicis. For the purpose of analysis the contractions are recorded on charts at two different speeds. A fast recording is made at a speed of 5 mm per second on a Mingograf ink-jet recorder with a frequency response up to 500 Hz. At this speed it is possible to follow the pattern of the tetanic contraction, including the element of fade, the radial arterial pressure and the electrocardiogram which are recorded simultaneously. The slow recording of the tetanic and single twitch contractions are made on a Brush Clevite recorder or similar instrument at a chart speed of 5 mm/min to illustrate the overall pattern of the responses. The contour of the tetanic contraction is analysed from the fast record and special attention is paid to the peak height as an expression of tetanic transmission and the tetanic fade expressed as the tetanic-tension ratio. The tetanic-tension ratio is defined as the percentage of the amplitude of the tetanic contraction at the end of each one-second burst of tetanic stimulation compared with the initial peak amplitude of the tetanic contraction (de Jong & Freund, 1967). In the control state the tetanus is well maintained and the tetanic-tension ratio is virtually 100%.

Such analyses are tedious, time-consuming and relatively inaccurate. Fortunately the data lend themselves to computer handling on-line in real-time and a suitable computer program as shown in Figure 1 has been described for the purpose (Perry, Worsley, Sugai & Payne, 1975). The program allows the on-line real-time analysis of a range of variables including twitch height, maximum slope of the twitch and twitch pulse widths, peak height of tetanic contraction, end height of tetanic contraction, the tetanic-tension ratio and the percentage tetanic transmission. The program has been used to study the pattern of action of neuromuscular blocking drugs and similar programs have particular value in the assessment of pharmacokinetic activity.

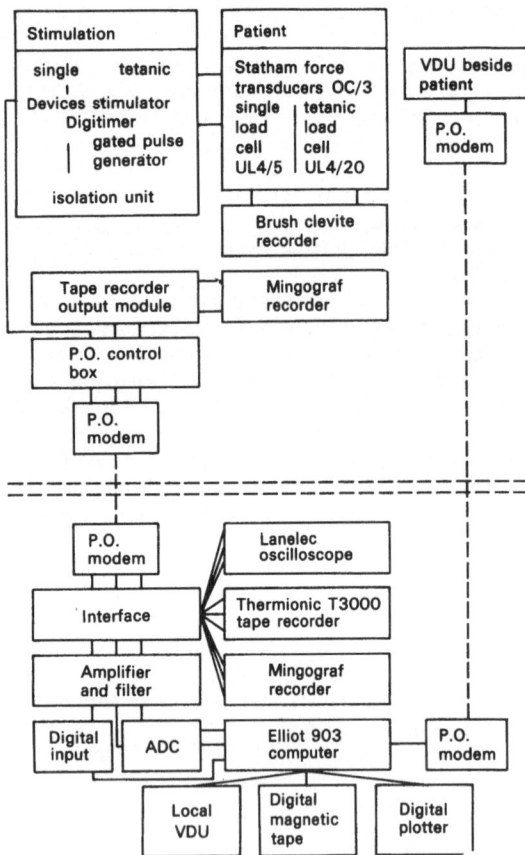

Figure 1 Schematic diagram of the arrangements for the computer analysis of neuromuscular blockade.

The advantages of the tetanic response over the single twitch can be exemplified by simultaneous recordings obtained in three different situations. First, the onset of full block of the tetanic response is more rapid than that of the single twitch so that intubation can be accomplished as soon as the tetanic contractions have disappeared (Figure 2). Second, exposure to 1–2% halothane during recovery from competitive neuromuscular block enhances blockade of the tetanic response and re-establishes fade, whereas the single twitch is unaffected (Figure 3). Thus an assessment based on the single twitch response would not have revealed this effect. Third, in patients given neostigmine the tetanic response revealed the drug's known neuromuscular action as manifested by reduced peak contractions and marked tetanic fade, which persisted for up to 20 min. In contrast no evidence of block was shown by the single twitch contractions which in fact were augmented by neostigmine. Further a sub-paralysing dose of gallamine antagonised the tetanic block and reversed the augmentation of the single twitch (Figure 4).

Electromyography

Despite the expressed preference of most research workers for the recording of evoked mechanical activity in the study of neuromuscular events there are others who favour the use of the compound muscle action potential.

One of the earliest uses of electromyography for the assessment of neuromuscular blocking drugs was made by Churchill-Davidson & Richardson (1952) who measured hypothenar muscle activity in the hand to evaluate the action of decamethonium. For measurement of muscle power the ulnar nerve was stimulated supramaximally at the wrist or elbow and the total muscle action potential detected with skin electrodes held in position by suction and contact made with electrode jelly. The action potential was displayed on an oscilloscope after suitable amplification and photographed for subsequent measurement of height of the response. Results were expressed as a percentage of the control and plotted accordingly.

A similar approach was adopted by Desmedt (1962) who has used electromyography extensively in his studies of neuromyopathies but who has reservations about restricting his work to electromyographic measurements and argued that it was essential for the proper study of neuromuscular disorders that evoked electrical and mechanical responses should be recorded simultaneously. Similar reservations were expressed by Katz (1965) who carried out a comparison of electrical and mechanical recording of spontaneous and evoked muscle activity and concluded that the mechanical response to muscle stimulation offered the most satisfactory means of assessing neuromuscular block. But it should be noted that in this particular study the mechanical activity of the small muscles of the hand were being compared with the integrated electromyogram of the oblique-transversus group of abdominal muscles.

This view was not shared by de Jong & Freund (1967) who were of the opinion that in testing for neuromuscular function EMG and muscle tensions could be used interchangeably. Subsequently Katz seemed to modify his attitude when he chose to study the effects of suxamethonium and tubocurarine on various muscle responses by means of electromyographic and mechanical methods which he described in detail (Katz, 1973). In this study he noted that the presence or absence and magnitude of fade and post-tetanic potentiation depended, among other factors, on whether electrical or mechanical responses were used for the assessment but nevertheless by recording both, certain clear differentiations could be made.

Further support for the use of electromyographic techniques has come from Epstein and his colleagues on the grounds that electromyography avoids the difficulties encountered with mechanical recordings

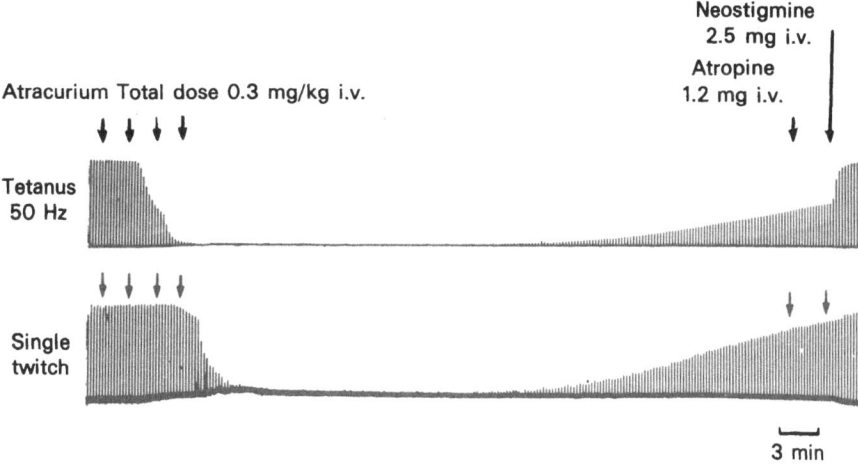

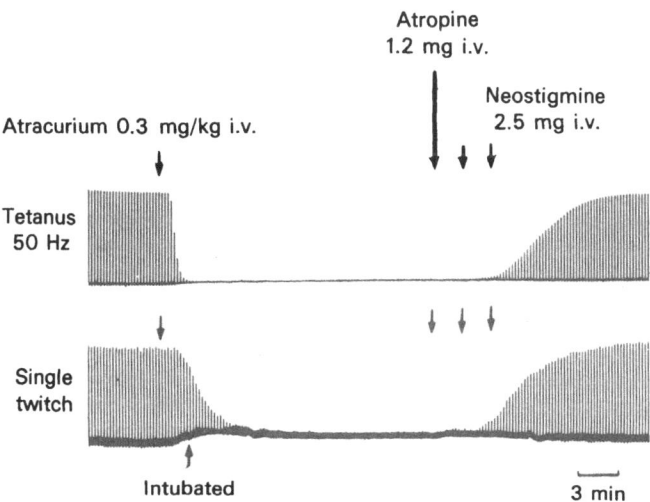

Figure 2 Recordings of the tetanic and single twitch responses of the adductor pollicis muscle from two anaesthetized patients who received atracurium in divided and single doses. Top tracings show rapid antagonism by neostigmine when recovery of tetanic response had reached 50%. Lower tracings show that intubation was accomplished within 2 min of administration of atracurium, 20 min later, complete block was reversed by neostigmine.

such as the proper direction of the force, the variations in loading and the effects of small changes in the angle of the force as well as problems of obtaining a constant resting tension and a true isometric system. In addition electromyographic techniques allow a large number of motor units to be sampled with either surface or bare needle electrodes and maintenance of a constant EMG waveform has not been a problem (Epstein & Epstein, 1973). Further-

more the inconvenience of having to photograph oscilloscope tracings can be avoided by making use of a specially developed recording system for which is claimed the advantages of faithful reproduction of high speed events, ease of use, economy of material and accessibility of large amounts of data (Epstein, Epstein & Lee, 1973).

It is probably true that in the hands of experts the EMG offers certain advantages but in the absence of

160

Tubocurarine 0.5 mg/kg

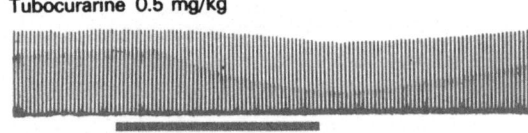

2% halothane for 10 min

Dimethyl tubocurarine 0.1 mg/kg

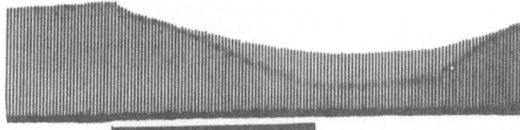

2% halothane for 10 min

Gallamine 0.8 mg/kg

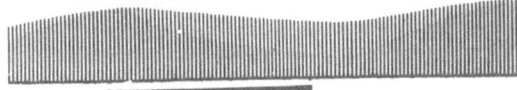

2% halothane for 10 min

Figure 3 Tracings from three anaesthetized patients showing the tetanic responses of the adductor pollicis muscles during recovery from neuromuscular blockade by tubocurarine, dimethyl tubocurarine and gallamine. Administration of 2% halothane for 10 min (solid bar line) caused an increase in fade (seen as the lighter lines) with a reduction in the peak height of the tetanic contraction. The effects were reversed when the halothane was turned off.

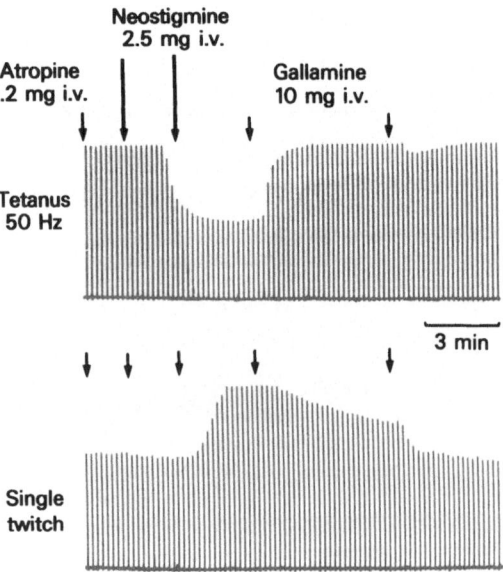

Figure 4 Tracings from an anaesthetized patient showing neuromuscular block of the tetanic response after two doses of neostigmine preceded by atropine and the potentiation of the single twitch. Gallamine antagonized the neuromuscular block of the tetanic response and reversed the potentiation of the single twitch.

special expertise most workers will continue to rely on mechanical recordings of the indirectly evoked muscle contraction.

Factors influencing the action of neuromuscular blocking agents

It is important from the point of view of patient safety that the factors which may modify the action of neuromuscular blocking drugs are properly understood since the lack of such knowledge could lead to operative and post-operative complications.

Route of administration

An important factor in the quantitative assessment of these drugs is the route of administration which may influence the intensity and duration of the response. For example, the more rapid the intravenous administration of a given dose the greater the intensity of the effect (Foldes, 1957). Furthermore after repeated administration of suxamethonium and decamethonium, tachyphylaxis may develop as manifested

by a progressively diminishing effect. In contrast competitive blocking agents usually show an enhanced effect due to accumulation. Since neuromuscular blocking drugs are virtually all highly ionised compounds absorption through the gut is minimal so that oral dosage is excluded. Although theoretically any parenteral route of administration is acceptable, a drug under investigation is usually given intravenously either as a single bolus or as a continuous infusion especially if the drug is a short acting agent like suxamethonium. An alternative approach is to use the divided dose technique now widely exploited and which has proved particularly useful in the study of the onset of action of the new blocking drug atracurium (Payne & Hughes, 1981).

Variations in sensitivity

Another factor is the variation in sensitivity to specific neuromuscular blocking agents that occurs between different muscles, and conversely the variation in response of the same muscles to different drugs, and the position is further complicated by species difference. It is therefore of fundamental importance to ensure that when neuromuscular blocking drugs are being studied such variations are fully recognised and they have in fact been widely studied. Paton & Zaimis

(1950) reported that the tibialis, a 'white' muscle was more sensitive to decamethonium than the soleus, diaphragm or intercostal muscles, all 'red' muscles. Conversely, the tibialis muscle is less sensitive than the soleus muscle and the diaphragm to tubocurarine (Paton & Zaimis, 1951; Jewell & Zaimis, 1954). However Alderson & Maclagan (1964) found that the difference in sensitivity between the diaphragm and tibialis muscles would be considerably reduced by abolishing the temperature difference which normally exists between the warmer diaphragm muscle and the cooler limb muscles.

Temperature

Lowering of muscle temperature increases the magnitude of a depolarising block and prolongs its action. In contrast cooling reduces the magnitude of the block produced by competitive agents but leaves the duration of the block almost unaltered (Bigland, Goetzee, Maclagan & Zaimis, 1958; Cannard & Zaimis, 1959; Alderson & Maclagan, 1964). An increase in the effectiveness of acetylcholine could explain the action of cooling on both types of block. Repolarisation of the post-synaptic membrane following the action of acetylcholine may be slowed by cooling (Bigland *et al.*, 1958). Such an action would enhance the paralysing effect of depolarising agents but reduce that of the competitive blockers. Based on these findings it is clear that the temperature of muscles should be maintained at body temperature (37°C) during the assessment of neuromuscular function.

Rate of stimulation

During monitoring of neuromuscular transmission the rate of stimulation is an important consideration since the frequency of stimulation increases the intensity of block both by depolarising and competitive agents (Preston & Van Maanan, 1953; Wislicki 1958). In this context tetanic stimulation is preferable to single twitch stimulation since with tetanus the acetylcholine is fully mobilised as it is released and any prejunctional effects are reflected in the degree of tetanic fade. The single twitch response is inadequate for this purpose since the amount of acetylcholine released is greatly in excess of that required for neuromuscular transmission and Paton & Waud (1967) have shown that before neuromuscular block of the single twitch becomes apparent the drug must occupy about 80% of the cholinergic receptors.

Acid-base balance

Experiments performed to investigate the effects of changes in acid-base balance on neuromuscular blockade have given conflicting results which are probably due to the widely differing experimental techniques employed. In general, neuromuscular blockade by tubocurarine is enhanced by acidosis but antagonised by alkalosis (Maclagan, 1976). Effects on dimethyl tubocurarine, gallamine, alcuronium, suxamethonium and decamethonium appear to be altered in the opposite direction. Various explanations are given for these differences including such factors as changes in muscle blood flow, drug distribution and ionization of the drug and the receptors. More recently, Hughes & Chapple (1980) have demonstrated that the non-enzymic inactivation of a novel competitive blocking agent atracurium is increased by raising the plasma pH and there is some evidence this may also be true in anaesthetised man (Payne & Hughes, 1981).

Drug interactions

In recent years more information has become available on the interaction of neuromuscular blocking agents with other drugs used in the treatment of surgical patients. Theoretically the simplest interaction at the myoneural receptor is the ability of anticholinesterase compounds such as neostigmine to reverse the competitive blocking action of drugs like curare. In this instance neostigmine acts by combining with the enzyme cholinesterase to prevent it destroying the acetylcholine released at the nerve endings. The accumulation of acetylcholine in turn competes with tubocurarine and similar drugs to displace them from the receptor site. In practice the situation is more complicated; first, the response is related to the existing degree of neuromuscular block and second, it is dose dependent. Thus it is possible to enhance rather than to antagonise the block and it may well be that the so-called neostigmine resistant curarisation occasionally reported in the postoperative period is in fact a neostigmine induced neuromuscular block. The fact that neostigmine and similar drugs can cause neuromuscular block has been known for many years (Briscoe, 1936, 1937; Brennan, 1956) but it is only recently that it has been highlighted in man (Payne, Hughes & Al-Azawi, 1980).

Again the principles have been well established that depolarising and competitive neuromuscular blocking agents are mutually antagonistic and that anticholinesterase drugs will not antagonise neuromuscular block caused by depolarising drugs. In practice however it can be shown that after repeated doses of suxamethonium and decamethonium, neostigmine and edrophonium will restore normal transmission at the neuromuscular junction. This alteration in response is presumably related to the change in pattern of neuromuscular block that has been demonstrated repeatedly with the depolarising blocking drugs. Apart from the development of tachyphylaxis which may be a component of the changing response it is clear that after repeated doses of suxamethonium and decamethonium the behaviour of the response becomes more readily identified with the pattern of competitive block. Neostigmine block itself must be classified as a depolarising block as witnessed by its enhancement by suxamethonium and its antagonism by gallamine. Of further interest is the prolongation of the block after suxamethonium the duration of which may be extended beyond thirty minutes (Payne *et al.*, 1980).

The matter is further complicated by the fact that general anaesthetics like ether (Paton & Zaimis, 1951) and halothane (Miller, Way, Dolan, Stevens & Eger, 1972; Hughes & Payne, 1979) significantly enhance the effect of neuromuscular block with competitive blocking agents. Furthermore intravenous agents such as thiopentone and diazepam have a potentiating effect on the same agents and in the case of thiopentone this action may be added to the non-specific muscle relaxant properties of the drug, a property that was once frequently used by anaesthetists to obtain profound relaxation for short periods for example for the closing of the peritoneum.

Of clinical importance is the interaction of the aminoglycoside antibiotics with neuromuscular blocking agents (Pittinger & Adamson, 1972). The mechanism of action has not been clearly defined but a mixture of competitive and depolarising block is often seen with the result that the response to neostigmine is scarcely predictable. There is some evidence that these antibiotics act both by competition and by reducing or preventing the release of acetylcholine an action similar to that of magnesium. The similarity to magnesium is further emphasised by the fact that calcium ions which antagonise the action of magnesium can also relieve antibiotic paralysis.

Genetic deficiencies

Apart from drug interactions certain genetic deficiencies and some disease states may distort the normal response to neuromuscular blocking drugs. Of the genetic disturbances an abnormally low cholinesterase activity may manifest itself as a prolonged apnoea in response to a normal dose of suxamethonium. Three genetically determined cholinesterases have now been described on the basis of the dibucaine (cinchocaine) inhibition test which measures the ability of dibucaine to inhibit serum cholinesterase activity. The first represents normal individuals in whom 80% of the activity of their serum cholinesterase is inhibited. In 3% of the population who form the second group about 62% inhibition occurs and in the third group, probably about 1 in 5,000 of the population the inhibition of the serum cholinesterase does not exceed 16%. It is this third

group who give rise to the clinical problem of prolonged apnoea after suxamethonium although the condition may also be seen in patients with liver disease or dietary deficiency.

A second genetic disturbance even more important to the anaesthetist because of its high mortality is a metabolic disorder of unknown aetiology which gives rise to malignant hyperthermia. The syndrome which has been described in pigs as well as in man is usually triggered by some external factor such as stress or a high environmental temperature. However the commonest triggering agents are general anaesthetics and neuromuscular blocking drugs and the first indication of trouble may be the development of prolonged muscle rigidity rather than the usual relaxation after suxamethonium has been used for intubation. The disturbance is familial and thought to be an autosomal dominant myopathy. Identification of potential victims is difficult but a family history of anaesthetic problems should arouse suspicion. Serum creatine phosphokinase levels may be elevated in susceptible patients and some show an increased incidence of short duration polyphasic action potentials on routine electromyography.

Disease states

The classical disease state associated with skeletal muscle relaxation is myasthenia gravis and much of the current understanding of the disease mechanisms can be attributed to the accumulated experience of neuromuscular block with depolarising and competitive blocking agents. In particular the resistance of myasthenic patients to large doses of decamethonium contrasts markedly with their susceptibility to small doses of tubocurarine (Churchill-Davidson & Richardson, 1952). This difference in the response to depolarising and competitive blocking agents has formed the basis not only for diagnostic tests to confirm the presence of the disease but also for its routine management with neostigmine and atropine. It has also helped to define more accurately the site of the disease process. Results obtained from electrophysiological studies on myasthenic patients show that the action potentials and muscle contractions gradually wane during repetitive excitation and that if a brief tetanus is applied the muscles exhibit a characteristic post-activation exhaustion when single test shocks are given at short intervals. This pattern is almost identical with that obtained from muscles treated with hemicholinium which causes a reduction in the amount of acetylcholine released at nerve endings. This suggests that some disturbance of the normal pre-synaptic mechanisms is a fundamental component of the disease.

A syndrome of readily induced fatigue and progressive muscle weakness similar to that found in myasthenic patients has been observed in patients with malignant disease particularly that of the lung. Such patients are equally sensitive to tubocurarine but unlike those with myasthenia gravis they may also be sensitive to depolarising drugs. This sensitivity may be reversed by anticholinesterases which however have little effect on the muscle weakness itself. The condition usually improves once the malignancy has been removed much in the same way as the myasthenic patient sometimes responds to thymectomy.

A third group of patients with a marked change in sensitivity need to be remembered. Electromyographic studies have shown that premature and newborn babies have a pattern of neuromuscular transmission not unlike that seen in myasthenic patients. These infants, who are very sensitive to tubocurarine, tolerate very large doses of suxamethonium and when block does occur it can be reversed by anticholinesterases.

Finally there is a wide range of myopathic and neurogenic diseases as well as some endocrine disturbances that may give rise to abnormal and often unpredictable responses to neuromuscular blocking drugs. No specific tests are available to determine the pattern of response to be expected when particular neuromuscular blocking drugs are used in such patients.

Conclusion

The outstanding feature of any scrutiny of the literature of neuromuscular block is the obvious conflict of opinion that exists about almost every aspect of neuromuscular transmission. This is all the more remarkable since the neuromuscular junction is a fairly circumscribed physiological unit which has been well defined and the differences can probably be related to the lack of uniformity in the methods of assessment used by different investigators. The problem is that attempts have been made to interpret events on the basis of results obtained either by different methods of study or by the same method but under different conditions. For example, electromyographic and mechanical methods of assessment do not measure the same variable and even when purely mechanical techniques are used there may be quantitative and qualitative differences between the single twitch and the tetanic response. Furthermore the restriction of the investigation to one particular technique will not necessarily resolve the problem. In the case of tetanic stimuli the pattern of the response will vary with such factors as the frequency of the stimulation and the duration of its application.

Ideally what is needed in the assessment of neuromuscular block is agreement between workers in the field about a uniform pattern of investigation to be applied in all studies of new drugs, and the technology and the expertise are now available to provide completely standardised methods. Where investigators believe that a different approach might offer certain advantages the new approach should be compared with the standard methods. In the absence of such agreement editors of scientific journals should ensure that authors provide enough detail about their methods to allow other workers to repeat experiments which purport to show patterns of drug action that differ from the accepted response.

References

ALDERSON, A.M. & MACLAGAN, J. (1964). The action of decamethonium and tubocurarine on the respiratory and limb muscle of the cat. *J. Physiol. (Lond.)*, **173**, 38–56.

ALI, H.H., UTTING, J.E. & GRAY, C. (1970). Stimulus frequency in the detection of neuromuscular block in humans. *Br. J. Anaesth.*, **42**, 967–978.

BERNARD, C. (1851). Action de Curare et de la Nicotine sur le systeme Nerveux et sur le systeme Musculaire. *Compt. rend. Soc. Biol.*, **2**, 195.

BENNETT, A.E. (1941). Curare: a preventive of traumatic complications in convulsive shock therapy. *Am. J. Psychiat.*, **97**, 1040–1060.

BIGLAND, B., GOETZEE, B., MACLAGAN, J. & ZAIMIS, E. (1958). The effect of lowered muscle temperature on the action of neuromuscular blocking drugs. *J. Physiol. (Lond.)*, **141**, 425–434.

BIGLAND, B. & LIPPOLD, O.C.J. (1954). Motor unit activity in the voluntary contraction of human muscle. *J. Physiol. (Lond.)*, **125**, 322–335.

BODMAN, R.I. (1952). Evaluation of two synthetic curarizing agents in conscious volunteers. *Br. J. Pharmac. Chemother.*, **7**, 409–416.

BRENNAN, H.J. (1956). Dual action of suxamethonium chloride. *Br. J. Anaesth.*, **28**, 159–168

BRISCOE, G. (1936). Shift in optimum rate of stimulation due to prostigmine. *J. Physiol. (Lond.)*, **86**, 48P.

BRISCOE, G. (1937). Optimum stimulation rates for red and white skeletal mammalian muscles, and shift in rates produced by the eserine group. *J. Physiol. (Lond.)*, **90**, 10P.

CANNARD, T.H. & ZAIMIS, E. (1959). The effect of lowered muscle temperature on the action of neuromuscular blocking drugs in man. *J. Physiol. (Lond.)*, **149**, 112–119.

CHURCHILL-DAVIDSON, H.C. & RICHARDSON, A.T. (1952). Decamethonium iodide (C 10): some observations on its action using electromyography. *Proc. Roy. Soc. Med.*, **45**, 179–185.

COOKSON, J.C. & PATON, W.D.M. (1969). Mechanisms of

neuromuscular block. *Anaesthesia*, **24**, 395–416.

DALE, H.H. & FELDBERG, W. (1934). The chemical transmission of secretory impulses to the sweat glands of the cat. *J. Physiol.*, **82**, 121–128.

DALE, H.H., FELDBERG, W. & VOGT, M. (1936). Release of acetylcholine at voluntary motor nerve endings. *J. Physiol.*, **86**, 353–380.

DE JONG, R.H. & FREUND, F.G. (1967). Characteristics of the neuromuscular block with succinylcholine and decamethonium in man. *Anesthesiology*, **28**, 583–591.

DESMEDT, J.E. (1962). Donnees recentes sur la pathogenie de la myasthenie grave. *Bull. de l'Academie Royale de Medicine de Belgique*, **7**, 213–267.

EPSTEIN, R.M., EPSTEIN, R.A. & LEE, A.S.J. (1973). A recording system for continuous evoked electromyography. *Anesthesiology*, **38**, 287–289.

EPSTEIN, R.A. & EPSTEIN, R.M. (1973). The electromyogram and the mechanical response of indirectly stimulated muscle in anaesthetized man following curarization. *Anesthesiology*, **38**, 212–223.

FOLDES, F.F. (1957). Fate of muscle relaxants in man. *Acta anaesth. Scand.*, **1**, 63–79.

GISSEN, A.J. & KATZ, R.L. (1969). Twitch, tetanus and post-tetanic potentiation as indices of nerve-muscle block in man. *Anesthesiology*, **30**, 481–487.

GRIFFITH, H.R. & JOHNSON, G.E. (1942). The use of curare in general anaesthesia. *Anesthesiology*, **3**, 418–420.

HUGHES, R. & CHAPPLE, D.J. (1980). Experimental studies with atracurium, a new neuromuscular blocking agent. *Br. J. Anaesth.*, **52**, 238P.

HUGHES, R. & PAYNE, J.P. (1979). Interaction of halotnane with non-depolarizing neuromuscular blocking drugs in man. *Br. J. clin. Pharmac.*, **7**, 485–490.

JEWELL, P.A.. & ZAIMIS, E. (1954). A differentiation between red and white muscle in the cat based on responses to neuromuscular blocking agent. *J. Physiol. (Lond.)*, **124**, 417–428.

JOHANSEN, S.H., JORGENSEN, M. & MOLBECH, S. (1964). Effect of tubocurarine on respiratory and non-respiratory muscle power in man. *J. appl. Physiol.*, **19**, 990–994.

KATZ, R.L. (1965). Comparison of electrical and mechanical recording of spontaneous and evoked muscle activity. *Anesthesiology*, **26**, 204–221.

KATZ, R.L. (1973). Electromyographic and mechanical effects of suxamethonium and tubocurarine on twitch, tetanic and post-tetanic responses. *Br. J. Anaesth.*, **45**, 849–859.

MACLAGAN, J. (1976). Competitive neuromuscular blocking drugs. In *Neuromuscular Junction.* ed Zaimis, E., pp 462–467 Berlin: Springer-Verlag.

MAPLESON, W.W. & MUSHIN, W.W. (1955). Relaxant action in man. *Anaesthesia*, **10**, 265–278.

MILLER, R.D., WAY, W.L., DOLAN, W.M., STEVENS, W.C. & EGER, E.I. (1972). The dependence of pancuronium and d-tubocurarine-induced neuromuscular blockades on alveolar concentrations of halothane and Forane. *Anesthesiology*, **37**, 573–581.

MUSHIN, W.W., WIEN, R., MASON, D.F.J. & LANGSTON, G.T. (1949). Curare-like actions of tri-(diethylaminoethoxy) benzene triethyliodide. *Lancet*, **i**, 726–728.

ORGANE, G., PATON, W.D.M. & ZAIMIS, E.J. (1949). Preliminary trials of bistrimethyl ammonium decane and pentane diiodide (C.10 and C.5) in man. *Lancet*, **i**, 21–23.

PATON, W.D.M. & WAUD, D.R. (1967). The margin of safety of neuromuscular transmission. *J. Physiol.*, **191**, 59–90.

PATON, W.D.M. & ZAIMIS, E.J. (1948). Clinical potentialities of certain bisquaternary salts causing neuromuscular and ganglionic block. *Nature*, **162**, 810.

PATON, W.D.M. & ZAIMIS, E.J. (1950). Actions and clinical assessment of drugs which produce neuromuscular block. *Lancet*, **ii**, 568–570.

PATON, W.D.M. & ZAIMIS, E.J. (1951). The action of d-tubocurarine and of decamethonium on respiratory and other muscles in the cat. *J. Physiol. (Lond.)*, **112**, 311–331.

PAYNE, J.P. & HOLMDAHL, M.H. (1959). The effect of repeated doses of suxamethonium in man. *Br. J. Anaesth.*, **31**, 341–347.

PAYNE, J.P. & HUGHES, R. (1981). Evaluation of atracurium in anaesthetized man. *Br. J. Anaesth.*, **53**, 45–54.

PAYNE, J.P., HUGHES, R. & AL-AZAWI, S. (1980). Neuromuscular blockade by neostigmine in anaesthetized man. *Br. J. Anaesth.*, **52**, 69–76.

PERRY, I.R., WORSLEY, R., SUGAI, N. & PAYNE, J.P. (1975). The use of a digital computer for the on–line real-time assessment of neuromuscular blockade in anaesthetized man. *Br. J. Anaesth.*, **47**, 1097–1100.

PITTINGER, C. & ADAMSON, R. (1972). Antibiotic blockade of neuromuscular function. *Pharmac. Rev.*, **12**, 169–184.

POULSEN, H. & HOUGS, W. (1957). The effect of some curarizing drugs in unanaesthetized man, 1. *Acta anaesth. Scand.*, **1**, 15–39.

PRESTON, J.B. & VAN MAANAN, E.F. (1953). Effects of frequency of stimulation on the paralysing dose of neuromuscular blocking agents. *J. Pharmac. exp. Ther.*, **107**, 165–171.

ROBERTS, D.V. & WILSON, A. (1969). Physiology of neuromuscular transmission. In *Electromyography in diagnosis and treatment of myasthenia gravis*, ed Green, R., pp 14–19. London: William Heinemann.

SUGAI, N., HUGHES, R. & PAYNE, J.P. (1973). The use of tetanic and single twitch stimuli to assess neuromuscular block in man. *Br. J. Anaesth.*, **45**, 642–643.

THESLEFF, S. (1952). An investigation of the muscle-relaxing action of succinyl-choline-iodide in man. *Acta physiol. Scand.*, **25**, 348–367.

TYRRELL, M.F. (1969). The measurement of the force of thumb adduction. *Anesthesia*, **24**, 626–629.

WEST, R. (1932). Curare in man. *Proc. Roy. Soc. Med.*, **25**, 1107–1116.

WISLICKI, L. (1958). Effects of rate of stimulation and of fatigue on the response of neuromuscular blocking agents. *Br. J. Pharmac.*, **13**, 138–143.